Office-Based Gynecologic Surgical Procedures

Jonathan D. Emery
Marie Fidela R. Paraiso
Editors

Office-Based Gynecologic Surgical Procedures

Springer

Editors
Jonathan D. Emery, M.D.
Department of Obstetrics
and Gynecology
Cleveland Clinic
Willoughby Hills, OH, USA

Marie Fidela R. Paraiso, M.D.
Cleveland Clinic Lerner College of Medicine
at Case Western Reserve University
Cleveland, OH, USA

Center for Urogynecology and Reconstructive
Pelvic Surgery, Obstetrics, Gynecology
and Women's Health Institute
Cleveland Clinic
Cleveland, OH, USA

Glickman Urological and Kidney Institute
Cleveland Clinic
Cleveland, OH, USA

ISBN 978-1-4939-1413-5 ISBN 978-1-4939-1414-2 (eBook)
DOI 10.1007/978-1-4939-1414-2
Springer New York Heidelberg Dordrecht London

Library of Congress Control Number: 2014949264

Printed on acid-free paper

Springer is part of Springer Science+Business Media (www.springer.com)

Preface

Recent trends in medicine have begun to allow for advances in surgical procedures: what were previously surgical procedures performed in the operating room have been transitioned to the ambulatory surgery center and ultimately to the office setting. This movement has been driven by several forces: improvements in technology with smaller caliber instruments; patient's desire for lesser invasive procedures; rising health care costs with the ability to decrease expenses by performing procedures in less resource-intensive settings. National organizations such as the Advisory Board Company and the American Hospital Association have noted this shift away from inpatient to outpatient surgery. Since the late 1990s, greater than 60 % of surgical procedures in the United States were being performed in the outpatient setting.

With this shift in the provision of surgical care in this country, our specialty of gynecology has been fortunate to be a leader in outpatient surgery. In the past 10 years, however, the shift has continued to evolve to the office setting. Gynecologists have been performing office-based procedures for years: colposcopy with cervical biopsy, endometrial biopsy, vulvar biopsy and excision to name a few. Improved technology, however, has allowed for further transition to the office-based setting for more diagnostic and even therapeutic procedures. Hysteroscopic sterilization is a perfect example of this trend.

The recent growth in office-based gynecologic surgeries cannot be accomplished without a clear vision for patient safety. In the United States, governmental agencies and national specialty societies, including the American Congress of Obstetrics and Gynecology, have made patient safety a top priority. Clearly, the transition to office-based gynecologic surgeries must be achieved with patient safety as a primary focus; patient satisfaction is a secondary focus when developing an office-based surgical program. This book has two chapters which address these concerns. Identifying the appropriate patient for an office surgery and then putting in place policies and protocols that emphasize and mandate safe practices will ensure continued success and further advancement of office-based surgery. Also included are chapters ranging from long-standing procedures as well as newer techniques adapted to the office. Each chapter contains advice and some "tips and tricks" that will allow gynecologists and women's health specialists to successfully establish these procedures in their offices.

A number of excellent and well-regarded texts of gynecologic surgery as well as office gynecology are currently available. There are not, however, texts that deal with the specifics of office-based gynecologic surgery: that is what makes this book unique. Our goal for this textbook is to provide gynecologists and women's health specialists the specifics needed to begin to perform both basic and advanced gynecologic surgeries in the office—from start to finish. As gynecologists, we have the distinctive opportunity to continue to advance minimally invasive procedures that can make a significant impact on a women's health, all the while done in the safe and comforting environment of our offices. Our patients deserve the best care from us and we hope this text will continue to allow gynecologists to put "Patients First."

Willoughby Hills, OH, USA Jonathan D. Emery, M.D.
Cleveland, OH, USA Marie Fidela R. Paraiso, M.D.

Contents

1 **Pre-procedure Patient Evaluation and Management** 1
May Hsieh Blanchard

2 **Getting Started in Office-Based Gynecologic Procedures: Office Set-up, Procedural Implications and Ensuring Patient Safety** 9
Natalie A. Bowersox and Jonathan D. Emery

3 **Informed Consent** 25
Ruth M. Farrell and Cristie M. Cole

4 **Anesthesia and Analgesia for Office Gynecological Procedures** 35
Nicholas Marcanthony, Sharon Marcanthony, and Englok Yap

5 **Basic Gynecologic Procedures** 51
M. Jean Uy-Kroh

6 **Saline Infusion Sonohysterography** 71
Jamie Stanhiser and Rebecca Flyckt

7 **Office Diagnostic Hysteroscopy** 85
Jonathan D. Emery

8 **Hysteroscopic Tubal Sterilization** 101
Jonathan D. Emery

9 **Office Operative Hysteroscopy: Polyp and Submucosal Fibroid Removal** 117
Mona E. Orady and Rakshanda Aslanova

10 **Office-Based Global Endometrial Ablation** 133
Margaret L. McKenzie and Monique Yoder

11 **Cystoscopy** 143
Audra Jolyn Hill and Marie Fidela R. Paraiso

12 **Urodynamic Testing** 149
Nathan Kow and Marie Fidela R. Paraiso

13 **Peri-urethral Injections** 163
Megan E. Tarr

14 Trigger Point Injections for Pelvic Pain 179
Jeannine M. Miranne and Amy J. Park

15 Colposcopy 191
Robert J. Kim

16 Loop Electro-Excision Procedure (LEEP) 211
Kimberly L. Levinson and Chad M. Michener

17 Vulvar Biopsy and Excision/Ablation 221
Sarah Goodrich and Mehdi Kebria

Index 229

Contributors

May Hsieh Blanchard, M.D., F.A.C.O.G. Department of Obstetrics, Gynecology and Reproductive Sciences, University of Maryland School of Medicine, Baltimore, MD, USA

Natalie A. Bowersox, M.D. Department of Obstetrics and Gynecology, Fairview Hospital, Brunswick, OH, USA

Cristie M. Cole, J.D. Department of Bioethics, Cleveland Clinic, Cleveland, OH, USA

Jonathan D. Emery, M.D. Department of Obstetrics and Gynecology & Women's Health Institute, Cleveland Clinic, Willoughby Hills, OH, USA

Ruth M. Farrell, M.D., M.A. Departments of Obstetrics & Gynecology and Bioethics, Cleveland Clinic, Cleveland, OH, USA

Rebecca Flyckt, M.D. Department of Obstetrics and Gynecology & Women's Health Institute, Cleveland Clinic, Cleveland, OH, USA

Sarah Goodrich, M.D. Department of Gynecologic Oncology, Cleveland Clinic, Cleveland, OH, USA

Audra Jolyn Hill, M.D. Department of Obstetrics and Gynecology & Women's Health Institute, Cleveland Clinic, Cleveland, OH, USA

Mehdi Kebria, M.D. Department of Obstetrics and Gynecology, Cleveland Clinic, Cleveland, OH, USA

Robert J. Kim, M.D. Department of Obstetrics and Gynecology, John A. Burns School of Medicine, University of Hawaii, Honolulu, HI, USA

Nathan Kow, M.D. Department of Obstetrics and Gynecology & Women's Health Institute, Cleveland Clinic, Cleveland, OH, USA

Kimberly L. Levinson, M.D., M.P.H. Department of Obstetrics and Gynecology & Women's Health Institute, The Cleveland Clinic, Cleveland, OH, USA

Nicholas Marcanthony, M.D. Department of Anesthesiology, Cleveland Clinic, Cleveland, OH, USA

Anesthesiology Institute, Cleveland Clinic Wooster, Cleveland Clinic, Cleveland, OH, USA

Sharon Marcanthony, M.D. Department of Obstetrics and Gynecology & Women's Health Institute, Cleveland Clinic, Wooster, OH, USA

Margaret L. McKenzie, M.D., M.S. Department of Obstetrics and Gynecology & Women's Health Institute, Cleveland Clinic, Cleveland, OH, USA

Chad M. Michener, M.D. Department of Obstetrics and Gynecology & Women's Health Institute, Cleveland Clinic, Cleveland, OH, USA

Jeannine M. Miranne, M.D. Section of Female Pelvic Medicine and Reconstructive Surgery, MedStar Washington Hospital Center/Georgetown University School of Medicine, Washington, DC, USA

Mona E. Orady, M.D. Department of Obstetrics and Gynecology & Women's Health Institute, Cleveland Clinic, Cleveland, OH, USA

Rakshanda Aslanova, M.D. Department of Obstetrics and Gynecology, Faculty of Medicine, Trakya University, Cleveland, Edirne, Turkey

Marie Fidela R. Paraiso, M.D. Cleveland Clinic Lerner College of Medicine at Case Western Reserve University, Cleveland, OH, USA

Center for Urogynecology and Reconstructive Pelvic Surgery, Obstetrics, Gynecology, and Women's Health Institute, Cleveland Clinic, Cleveland, OH, USA

Glickman Urological and Kidney Institute, Cleveland Clinic, Cleveland, OH, USA

Amy J. Park, M.D. Section of Female Pelvic Medicine and Reconstructive Surgery, MedStar Washington Hospital Center/Georgetown University School of Medicine, Washington, DC, USA

Department of Urology, Section of Female Pelvic Medicine & Reconstructive Surgery, MedStar Washington Hospital Center/Georgetown University School of Medicine, Washington, DC, USA

Jamie Stanhiser, M.D. Department of Obstetrics and Gynecology, Cleveland Clinic Foundation, Cleveland, OH, USA

Megan E. Tarr, M.D. Department of Obstetrics and Gynecology, Cleveland Clinic, Cleveland, OH, USA

M. Jean Uy-Kroh, M.D. Department of Obstetrics and Gynecology, Cleveland Clinic, Cleveland, OH, USA

Englok Yap, M.D. Cleveland Pain Management and Acupuncture LLC, Beachwood, OH, USA

Monique Yoder, M.D. Women's Health Institute, Cleveland Clinic Foundation, Cleveland, OH, USA

Pre-procedure Patient Evaluation and Management

1

May Hsieh Blanchard

The volume of surgical procedures being performed in the United States continues to rise (Fig. 1.1) [1]. The striking change, however, is in noting the setting in which the change is occurring most rapidly. From 1996 to 2006, the growth in number of procedures being done in freestanding centers was much greater than in hospital-based ambulatory surgery centers. In fact, the trend in the rate of procedures performed in hospital-based centers was flat, while the rate of visits to freestanding ambulatory surgery centers increased about 300 % in that decade (Fig. 1.2). In the twenty-first century, many gynecologic procedures once performed only in the hospital operating room are now finding their place in the office (office-based surgery, OBS) setting. Some of the benefits of moving away from the traditional operative arena to the physician's office include decreased cost to the patient (particularly for procedures not covered by insurance, or at a high deductible), ease of access and scheduling (avoiding the complexity of booking into general surgical suite time), and improved physician reimbursement (Table 1.1) [2].

Furthermore, patients intimidated by the thought of having to go to the "hospital" for "surgery", may be somewhat comforted and calmed at the prospect that the same procedure can be done by the physician she knows and trusts in the reassuring environment of the office where she receives her routine gynecologic care.

Establishing an office-based surgery component to one's practice, however, should not be embarked upon without serious consideration of the possible pitfalls. Thoughtful planning and consideration must be given to the risks of complications inherent in any surgical procedure, but then also the implications of how one will manage those complications in the setting of the office. As with current scrutiny of volumes of surgical cases and their proposed reflection on the skills maintained by the surgeon, an office-based surgery practice may be less efficient if more complex procedures are done infrequently, such that the staff is less familiar with the steps of the procedure. An office procedure complication can derail the physician's schedule if in the midst of a busy office day, and any delays in the ability to access emergency backup can unnerve even the most capable clinician. Strict policies and protocols for staffing, facilities, equipment, standards (sterilization, postoperative observation, appropriate post-anesthetic milestones), and patient flow and workflow can help to minimize the hazards due to inconsistencies. One of the advantages of the out-patient or office setting is that there is little to no external regulatory requirement. This is also one of the drawbacks and cause for concern: lack of external oversight puts more of the onus of maintaining quality control, auto-policing, and upholding standards on the physician and the office staff.

M.H. Blanchard, M.D., F.A.C.O.G. (✉)
Department of Obstetrics, Gynecology & Reproductive Sciences, University of Maryland School of Medicine, 11 S. Paca Street, Suite 400, Baltimore, MD 21201, USA
e-mail: mblanchard@fpi.umaryland.edu

J.D. Emery and M.F.R. Paraiso (eds.), *Office-Based Gynecologic Surgical Procedures*,
DOI 10.1007/978-1-4939-1414-2_1, © Springer Science+Business Media New York 2015

Fig. 1.1 Ambulatory surgery visits and discharges of hospital inpatients with procedures: United States, 1996 and 2006 (revised)

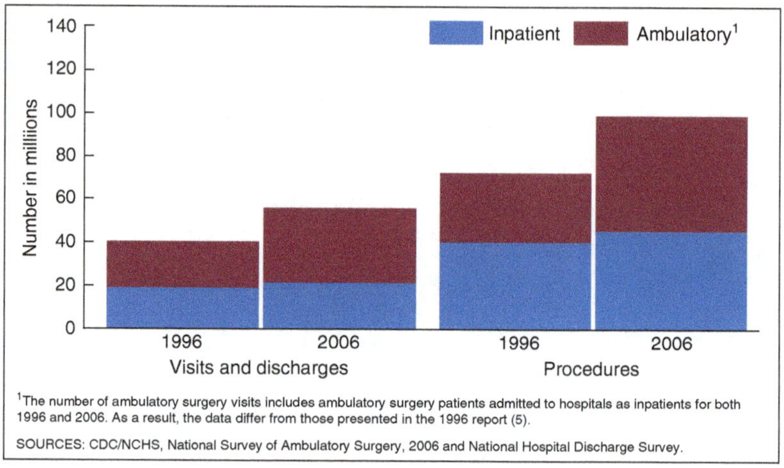

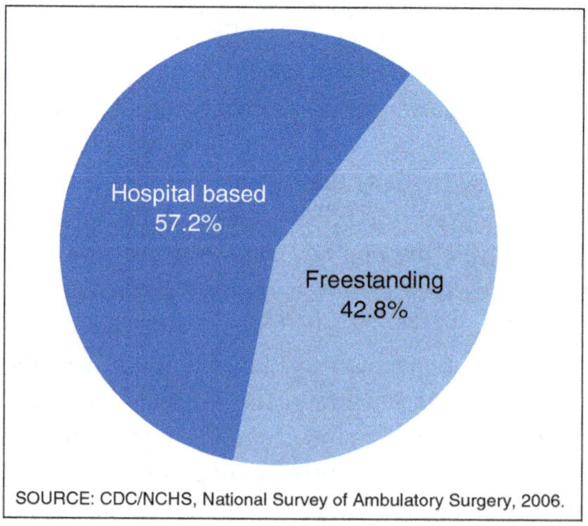

Fig. 1.2 Rates of ambulatory surgery visits by facility type: United States, 1996 and 2006

Table 1.1 2014 Physician Fee Schedule Search, National Payment Amount (www.cms.gov)

HCPCS code	Short description	Non-facility price (office-based surgery) ($)	Facility price (hospital/ASC) ($)
58565	Hysteroscopy sterilization	1,874.61	450.29
58353	Endometr ablate thermal	1,009.13	227.47
58555	Hysteroscopy dx sep proc	309.15	198.10
57461	Conz of cervix w/scope leep	327.06	196.31
57460	Bx of cervix w/scope leep	288.73	170.16
52000	Cystoscopy	203.12	128.60

HCPCS Healthcare Common Procedure Coding System, *ASC* Ambulatory Surgery Center

After all of the considerations for setting up the office-based surgery program, obtaining the best equipment, training the staff, establishing protocols, and transferring the surgical skill set from the operating room to the office procedure room, these well-laid out plans will be for naught if adequate attention and respect are not devoted toward ensuring appropriate patient selection, pre-procedure evaluation, and management. Selecting the right patient for office-based surgery is of paramount importance as not all patients are candidates for office-based surgery.

Patient Selection

Success of the office-based surgery program requires appropriate patient selection. The patient should be counseled and educated appropriately so as to have reasonable expectations regarding what the procedure will accomplish, an understanding of the procedure itself, risks of the procedure, anticipated outcomes (immediate and long-term), pain during the procedure and immediately afterward, an understanding that the patient will have some level of awareness during the procedure, and the anticipated immediate post-procedural course.

Unrealistic expectations begin with patients' perceptions that ambulatory surgery procedures are "routine" or "minor." On the contrary, invasive procedures that were performed on an inpatient basis only a few years ago are now performed on an outpatient basis. Physicians may also view outpatient procedures as "routine," making them less apt to spend as much time educating an outpatient about possible complications as they would an inpatient. Patients may expect to walk out of the ASC [ambulatory surgery center] or hospital-based unit pain-free immediately after surgery [3].

The patient must be willing and able to comply with preop medical/drug therapy (e.g., hormonal thinning of the endometrial lining prior to endometrial ablation), as well as postoperative requirements (e.g., effective contraception for 3 months after hysteroscopic sterilization until tubal occlusion can be confirmed).

Patient history. As part of the initial evaluation of the patient, it is assumed that a complete history is obtained, including:

- Past medical history
  - Medical complications/comorbidities
    - Hypertension, pulmonary disease, sleep apnea, diabetes, renal disease, liver disease, neurologic disease
    - Anxiety, depression
    - History of severe vagal reactions
    - Developmental delay (impact on ability to comply with pre-/intra-/post-procedural instruction)
  - Consider risk factors such as age, obesity, exercise capacity, diagnosis of obstructive sleep apnea (particularly in the patient undergoing conscious sedation)
  - Current medications (including over-the-counter and herbal preparations)
    - Discontinue nonsteroidal anti-inflammatory drugs (NSAIDs) for 2–3 days before surgery, substituting acetaminophen if necessary. Vitamin E and some herbal agents, such as ginkgo, can also prolong bleeding times and should be avoided before surgery.
    - For most patients, the risk of thrombotic events from discontinuing antithrombotic agents (e.g., aspirin, clopidogrel, warfarin) outweighs any increased risk of bleeding with their continued administration [4, 5]. Patients who are taking aspirin for primary prevention of cardiovascular disease or for an indication other than antiplatelet therapy (such as pain control), should discontinue aspirin 7–10 days before surgery.
  - Allergies (reactions to medication, latex, iodine, local anesthetics)
    - In addition to allergies (or reported allergies) to medications, inquire about reactions to latex, iodine, local anesthetics, and adhesive tape. Reactions to these items used commonly in the office setting may resemble allergies. Reactions including psychomotor or anxiety-related actions, vasovagal syncope, and sympathetic

stimulation can simulate allergic reactions. Reports of dyspnea, syncope, light-headedness, and hypotension may be associated with both allergic and non-allergic reactions. However, signs such as wheezing, pruritus, angioedema are suggestive of true allergic reaction.

Psychomotor reactions—Psychomotor reactions or anxiety-related symptoms include hyperventilation (manifested by dyspnea and tachypnea), paresthesias in the fingers or peri-oral area, dizziness, palpitations, tachycardia, nausea, or simply "not feeling good" [6, 7].

Vasovagal syncope—Vasovagal syncope is usually associated with bradycardia (rather than tachycardia) and pallor (rather than flushing). These differences can be helpful in distinguishing it from anaphylaxis.

Sympathetic stimulation—Tachycardia, hypertension, anxiety, and palpitations may be caused by the release of endogenous catecholamines in response to pain. In addition, the vasoconstrictor epinephrine is sometimes added to local anesthetic solutions for the purposes of reducing bleeding, potentiating the degree of local anesthesia achieved, limiting the total dose required, and minimizing systemic absorption of the local anesthetic [8, 9]. Although the amount of epinephrine in these preparations is too small to induce significant systemic responses in most normal subjects, or in those with heart disease, high blood pressure, hyperthyroidism, or on tricyclic antidepressants [8–10], it is still possible that some patients are very sensitive to its actions.

- Obstetric history
- Gynecologic history
  - Menstrual history

    History of heavy menses (consider screening for von Willebrand disease, particularly if the patient reports a history of post-partum hemorrhage, or excessive bleeding associated with previous surgery or dental work)
  - Current reproductive status

    If menopausal, any abnormal bleeding or atrophy complaints
  - Anatomic anomalies

    Cervical stenosis

    Previous cervical procedures (cerclage, cryotherapy, LEEP/cold knife cone biopsy, laser)

    Mullerian anomaly

    Anatomic abnormalities (fibroids, synechiae)
  - History of sexually transmitted infections (STI) or pelvic inflammatory disease (PID)
- Surgical history
  - Presence of a pacemaker (consider when using electrocautery)
  - History of bleeding diathesis in the patient herself or a family member (see also menstrual history)
  - Depending on type of office procedure, specifics of previous uterine surgery

    Cesarean section

    Myomectomy

    Dilatation and Evacuation (D&E)

    Dilatation and Curettage (D&C)
  - History of acute procedure anxiety

    Consideration of anxiolytic medication
- Family history
  - Bleeding history
  - Complications associated with anesthesia
- Social history
  - Smoking, alcohol, and illicit drug use
  - Avoid alcoholic beverages for 48 h before surgery; they also may increase bleeding.

Physical Exam

In addition to the standard gynecologic exam, including assessment for thyromegaly, cardiac and pulmonary abnormalities, and evaluation of habitus, the physical exam is a critical aspect of patient selection and maximizing success of the planned office-based surgical procedure. A key area to note is the patient's level of anxiety and ability to comply with even the basic gynecologic exam. In particular, a patient who has such anxiety that placement of a small speculum is challenging and requires significant counseling and "hand-holding" is not likely able to tolerate an office procedure that requires tolerance of a prolonged exam with discomfort, no matter how much the patient may desire to cooperate. Patients with a history of sexual abuse or trauma may involuntarily spasm or tense their pelvic floor musculature, despite acknowledgment that the exam and/or procedure is beneficial. Patients with vulvodynia or vaginismus may similarly be intolerant of office procedures.

Additional physical findings that may limit the success of office-based gynecologic procedures include enlarged or irregularly-shaped uterus, which may severely displace the location of the cervix and limit accessibility to the endometrial cavity. Cervical patency, which may be limited by previous surgery or menopausal status, should be assessed prior to attempting an in-office procedure. Furthermore, redundant vaginal walls or extreme obesity may prevent adequate retraction necessary for cervical or intrauterine access.

Finally, consider limitations of mobility and range of motion at the hips and knees, particularly in geriatric patients. Utilizing medical assistant aid in supporting a leg that cannot be flexed at the knee due to joint replacement may be feasible during such quick exams as obtaining a pap smear or culture swab; any procedure with its commensurate risk of complications requires a more reliable way to stabilize and secure the patient's extremities, so as to avoid potential injury to the patient or staff. Some patients with vasculopathy may also complain of leg cramps when having to maintain legs in stirrups, which could interfere with time-dependent procedures such as endometrial ablation.

Laboratory

In general, routine preoperative laboratory tests in healthy patients do not improve outcomes and are unnecessary. If the patient has known chronic illness, verifying that her medical management is optimized prior to the planned procedure is prudent. This may be done via targeted laboratory tests in the office (TSH, hemoglobin A1C, serum creatinine, hemoglobin/hematocrit), or in conjunction with the patient's internist. If excessive bleeding is anticipated in a patient with anemia, a preoperative hemoglobin may be of benefit. As a whole, routine tests such as electrolytes, blood glucose, liver function tests, coagulation profile, ECG, or chest X-ray, are not recommended for the healthy patient with normal function and capacity.

The exception is that rather than relying only on history, pregnancy testing should be performed in all reproductive-aged women prior to surgery. In addition to providing a safety check prior to starting an invasive procedure, a negative result contributes safeguards from a medico-legal standpoint. The prevalence of unrecognized pregnancy was illustrated in a prospective study that performed pregnancy tests on all women of childbearing potential (defined as menstruating women without prior hysterectomy or tubal ligation) scheduled for ambulatory surgery [11]. Testing revealed seven previously unrecognized pregnancies in 2,056 women (0.3 %), including two patients scheduled to undergo fertility procedures. All of the pregnant women cancelled or postponed their procedures.

Special Considerations

Management of Thrombotic Risk

The primary consideration when preparing a patient taking blood-thinning agents for office-based surgery is: *what is the thrombotic risk if anticoagulation is stopped*? versus *what is the bleeding risk if anticoagulation is continued*? In patients with high thrombotic risk (i.e., stroke within 3 months [12]), the surgeon should consider the urgency of the proposed surgery, and whether waiting 6–9 months is acceptable to allow the patient's thrombotic risk stratification to improve. Conversely, gynecologic procedures such as dilation and curettage, and even abdominal hysterectomy, are considered low bleeding risk procedures (2-day risk of major bleed of 0–2 % [13]), such that the gynecologic procedures that would be performed in the office setting are low bleeding risk even if anticoagulation is continued.

In the context of these considerations and the risk-benefit analysis is to contemplate the specific procedure to be performed. The inherent risk for bleeding is clearly different when performing endometrial biopsy or cystoscopy, as compared to LEEP or vulvar biopsy.

Additional considerations. The "*office* set-up" and policies are discussed in Chap. 2, but there are some items worth underscoring and remembering as they pertain to patient selection and optimization of "*patient* set-up". Consider whether there are some "absolutes" in the preprocedural protocol and work-up. Establish protocols and adhere to them (e.g., always check a pregnancy test). Exceptions can be incorporated (e.g., no pregnancy test in those patients older than 65 years of age, or after tubal ligation), but should not be provider-dependent or based on assumptions. Consider defining rules on doing the procedure immediately at the patient's first visit to the office, as compared to requiring "mandatory" one or two pre-op appointment(s) first. Anticipate there will be questions, even if the patient has done her "homework", or comes into the office determined on a certain procedure. Oftentimes, the patient's source of information may be unreliable or anecdotal; send the patient home with written materials and return for preop counseling and review.

Adequate preparation (nothing by mouth, medications or preparation such as misoprostol or laminaria) is necessary for the planned procedure to be successful. Consider the patient's ability to be compliant with preoperative medical therapy (including medical therapy of the endometrium, vaginal estrogen therapy in a postmenopausal patient).

Consider adequacy of the consent process and comprehension (see Chap. 3 for details regarding "Informed Consent"). The office must have adequate and timely interpreter services available. If a "language line" interpreter is being used, verify that there are telephone jacks and hands-free equipment available in the procedure room(s). Many localities have rules pertaining to the use of "certified" interpreters (e.g., sign language interpreters specific to the patient's language who are also able to speak English). Family members should not be relied upon as interpreters.

Consider post-procedure management protocols. Each specific chapter will review post-procedure management and instructions specific to the procedure. However, there should be clearly written instructions for the patient to take home, with listing of common symptoms (such as mild nausea, constipation, anticipated level of pain), as well as indications for seeking medical care emergently. Anticipate how the patient will get home. Particularly in urban settings, public transportation may be the patient's only mode of transportation, and accounting for special travel arrangements after an office-based procedure should parallel what occurs in the hospital setting, especially when the procedure is performed under any level of sedation.

Conclusion

Office-based gynecologic procedures provide the opportunity for patients to receive treatment and evaluation in a lower-anxiety, familiar setting while also avoiding the many logistical hurdles involved in performing the same procedures in the operating room. Additionally, surgeons have the added benefit of recouping costs at a significantly higher rate than in regulated hospital settings. However, the most critical component for a successful office-based procedure program is appropriate patient selection and evaluation. The evaluation of the patient is similar to that of any preoperative assessment, but the patient selection component requires that the physician considers other factors that come into play when performing invasive procedures on the patient who is awake, in an environment where emergency services may not be immediately available. Adhering to written protocols and established practices, in addition to prudent risk-consideration and management in patient selection will allow for a safe, positive experience for both the patient and her physician.

References

1. Cullen KA, Hall MJ, Golosinskiy A. Ambulatory surgery in the United States, 2006. National health statistics reports; no. 11. Revised. Hyattsville, MD: National Center for Health Statistics; 2009.
2. www.cms.gov, 2014 Physician Fee Schedule Search, National Payment Amount.
3. Goldberg-Alberts AL, Solomon RP. A primer on risk management for ambulatory surgery. J Ambul Care Manage. 1997;20(3):72–90.
4. Kovich O, Otley CC. Thrombotic complications related to discontinuation of warfarin and aspirin therapy perioperatively for cutaneous operation. J Am Acad Dermatol. 2003;48(2):233–7.
5. Alcalay J, Alkalay R. Controversies in perioperative management of blood thinners in dermatologic surgery: continue or discontinue? Dermatol Surg. 2004;30(8):1091–4.
6. Dower Jr JS. A review of paresthesia in association with administration of local anesthesia. Dent Today. 2003;22:64–9.
7. Fiset L, Milgrom P, Weinstein P, et al. Psychophysiological responses to dental injections. J Am Dent Assoc. 1985;111:578–83.
8. Cawson RA, Curson I, Whittington DR. The hazards of dental local anaesthetics. Br Dent J. 1983; 154:253–8.
9. Chernow B, Balestrieri F, Ferguson CD, et al. Local dental anesthesia with epinephrine. Minimal effects on the sympathetic nervous system or on hemodynamic variables. Arch Intern Med. 1983;143:2141–3.
10. Latronica RJ, Goldberg AF, Wightman JR. Local anesthetic sensitivity. Report of a case. Oral Surg Oral Med Oral Pathol. 1969;28:439–41.
11. Manley S, de Kelaita G, Joseph NJ, Salem MR, Heyman HJ. Preoperative pregnancy testing in ambulatory surgery. Incidence and impact of positive results. Anesthesiology. 1995;83(4):690–3.
12. Douketis JD, Spyropoulos AC, Spencer FA, et al. Perioperative management of antithrombotic therapy: Antithrombotic Therapy and Prevention of Thrombosis, 9th ed: American College of Chest Physicians Evidence-Based Clinical Practice Guidelines. Chest. 2012;141(2 Suppl):e326S.
13. Spyropoulos AC, Douketis JD. How I treat anticoagulated patients undergoing an elective procedure or surgery. Blood. 2012;120:2954–62.

Getting Started in Office-Based Gynecologic Procedures: Office Set-up, Procedural Implications and Ensuring Patient Safety

2

Natalie A. Bowersox and Jonathan D. Emery

Introduction

As more minimally invasive gynecologic procedures move from the operating room to the office setting, physicians are responding by offering previously hospital or ambulatory surgery-based procedures in their offices. The reasons for this seem to be related to the physician, the patient, and the payer due to better reimbursement and the convenience of the office. After a patient has been scheduled in the office setting, they have the right to expect the same level of safety and structure that occurs in a hospital setting and studies have supported this [1, 2]. This chapter will discuss the establishment of an office-based program for minimally invasive gynecologic procedures which include creating a procedure room, instituting proper documentation, including the use of checklists, as well as issues surrounding compliance, all in the hopes of creating a culture of patient safety and satisfaction in the office setting when instituting an in-office gynecologic surgery program.

N.A. Bowersox, M.D. (✉)
Department of Obstetrics and Gynecology & Women's Health Institute, Fairview Hospital, 3574 Center Road, Brunswick, OH 44212, USA
e-mail: bowersn@ccf.org

J.D. Emery, M.D.
Department of Obstetrics and Gynecology & Women's Health Institute, Cleveland Clinic, 2550 SOM Center Road, Suite 100, Willoughby Hills, OH 44094, USA
e-mail: emeryj@ccf.org

Office Set-up

Designating the Right People and the Right Place

To start, a room or rooms should be designated within the office specifically dedicated to the procedures to be performed. This space should be large enough to allow for access to the patient during the office-based procedure, and to accommodate all equipment needed to perform the procedure (Fig. 2.1). This may be in the same area where the provider sees patients, or in a separate area designated for procedures only, dependent on specifics of the office practice. With this, the necessary equipment should optimally be designated only for these rooms to reduce the possibility that the equipment needed for a specific procedure would be unexpectedly unavailable, damaged, or missing. Adequate lighting is imperative. This would include a high-intensity, adjustable examining light source, either mounted with an extended arm or portable so as to allow adequate lighted exposure during procedures, whether external or vaginal. Baggish [3] recommends an electrically controlled examination bed in order to assist in optimally positioning the patient.

An individual or group of individuals specifically dedicated to office procedures should manage the set-up and maintenance of the room itself. This way, a "team" for office procedures is established and is familiar with what needs to

J.D. Emery and M.F.R. Paraiso (eds.), *Office-Based Gynecologic Surgical Procedures*, DOI 10.1007/978-1-4939-1414-2_2, © Springer Science+Business Media New York 2015

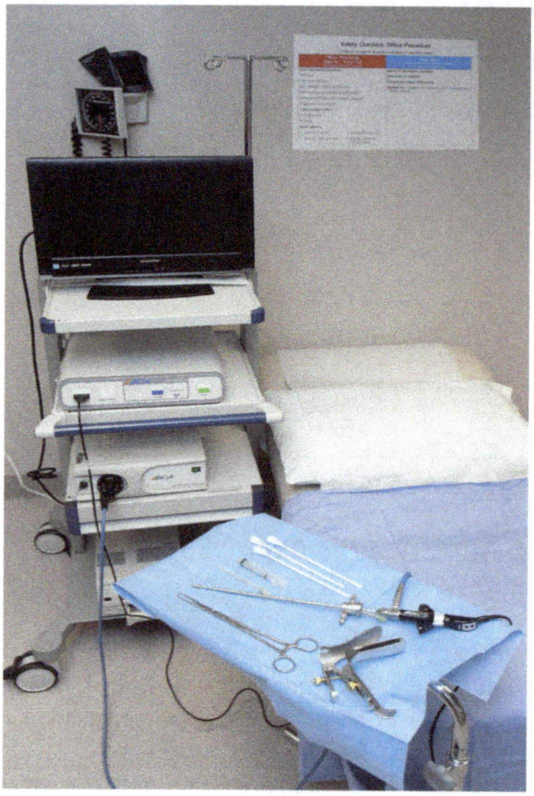

Fig. 2.1 Example of procedure room set-up for office-based surgery

be done prior to, during, and after a procedure. This would also ensure that equipment is available, functioning, sterilized (when needed) and ready to go. The office team may include medical assistants (MA) and/or nurses depending on the scope of practice required. If medication is to be given, either orally, intramuscularly or intravenously, then availability of a nurse is recommended. Office managers or other administrative personnel should be included to help ensure appropriate oversight and compliance as needed. Also, one of the team members should be responsible for documentation before, during, and after the procedure to delineate performance of necessary items of the surgical checklist, referenced below.

A physician must always be readily available before and after the procedure as well. This is of primary importance for safety in the office. If a physician is not present in the office, for instance, pre-procedural medications or anesthetics should not be given in case allergic or other related complications were to occur. The physician is the designated "team leader" and must be accountable to the office staff and to the patients. Ideally, the physician will be in the office setting until all the patients who underwent procedures that day safely leave the office.

Equipment

Performance of office-based surgical procedures requires certain equipment be available in order to perform each procedure as well as have specific supplies readily available in case problems or complications occur during the procedure. A basic list of equipment needed to perform any office procedure is listed in Table 2.1. Most gynecology offices will have many of the suggested pieces of equipment available; however, supplies should be checked prior to each procedure, or optimally at the beginning of each week to assure sterilization of needed equipment is undertaken and to prevent mishaps during the procedure.

For the more invasive procedures (hysteroscopy, both diagnostic and operative, global endometrial ablation, hysteroscopic sterilization, cystoscopy, urodynamics, and colposcopy with LEEP), procedure-specific equipment will need to be purchased or leased. While this process will be physician and office dependent, several points must be considered. First, the physician must be certain to be appropriately trained and credentialed in the procedure (see below). Also, the specifics of certain types of equipment (that of a certain brand or manufacturer) will depend upon both physician preference and cost: use of a certain brand at the hospital where the physician operates may be too costly or unavailable for the office so it may be important to see if a more affordable option is available that provides the same level of effectiveness and safety. Maintenance, sterilization requirements, and associated costs also need to be considered. Overall expense to the office practice needs to be evaluated as well, many times in conjunction with an office manager or financial consultant.

Table 2.1 Basic office supplies for performance of office-based gynecologic surgery

• Sterile and nonsterile gloves
• Antiseptic/cleansing solution (such as betadine or baby shampoo)
• Cotton swabs
• Pads or fluid drapes (such as chux pads)
• Speculum (variety of sizes and types)
• Tenaculum
• Dilator(s) or dilator probes
• Specimen containers
• Basin
• Appropriate suture
• Needle driver
• Scissors
• Forceps
• Syringes and appropriate needles for local anesthetics
• Normal saline

When considering which procedure-specific equipment is needed, it is important to decide whether disposable instruments will be used or whether the use of sterilization equipment will be needed for cleaning and sterilization of reusable equipment, especially the hysteroscope or cystoscope. The care and maintenance of instruments must be maintained according to the manufacturer's instruction manual and serviced by the specific vendor to ensure equipment is maintained properly to maximize its use and shelf life if disposable instruments are not being used. Improper handling or sterilization of the expensive scopes can lead to equipment damage such as condensation of fluid within the lens. Mishandling of light cords or electrical equipment can lead to damage and/or breakage with increased costs for repair or replacement.

If ultrasound is being utilized in the office, either alone or for use with saline infusion sonography, acquisition of necessary ultrasound machines is needed as well as that needed for appropriate disinfecting and sterilization of the transvaginal probe. Image capture and storage also needs to be addressed as well as if appropriate office or ultrasound site credentialing from a national organization such as American Institute of Ultrasound Medicine (AIUM) is desired or required.

While physicians must be appropriately credentialed and trained in the procedure(s) to be performed in the office setting, it is important that the physician and the office team review information about any new procedure or device being used. Stumpf recommends that all members of the team be acquainted with and knowledgable about new equipment (and for some office nurses and medical assistants, hysteroscopy and cystoscopy, for example, will be new equipment and procedures *for them*) and should be aware of safety features, warning mechanisms, and alarms on the device [2]. For example, it has been shown that serious complications occurred with use of global endometrial ablation devices when there was nonadherence to manufacturer's protocols or when the safety features of the devices were "over-ridden" [4]. Nurses and medical assistants should read and periodically review manufacturer's instructions and have them available for all team members should questions about the procedure arise.

Sterilization

In terms of sterilization, the initial decision is to determine if this is to be done in the office itself or sent to an outside vendor for processing and sterilization. If the process is to be done by an outside vendor, the surgeon and staff need to be aware of scheduling and stocking of equipment in order to ensure needed equipment such as the cystoscope or hysteroscope is clean and available. If this is done in the office, who will be completing this, and how will they be kept in compliance for maintaining the instruments? Some institutions have specific protocols that are followed in regards to sterilization (see policy for your specific institution) but stand-alone offices will need to have one.

The ultimate goal of disinfection and sterilization in office surgical practices is to reduce rates of health care-associated infections through appropriate use of both disinfection and sterilization [5]. Therefore, the type of sterilization should be addressed first. Once this has been decided, keep in mind that is important to always clean first, then disinfect or sterilize [6]. This

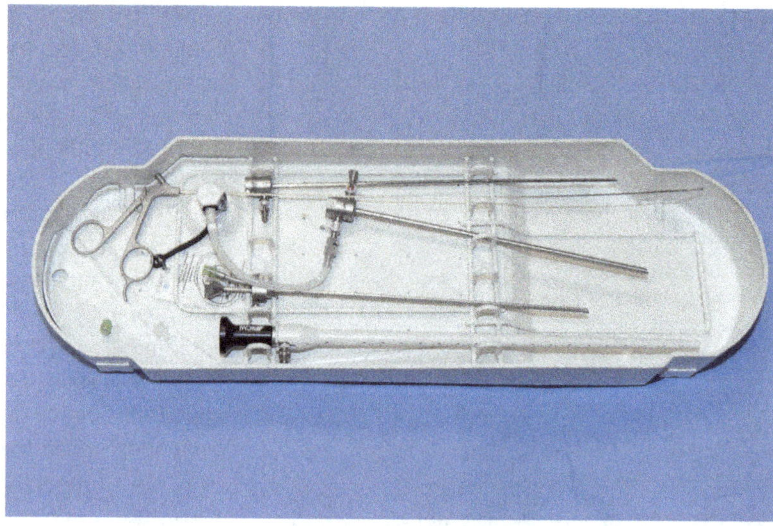

Fig. 2.2 Example of disassembly of an office hysterocope prior to sterilization

includes removing visible tissue and fluids to allow for the removal of microorganisms and organic matter. Shortly after use, take apart the equipment for cleaning and reassemble it on the field. Sterilize all moving parts in the open position to ensure proper cleaning. If there is a question about how an instrument should be cleaned, it is suggested to first follow the manufacturer's guidelines to avoid damaging an instrument or shortening its usefulness due to unnecessary wear and tear from improper maintenance.

All endoscopes should be disconnected and disassembled and cleaned with an enzymatic cleaner that is suitable with the cystoscope or hysteroscope (Fig. 2.2). Cleaning is needed before disinfection or sterilization. Also, single piece, reusable medical equipment such as single tooth tenaculum, Allis clamp or uterine sound should also be sterilized: each office will need to decide if it will sterilize each piece individually or as a procedure "set" and follow its own policy. Also, quality control and monitoring of sterilization equipment and of infection control is recommended and should be monitored and reviewed by the Medical Director (see below). Lastly, local and state standards and policies should be reviewed relative to the office location as well as compliance with Joint Commission on Accreditation of Healthcare Organizations (JCAHO) and Occupational Safety and Health Administration (OSHA) requirements.

If sterilization will be done in the office there are several types of sterilization techniques to consider, and the choice should be determined by what is most readily available and appropriate for each office. Time, space, and cost are factors to determine when considering set-up of sterilization system. Also, the office should be certain to utilize a Food and Drug Administration (FDA)-cleared liquid chemical sterilant and high-level disinfectant that can be used to reprocess office endoscopes and other equipment [5]. Below is a brief summary of common sterilization processes as outlined by Bradley and Fluharty [6].

Steam Sterilization

Steam is the preferred method for sterilizing critical medical and surgical instruments that are not damaged by heat, steam pressure, or moisture (CDC). Sterilization using steam is hazardous to telescopes and light cables unless they are wrapped for prevacuum sterilization or are flash sterilized when they are unwrapped. The prevacuum step takes about 45 min and is a multistep process. The flash sterilization is performed at high temperatures and high pressures. A drying phase may be added. Equipment must then be used immediately after sterilization. The equipment must be handled carefully because it is very hot.

Steris

Steris systems are becoming more popular due to the ability to rapidly disinfect equipment. Instruments are immersed in the buffered solution of 35 % peracetic acid and then treated in a high-agitation system. The time from start to finish is around 30 min. Instruments need to be used immediately after sterilization. The Steris system works by a combination of hydrogen peroxide combined with a low-temperature gas plasma system that produces low temperatures (50–104 °F).

Ethylene Oxide Gas Sterilization

Sterilization with ethylene oxide takes about 12 h to complete. Instruments must be totally dry when employing this method. All instruments must be properly aerated to remove residual toxic gas. Many health care facilities are starting to require other methods of sterilization as this method is restricted in some communities.

Single-use equipment, such as catheters for urodynamics, hysteroscopic sterilization catheters (microcoils), and loops for electo-excision procedures, should be used once and then disposed of in appropriate hazardous waste containers. If transvaginal ultrasound equipment is used with saline infusion sonography (SIS), appropriate cleaning and disinfection of the transvaginal probe is needed. Disposable single-use endovaginal probe covers have significant leakage rates and as such, the probe should undergo high-level disinfection of the probe between each use even if the probe cover appears intact [7].

Finally, standard office cleaning and disinfection should be undertaken after each office-based procedure to other equipment such as colposcopes (wiping down handles and dials), urodynamics equipment such as the urochair and other procedural office equipment.

Anesthesia and Analgesia

The next area to be addressed in regards to office set-up should be that of anesthesia and analgesia. This must be dictated by the type of procedure to be performed as well as input from the patient. The type of anesthesia used should never be altered due to limitations of equipment or personnel in the office setting. If the appropriate anesthesia needed for a specific case or a specific patient cannot be accommodated, then the case should be done in a more acute facility so it can be done safely and efficiently. With this in mind, the level of anesthesia (which includes light, moderate, or deep sedation) will dictate the equipment and the appropriate personnel needed for the case.

Once a procedure is scheduled in the office, it is necessary to first decide which level of anesthesia the office will provide, as the level of sedation needed for the procedure dictates specific protocols as listed below. The American Society of Anesthesiologists (ASA) has developed guidelines for sedation and these are discussed in more detail in Chap. 4. Level one includes the use of local anesthesia with minimal preoperative use of oral anxiolytics. Level two is moderate sedation, and level three is considered deep sedation or general anesthesia. A majority of the procedures in this text will likely need only local anesthetic with level-one sedation. On some occasions, level-two sedation may be needed. It is recommended by these authors that if sedation beyond level 2 is needed, consideration of assistance in office from an anesthesia related provider (Certified Registered Nurse Anesthetist (CRNA) or anesthiesiologist) be available during the procedure or consideration of performance of the procedure in an ambulatory surgery center (ASC) or monitored facility. The ability to rescue a patient from sedation is based on the level of anesthesia being used. Each office should develop a policy for emergency medication, resuscitation, and have the ability to rescue a patient from excessive medication. In the *Report of the Presidential Task Force on Patient Safety in the Office Setting* [5], it is recommended that these policies be based on ASA levels depending on the level of invasiveness.

Specifics for both local anesthetics and use of adjunct medications of analgesia or sedation are discussed more fully in Chap. 4. However, it is also advisable that gynecologic surgeons planning to perform in-office procedures review the document, "Practice Guidelines for Sedation and Analgesia by Non-Anesthesiologists" [8].

Use of Medications

In-office anesthesia and analgesia requires assessment of in-office medication use and safety. All medications necessary to complete a specific procedure need to be present and immediately available in the procedure room for use during an in-office surgery; this includes mediations that may be necessary to reverse or "rescue" any potential complications or oversedation. When a procedure will include a controlled medication, this must be stored, registered, and removed from a secure location. All medication use needs to be recorded and monitored with a medication log including the use of local anesthetics as well as controlled substances such as anxiolytics and medications used for pain relief. Medications need to be periodically checked for expiration dates to allow replacement as needed. It is frustrating to schedule an in-office surgery only to find that an important medication needed has passed its expiration date. The person(s) responsible for the medications needs to be present in the room during the procedure. Who this person is depends on the level of anesthesia that is being used. The responsible party ranges from nurse, CRNA, or anesthesiologist. The surgeon assumes responsibility for the first two. Once the procedure is complete, patient monitoring postoperatively will need to be correlated to the level of sedation achieved during the surgery. Many states are now requiring specific accreditation dependent upon if moderate sedation or deeper anesthesia is to be administered in office [9] and most states have regulations set forth by state pharmacy boards for specifics regarding use and distribution of in-office medication. Each physician is advised to avail him or herself of state and local guidelines regarding purchase, use, and storage of medications in the office setting.

Medication safety has been clearly recognized as a source of patient harm in the office setting [10]. One first step to overcome this potential problem is a clear process to assess patients' medications and allergies before beginning the procedure. While the advent of the computerized medical record has seemingly streamlined this process, a member of the office team should document medications and allergies prior to the start of the procedure as well as inform the surgeon and members of the team at the beginning of the procedure, such as during a procedural "time out". Use of standardized doses and schedules for each procedure are recommended. However, during or after the procedure and during urgent situations in the office, increased stress or the use of "verbal orders" may increase the possibility of error in prescribing and administering or monitoring medications [11].

Joint Commission has published Ambulatory Care National Safety Goals (NPSG) with specifics to medication safety in the ambulatory setting. In regards to medication safety, NPSG.03.04.01 *Improve the safety of giving medications* states," Label all medications, medication containers, and other solutions on and off the sterile field in perioperative and other procedural settings. Note that medication containers include syringes, medicine cups, and basins" [12]. This means that any medication, whether given orally, intravenously (IV), or intramuscularly (IM) to the patient before the procedure, used in a syringe during a procedure (such as with local anesthesia) or if given in oral, IV or IM in recovery after the procedure should have labels that include the following:

- Medication name
- Strength
- Quantity
- Diluent and volume (if not apparent from the container)
- Expiration date when not used within 24 h
- Expiration time when expiration occurs in less than 24 h

This can be done by a member of the surgical team, typically a registered nurse, with appropriate documentation and logging of in-office medications given. Documentation in the patient's medical record of administered medications given at any time during the procedure (preoperative, during the procedure or in recovery) must also be clearly recorded.

Recovery and Follow-up

Following the procedure, the patient should be taken to a designated recovery area where she can be monitored. A physician must be available in the office, and reasonably free of other duties to be able to respond to an emergency until the patient is discharged. Depending on the level of sedation used, the physician must be certified in basic life support (BLS) or advanced cardiovascular life support (ACLS) as well. In addition, any health care professional or staff involved in the office-based surgeries using sedation should be familiar with the office policy and procedure in the event of an emergency as well as the policy in the event of an office evacuation. Also, procedures to be followed in the event of a patient transfer to another medical facility (for a higher level of care) should be available for all office staff to ensure a safe and timely patient transfer.

Prior to the start of the procedure it is important to always confirm the patient has transportation to home. The discharge to home (or other facility) should be documented in the patient's medical record, and should include the time and date of discharge, and a description of the patient's medical condition at the time of discharge. It is also recommended to give the patient written discharge instructions, which should be given at an appropriate reading level and available in multiple languages if needed [10] and document in the medical record that this was done. These instructions should include guidelines to be followed by the patient and associated caregivers for postoperative wound care, medication use as well what to do in the event of a postoperative problem [13]. If the patient or potential home caregiver is unable to carry out these instructions, the patient's postoperative care may be compromised and hospital admission should be considered depending upon the procedure performed and the patient's medical comorbidities.

The patient should be given an appropriate follow-up appointment. Consideration of a follow-up phone call from the office within 24–48 h after discharge from the office (typically the next day) is suggested in order to assess the patient's status and to attempt to recognize possible complications; this call should also be documented in the patient's medical record. Again, office staff should be encouraged to have patients seek care, preferably at the office, for concerns or complications that occur during this time or at any time in the following days to weeks. Patients frequently have the expectation that office-based surgery will be "pain-free" or "without complications" since it is done in the office (a lower acuity environment) versus being done in a hospital (a higher acuity setting). Because of this, the physician and staff should be aware of this during preoperative and postoperative communication in order to better assess patient's concerns and to recognize and triage potential complications.

Procedural Considerations

Informed Consent

Informed consent is defined as permission granted in the knowledge of the possible consequences, typically that which is given by a patient to a doctor for treatment with full knowledge of the possible risks and benefits. That being said, Chap. 3 will discuss fully all aspects of informed consent, but here it is important to emphasize that this is an active process that occurs between the provider and the patient. The patient needs to be informed about what procedure is being performed, the equipment that is to be used, risks, benefits, and alternatives to this procedure so that they are properly engaged and educated about how the procedure will impact her health. The patient needs to be able to understand the risks in lay terms and be able to say them back to you. Keats notes that communication with patients in general should be undertaken in the context of her level of health literacy in terms of the ability of the patient to comprehend and understand what is being conveyed to her [10]. This should be a face-to-face discussion, preferably at a visit separate from the actual procedure time itself and informed consent should be obtained in writing. The informed consent document should be kept in the patient's medical record. If possible, provide the patients with educational material that they can take home with them or reference online. Be mindful, that any educational material for the patient should keep in mind her level of health literacy as well: ACOG has published guidelines for this [14] but most agree that educational material should be written at a fifth grade level. Also, encouraging your patients to keep a medical journal could be considered so that areas of concern can be addressed in a timely manner and questions that may come up after the patient leaves the office can be remembered and discussed at the next visit or just prior to their scheduled procedure. The informed consent process also allows for establishing a dialogue about the procedure that begins before and extends to after the office procedure has been performed.

Documentation

Documentation is the logical next issue that should be discussed and established, and perhaps the best place to start is at the beginning with a policy and procedure manual. The Medical Director should be the primary provider to establish a policy and procedure manual for the office, primarily to focus on patient safety practices [10] though other team members should be involved in establishing this manual.

Prior to any gynecologic surgical procedure being performed in the office, it is reasonable to develop a policy and procedure manual that outlines all the information that pertains to office-based surgery. This would include consent forms, checklists (see below), instructions for pre and postoperative care as well as other documents and required forms needed to assure patient safety [10]. This would include policies and required documents and standards from local and state agencies. Wortman has outlined various regulations and policies that govern office-based surgery across the United States [15] but bear in mind, each office (especially the Medical Director) should be aware of the requirements in her office jurisdiction. Specific national recommendations from accrediting agencies such as American College of Obstetricians and Gynecologists (ACOG) or the American Medical Association (AMA) should also be included. If the office practice is part of a larger hospital or hospital system, the manual may come from your institution and be adapted for the office, or can be derived from your office individually.

Tracking of patient results and follow-up is important for both the patient and the office staff. Office-based gynecologic procedures often require some form of follow-up that involves pathology results, need for further testing, possible referral or consultations as well as timing of appropriate follow-up: thus, gynecologists should have policy and procedures in place to track these actions efficiently and to ultimately improve patient safety [16]. After the procedure is completed, the office should have a standard procedure in place to track that results were both received *and* communicated with the patient. Failure to track this data may be a significant source of missed or delayed diagnosis and/or treatment with the potential for patient harm [10]. Gone are the days of "no news is good news" and patient communication of all results, both significant or benign, need to be communicated with the patient, ensuring it is done in a manner consistent with patient privacy laws.

Along with this, each patient should receive a copy of their rights and responsibilities. Another approach to this could also be using the Universal Patient Compact which outlines principles for partnership. Whichever way this is approached, the policy needs to be available and visible for your patients. Figure 2.3 lists an example from the National Patient Safety Foundation [17].

The Universal Patient Compact™

Principles for Partnership

As your healthcare partner we pledge to:

- Include you as a member of the team
- Treat you with respect, honesty and compassion
- Always tell you the truth
- Include your family or advocate when you would like us to
- Hold ourselves to the highest quality and safety standards
- Be responsive and timely with our care and information to you
- Help you to set goals for your healthcare and treatment plans
- Listen to you and answer your questions
- Provide information to you in a way you can understand
- Respect your right to your own medical information
- Respect your privacy and the privacy of your medical information
- Communicate openly about benefits and risks associated with any treatments
- Provide you with information to help you make informed decisions about your care and treatment options
- Work with you, and other partners who treat you, in the coordination of your care

As a patient I pledge to:

- Be a responsible and active member of my healthcare team
- Treat you with respect, honesty and consideration
- Always tell you the truth
- Respect the commitment you have made to healthcare and healing
- Give you the information that you need to treat me
- Learn all that I can about my condition
- Participate in decisions about my care
- Understand my care plan to the best of my ability
- Tell you what medications I am taking
- Ask questions when I do not understand and until I do understand
- Communicate any problems I have with the plan for my care
- Tell you if something about my health changes
- Tell you if I have trouble reading
- Let you know if I have family, friends or an advocate to help me with my healthcare

NPSF National Patient Safety Foundation®

Reviewed and reaffirmed for Patient Safety Awareness Week 2010

Fig. 2.3 National Patient Safety Foundation "principles for partnership"

Establishing a Climate of Patient Safety in Office Surgery

Medical Director

During the set-up of an office-based surgical practice, the office should appoint a physician as Medical Director as this is a requirement by ACOG and many national accrediting institutions [18]. This is crucial for leadership as well as assuring all office personnel are held accountable for all aspects of patient safety. This director will have the responsibility of making sure that all personnel involved in the office procedures, including any other physicians in the practice, are qualified and well-versed in their respective roles. A Medical Director would verify qualifications including credentialing, privileging, and accreditation, work to ensure safety, and have a thorough understanding of people, equipment, space, and supplies [19]. In addition, regular meetings with all stakeholders should be held to ensure that this is occurring and to troubleshoot any issues. Many of the aspects of the duties of the Medical Director are found in Table 2.2. If the office is a larger site, a Safety Officer appointed by the Medical Director should be considered as well. In addition, this person should also be notified of all complications and unanticipated outcomes as well as lead periodic audits and evaluations of procedures and policies. Finally, the Medical Director should be encouraged to seek and use national governmental and nongovernmental agencies to assure compliance and safety are maintained in the office (Table 2.3).

The Checklist

The use of checklists has been advocated in aviation and other sectors for many years but have become increasingly popular in medicine in the past 10 years especially after the publication of Atul Gawande's *The Checklist Manifesto* [20] for the simple reason that no matter how expert one is, studies show a well-designed checklist can improve outcomes and because medicine has become more complex such that procedures and safety require a "team-based" approach. For inpatient surgery, the "Safe Surgery Saves Lives" campaign by the World Health Organization (WHO) was shown to improve outcomes using a checklist [21]. While this approach was developed for inpatient surgery, many of the principles could be applied in office-based surgery as well. Also, the Joint Commission introduced the "Universal Protocol" which includes three crucial steps for ensuring patient safety: (1) pre-procedure verification, (2) marking the operative site and (3) performing a pause or "time out" before starting the procedure [12].

Utilizing the WHO checklist in the office setting means that a sign-in, time-out, and sign-out should be completed for each case as well, just as they are in the operating rooms at the hospital. On arrival to the office, the patient should have photo identification, insurance information, and any relevant medical information with them. In addition, prior to the start of any procedure or administration of any anesthesia, the "sign-in" is performed and includes verification of informed consent as well as review of medications and allergies. This should include all members of the team as well as the patient and should verify: correct patient (with two independent identifiers, typically name and date of birth), correct procedure, and correct site of the surgery. Included in this portion is the "marking the site" of surgery. All personnel involved as well as the timing and steps of this process should be documented during the surgery (Table 2.4). This is the time to verify that all medical information is correct and consistent, all teams members and the patient agree on the procedure to be performed as well as the location and side or site of the procedure. If a *side* is designated, this will need to be marked by the physician performing the procedure and verified with the patient (the left labia or the right Bartholin's gland). However, in the case of many office-based gynecologic procedures, "marking" the *site* of surgery, such as the cervix or uterus may not be feasible.

Table 2.2 Office surgical safety checklist

How to use the office surgical safety checklist
• Review the checklist with your entire surgical team. Assign each task to the appropriate staff member (e.g., patient's escort driver is confirmed by the front desk staff or the preoperative time-out is performed by the physician). This may vary from office to office.
• Assign one person (i.e., physician or nurse) as a checklist coordinator to be responsible for confirming the tasks on the list with the assigned individual.
• The checklist coordinator should confirm each task verbally with the appropriate office team member to ensure the appropriate procedures have been implemented and documented. If necessary, the checklist coordinator also can obtain initials from each of the assigned individuals to confirm completion of their respective tasks.
• If the task does not apply to the patient, the checklist coordinator should confirm this with the physician (e.g., the use of imaging may not apply to all patients).
• The checklist coordinator should stop the office surgery team from progressing to the next phase of the operation until all tasks have been appropriately addressed. Ideally, any team member should feel comfortable to stop the procedure if they have safety concerns.
• The office surgery team should debrief to discuss modifications for future uses of the checklist. Removing tasks is not recommended.
Preoperative checklist
• Meets office-based surgery requirements
• Meets American Society of Anesthesiologists (ASA) Physical Status I criteria or medically controlled ASA Physical Status II
• Prescreening verification that the patient is a candidate for an office-based procedure. Contraindications include but are not limited to:
– Personal or family history of adverse reaction to local anesthetic
– History of previous failure with local anesthetic or low pain threshold
– An acute respiratory process
– Failure to comply with preoperative dietary restrictions
– Substance abuse
– High-risk airway assessment
– Abnormal blood sugars
– Pregnancy (unless procedure is pregnancy related)
• Document appropriate workup, patient selection, and informed consent
• No change in medical condition since previous office visit
• Preoperative vital signs
• Current history and physical
• Review and record all medications taken previously that day
• Confirm nil per os (nothing by mouth-NPO) status
• Confirm preoperative instructions followed
• Review allergies
• Confirm patient has an escort driver
• Document no change in patient's medical condition
• Confirm presence of any indicated lab work (e.g., glucose level in a diabetic)
Intraoperative checklist
• Time-out (verify provider, patient, surgical site, and procedure)
• Record intraoperative medications
• If sedation implemented, monitor and document oxygen saturation, blood pressure, and level of alertness every 5 min
• For hysteroscopic procedures, record cavity assessment per manufacturer's guidelines
Postoperative checklist
• Record vital signs and ensure return to within 20% of baseline
• Document adequate level of consciousness, pain control, ability to tolerate liquids by mouth, and ability to void (if appropriate for the procedure)

(continued)

Table 2.2 (continued)

How to use the office surgical safety checklist
• Discharge instruction sheet that includes how to recognize a postoperative emergency and steps to follow should one occur after discharge (e.g., hemorrhage)
• Postoperative follow-up call within 48 h
• Schedule appropriate postoperative follow-up appointment
• Record long-term outcome
• Record complications

Reprinted with permission from American College of Obstetricians and Gynecologists. Report of the Presidential Task Force on Patient Safety in the Office Setting. Washington, DC: American College of Obstetricians and Gynecologists; 2010

Table 2.3 Important references for establishment of office-based gynecologic surgical practice

National Patient Safety Foundation	www.npsf.org
Joint Commission on Accreditation of Healthcare Organizations	www.jointcommission.org
Safety Certification in Outpatient Practice Excellence for Women's Health	www.scopeforwomenshealth.org
Accreditation Association for Ambulatory Healthcare	www.aaahc.org

Table 2.4 Example of safety checklist to use during office procedures

Office procedure
Sign-in/time-out
Pre-procedure checklist
1. Informed consent
2. Allergies
3. Equipment/supplies available
4. Site marked (as applicable)
5. Imaging and diagnostic test results
Procedural list:
Nursing/concerns
Team agrees
1. Correct patient
2. Correct procedure
3. Correct side and site
4. Correct position (as applicable)
Sign-Out completed prior to patient leaving procedure room
Post-procedure checklist
1. Name of procedure recorded
2. Specimens conformed and labeled
3. Equipment issues identified/addressed
4. Patient recovery issues and concerns for patient management

Finally, a "time-out" is performed before the procedure itself commences. This involves the entire office team—physician, nurse, MA, and any anesthesia personnel if present—and may be done after initiation of local anesthesia or IV sedation. This portion would also include administration of antibiotics, if needed. Then, a "sign-out" should be performed at the conclusion of the procedure to document for the team what was done, any specimens that were collected, properly labeled and to be sent to pathology and any issues with equipment, the anesthesia or the surgery itself that need to be documented. Also, if there are concerns about patient-specific recovery or discharge issues, these should be addressed at this time. An operative or procedure note should be completed at the end of the case similar to what is done at the hospital both for documentation and billing purposes. This operative report should also be available in the patient's medical record.

The American College of Obstetricians and Gynecologists Presidential Task Force on Patient Safety in the Office Setting recommends utilization of a checklist throughout the patient's journey through any office gynecologic procedure. An example of this checklist is shown in Table 2.2.

Emergency Preparedness in the Office

Each office should have an Emergency Plan in place in the event of an adverse event in the procedure room, or a problem in the office itself (weather, electrical, etc.). This plan should be included in the office policy and procedural manual and this should be clearly posted along with an evacuation route. An agreement with a local hospital should be established prior to performing any office procedures should the need to transport a patient arise. Ideally, the physician should have admitting privileges at the chosen hospital [15] and a specific office protocol for the office should be in place which clearly states the steps needed to easily accomplish this transfer.

Another aspect of office preparation is the periodic performance of drills and simulation to help prepare for, as Weiss and Swisher call, the "what-ifs" [19] and are effective for preparing the office team for the emergencies that could pose a risk to the patient [1]. It is recommended that these drills be performed at least quarterly so as to keep all members of the office focused on their roles, including interventions and communication among team members. After each drill, debriefing and feedback should be undertaken for continuous improvement. Areas for drills include uncommon but serious patient events such as respiratory arrest, myocardial infarction, major hemorrhage, syncope, and vasovagal reaction [10] as well as anaphylaxis and anxiety/panic attacks. Surgical fires are another uncommon but possible event in office-based surgery and should be addressed. In-office concerns would include surgical drapes and use of cautery: thus, training simulation and drills for prevention of and management of surgical fires is also critical. The Medical Director should be involved in and assist in developing drills: leading by example is tantamount in establishing a culture of safety in the office surgery setting. As Erickson recommends, "create a mock drill and try one. (Don't worry if it fails. Learn by doing)" [1]. This is certainly true and applicable—be prepared for staff resistance at first but typically all members of the team can become engaged in not only the drills but in complete patient safety as well.

Competency and Credentialing

As mentioned previously, it is imperative for patient safety that the physician be competent to perform the proposed surgical procedure in the office: maintaining appropriate credentialing as well as determining ongoing competence in office surgical procedures is recommended [10]. ACOG recommends that procedures initially performed only in the inpatient arena could be transitioned to the office setting after the physician has shown competency in "an accredited operating room setting" [1]. Typically, a gynecologic surgeon will be credentialed or be granted "privileges" to perform a surgical procedure at a hospital or surgery center based on appropriate training and education as well as documentation of surgical competence and/or attendance at an educational hands-on course. When first performing these procedures, many facilities require a "proctor" or preceptor to assist and be certain that the physician does have competence to perform the procedure. Only once a surgical procedure is mastered in the inpatient hospital setting, can consideration for transfer of the procedure to the office be undertaken. This is especially true when a new technology is introduced. Stumpf notes that any gynecologic surgeon who is incorporating a new surgical technique should be assisted or supervised by a more experienced provider until full competency is achieved [2]. It is suggested that a physician perform a minimum number of procedures successful (and unsupervised) in the inpatient hospital or ASC setting before transitioning to the office. These cases should be of varying difficulty in order that the surgeon acquires adequate experience and skills to negotiate these types of cases in the office. One approach to help with this is to perform the procedure in the operating room just as one would in the office: anesthesia should provide minimal IV sedation (or even monitored anesthesia care) with local anesthetics used as appropriate. Once she or he feels confident in performing the procedure can the move to an office-based procedure be undertaken. Lastly, once a physician is credentialed for the in-office procedure, periodic review of that surgeon's office surgical volume, outcomes, and complications should be undertaken to ensure an ongoing competency review [18].

Conclusion

As office-based procedures become increasingly utilized in gynecologic practice, it may be important to consider outcomes reporting for professionalism and safety similar to what is being done now in the hospitals as it is just a matter of time before the office-based procedures are held to the same standard of accountability and reporting as the hospitals currently are. Establishing an office-based gynecologic surgical practice requires detailed planning for office set-up with equipment and development of office policies. Also, training and practice for the office team will help to ensure preparation for not only a safe, smooth, and uneventful patent experience but also for unexpected events. With due diligence in both the establishment, maintenance and review of all office-based procedures, both the patient and the provider will benefit from thorough preparation, planning, and follow-through in the office-based gynecologic surgical practice.

References

1. Erickson TB, Kirkpatrick DH, DeFrancesco MS, et al. Executive summary of the American College of Obstetricians and Gynecologists Presidential Task Force on Patient Safety in the Office Setting: reinvigorating safety in office-based gynecologic surgery. Obstet Gynecol. 2010;115:147–51.
2. Stumpf PG. Practical solutions to improve safety in the obstetrics/gynecology office setting and in the operating room. Obstet Gynecol Clin North Am. 2008;35:19–35.
3. Baggish MS. Establishment of a hysteroscopy program. In: Baggish MS, Valle RF, Guedj H, editors. Hysteroscopy: visual perspectives of uterine anatomy, physiology and pathology. Philadelphia, PA: Lippincott Williams & Wilkins; 2007 [Chapter 13].
4. Brown J, Blank K. Minimally invasive endometrial ablation device complications and use outside of the manufacturers' instructions. Obstet Gynecol. 2012;120:865–70.
5. Center for Disease Control. Guidelines for disinfection and sterilization in healthcare facilities; 2008. [cited 2013 Dec 15]. Available from: http://www.cdc.gov/hicpac/Disinfection_Sterilization/17_00Recomendations.html.
6. Bradley LD, Fluharty S. Maintenance of equipment for hysteroscopy. In: Bradley LD, Falcone T, editors. Hysteroscopy: office evaluation and management of the uterine cavity. Philadelphia, PA: Mosby; 2009 [Chapter 5].
7. American Institute of Ultrasound Medicine. Guidelines for cleaning and preparing endocavity ultrasound transducers between patients [cited 2014 Jan 21]. Available from: http://www.aium.org/oficialStatements/27.
8. Practice guidelines for sedation and analgesia by non-anesthesiologists: an updated report by the American Society of Anesthesiologists Task Force on Sedation and Analgesia by Non-Anesthesiologists. Anesthesiology. 2002;96:1004–17.
9. Committee on Patient Safety and Quality Improvement. Patient safety in the surgical environment. Obstet Gynecol. 2010;116:786–90.
10. Keats JP. Procedures in the office setting patient safety in the obstetric and gynecology office setting. Obstet Gynecol Clin North Am. 2013;40:611–23.
11. Patient safety in the surgical environment. Committee opinion no. 464. American College of Obstetricians and Gynecologists. Obstet Gynecol. 2010;116:786–90.
12. Ambulatory Care National Safety Goals. [cited 2014 Jan 10]. Available from: http://www.jointcommission.org/assets/1/6/AHC_NPSG_Chapter_2014.pdf.
13. Goldberg-Alberts AL, Solomon RP. A primer on risk management for ambulatory surgery. J Ambul Care Manage. 1997;20:72–90.
14. American College of Obstetricians and Gynecologists. Health literacy. Committee opinion no. 491. Obstet Gynecol. 2011;117:1250–3.
15. Wortman M. Instituting an office-based surgery program in the gynecologist's office. J Minim Invasive Gynecol. 2010;17:673–83.
16. Tracking and reminder systems. Committee opinion no. 546. American College of Obstetricians and Gynecologists. Obstet Gynecol. 2012;120:1535–7.

17. National Patient Safety Foundation. [cited 2013 Sep 25]. Available from: http://www.npsf.org/.
18. Sclafani J, Levy B, Lawrence H, et al. Building a better safety net. Obstet Gynecol. 2012;120:355–9.
19. Weiss PM, Swisher E. Patient safety in the ambulatory OB/GYN setting. Clin Obstet Gynecol. 2012;55:613–9.
20. Gawande A. The checklist manifesto. New York, NY: Picador; 2009.
21. Haynes AB, Weiser TG, Berry WR, Safe Surgery Saves Lives Study Group, et al. A surgical safety checklist to reduce morbidity and mortality in a global population. N Engl J Med. 2009;360:491–9.

Informed Consent

3

Ruth M. Farrell and Cristie M. Cole

Introduction

Informed consent is a cornerstone of the ethical practice of medicine. Through the informed consent process, patients are able to make informed decisions about their healthcare and provide voluntary authorization to proceed with a recommended diagnostic or therapeutic procedure. The foundation of the informed consent process is grounded in a bioethical framework that recognizes patients' autonomy as a key value in the delivery of healthcare [1, 2].

Modern bioethics recognizes that a variety of frameworks may be utilized to analyze ethical challenges in clinical practice [3–5]. One of the leading bioethical frameworks is a principle-based approach centered on the concepts of autonomy, beneficence, non-maleficence, and justice [6, 7]. While each principle has an important role in the informed consent process, autonomy is the foundational principle from which to ensure that patients are prepared to make informed, voluntary choices about their healthcare. Autonomy describes an individual's right to self-determination and to make intentional choices about her life free from the controlling influence of others [7]. This concept stands in contrast to the previously accepted notion of paternalism. Under a paternalistic model of healthcare, the interests and opinions of the physician take precedence over those of the patient in healthcare decisions, most often driven by an underlying assumption about what decisions or actions she or he thinks are in the best interest of the patient. While guided by duties of beneficence and non-maleficence, such an approach to patient care is ethically problematic because it impinges on the patients' capacity and rights to exercise her rights of self-determination and autonomy. It also imparts other negative sequelae as this approach to patient care compromises healthcare quality, safety, and outcomes [8, 9]. As patients are most familiar with their values and beliefs, they are often best positioned to assess the impact that the risks and benefits of their medical choices will have on their immediate and long-term health and quality of life. This is particularly relevant in the practice of gynecology, where diagnostic and therapeutic interventions can have a direct, permanent, and significant effect on women's reproductive and sexual health, with far reaching ramifications for her health and well-being [10].

While an emphasis on autonomy empowers patients to actively engage in their own medical decisions, the physician's role is not minimized. Physicians generally control how the informed consent process unfolds. In this context, the focus on autonomy gives rise to physician

R.M. Farrell, M.D., M.A. (✉)
Departments of Obstetrics and Gynecology and Bioethics, Cleveland Clinic, 9500 Euclid Avenue, JJ-60, Cleveland, OH 44195, USA
e-mail: farrelr@ccf.org

C.M. Cole, J.D.
Department of Bioethics, Cleveland Clinic, 9500 Euclid Avenue, JJ-60, Cleveland, OH 44195, USA
e-mail: colec@ccf.org

J.D. Emery and M.F.R. Paraiso (eds.), *Office-Based Gynecologic Surgical Procedures*, DOI 10.1007/978-1-4939-1414-2_3, © Springer Science+Business Media New York 2015

obligations to take reasonable steps necessary to promote patient autonomy. When physicians undertake the informed consent process in an authentic and effective manner that fosters patients' autonomy, patients are enabled to make informed and voluntary medical decisions that best meet their personal and healthcare needs [11]. Without a mechanism to support the informed consent process, the patient is at risk for the medical and personal consequences for undergoing a procedure without having an adequate understanding of its limitations and implications. Alternatively, there is also the risk of the patient declining a recommended procedure, which would have otherwise been of benefit, without an adequate understanding of its utility.

Given the importance of informed consent in the practice of medicine, it is necessary for physicians to become familiar with the concept of informed consent and how to effectively facilitate the informed consent process with their patients. The growing role of outpatient procedures in gynecology requires physicians to understand the nuances of the informed consent process for procedures that traditionally would be performed in the operating room. In this chapter, we will discuss the ethical and legal aspects of informed consent, and the specific considerations for the informed consent process for outpatient gynecologic procedures.

Legal and Historical Aspects of Informed Consent

Prior to the 1900s, medical ethics literature made little, if any, reference to patient autonomy. Paternalism dominated medical practice, and the physician's primary duty was to preserve the health of the patient, generally superseding other values or obligations. Under this paradigm, the physician made decisions on behalf of the patient, and nondisclosure was often justified as protecting the patient from potential harm. The Hippocratic Writings and Percival's *Medical Ethics* directed physicians to exercise therapeutic privilege and avoid making disclosures that might be harmful or upsetting, a practice strongly discouraged in modern medical ethics [12]. Early editions of the American Medical Association's Code of Ethics adopted this position, instructing physicians against disclosure of information that might discourage or depress a patient unless "absolutely necessary" [13, 14]. Disclosure was valued only to the extent that it promoted a good medical outcome by encouraging patient compliance [12]. Even consent practices in the mid-nineteenth century were not demonstrative of patient choice [7].

Autonomy's influential role in the consent process was not recognized until the early 1900s, a change brought about by a series of legal cases that subsequently affected clinical practice. For centuries, the law has protected the fundamental right of every person "to complete immunity of his person from physical interference of others" through a claim of battery [15]. While the threat of liability may have prompted the existence of early consent practices, courts did not elucidate the philosophical weight of battery's fundamental premise in the clinical context until the twentieth century [7]. The earliest documented cases to do so were the 1905 cases *Mohr v. Williams* and *Pratt v. Davis* [15, 16]. The defendant physicians in each case were held liable for performing a surgical intervention without specific consent from the patient for that intervention. Reflecting the tenor of the medical profession at the time, the physicians' defense was that patients consented to any therapeutic intervention that the physician determined as appropriate; consent for a specific intervention was unnecessary. The courts in each case rejected this argument, instead emphasizing the importance of self-determination and need for consent for specific interventions.

However, it was not until after the 1914 case of *Schloendorf v. Society of NY Hospital* that courts throughout the country began to adopt the position articulated in earlier cases [17]. Citing *Mohr* and *Pratt*, this case established the concept that "[e]very human being of adult years and sound mind has the right to determine what shall be done with his own body; and a surgeon who performs an operation without his patient's consent commits an assault, for which he is liable in damages, except in cases of emergency where the patient is unconscious, and where it is necessary to operate before consent can be obtained." In subsequent cases, courts justified legal consent requirements by adopting without question the conclusions of *Schloendorf* and its reliance on self-determination as a natural right [7]. Initiating a shift in philosophical prioritization from paternalism to patient autonomy within medical practice, the courts firmly established the patient's right to participate in medical decision-making.

Building upon this foundation, courts in the 1950s and 1960s constructed a more robust consent process by imposing additional disclosure obligations on physicians before obtaining consent. The case of *Salgo v. Leland Standford, Jr. University Board of Trustees* focused on ensuring that the patient had sufficient information to make an "intelligent consent" to the proposed treatment [18]. Implicitly recognizing the competing obligations of the principles of beneficence, non-malfeasance and respect for patient autonomy, the court stated that a "certain amount of discretion must be employed consistent with the full disclosure of facts necessary to an *informed* consent." The court also determined that "necessary facts" encompassed the treatment's risks and alternatives. While the court relied on patient autonomy to justify imposing these new obligations, the final opinion left many questions unanswered regarding disclosure as part of the informed consent process. In the years to follow, the cases of *Salgo*: *Canterbury v. Spence*, *Cobbs v. Grant*, and *Wilkinson v. Vesey* helped clarify the concept of disclosure [19, 20]. The courts in these three cases collectively articulated standards of disclosure grounded in and measured by "the patient's right of self-decision." In rejecting a standard based on professional norms, the courts argued that disclosure obligations arose from the right of the patient to determine what to do with his or her own body, and it is this right that controls the scope of disclosure obligations.

Over the course of 70 years, the courts effectuated a new and dramatic emphasis on patient autonomy as a central guiding principle in medical ethics and practice. The landmark cases led to a dramatic shift about the role of physician and patient in medical decisions and informed consent. Changes were also taking place outside the courts. In subsequent years, additional changes made by both the American Medical Association and the American College of Obstetricians and Gynecologists supported a move towards adding principles of respect for human dignity, patient autonomy, and self-determination [21, 22]. The result of these changes was evident soon thereafter. By 1982, 85 % of physicians obtained written or oral consent for minor office surgeries, and almost all physicians obtained such consent before inpatient surgery or general anesthesia [9].

If the 1970s saw the rise of the legal doctrine of informed consent, the subsequent decades saw the evolution of an ethical concept of informed consent [11]. The legal constructs of informed consent had placed great emphasis on minimal requirements that had to be met for physicians to avoid liability [12, 19]. However, it became evident to physicians, legal scholars, and bioethicists that a rudimentary application of the legal doctrine failed to fully respect patient autonomy or fulfill physician obligations of beneficence and non-malfeasance [9, 12]. In response, the ethical concept of informed consent evolved in an attempt to address the shortcomings of an informed consent structured solely on concepts of legal protection of the healthcare provider [11]. This new model provided an approach to informed consent that focused on ensuring the patient would be able to make autonomous, voluntary choices about her medical options for the sake of her benefit [12, 23]. Thus, accepted current standards of informed consent include both legal and ethical functions, which are fulfilled through a process of clear and effective communication between a patient and her physician.

The Informed Consent Process

At its core, informed consent is a mechanism through which a patient's right to autonomous decision-making is operationalized in the therapeutic relationship. This takes place through an active dialog and exchange of information between a physician and patient. As part of the practice of medicine, a physician is charged with ensuring a patient is prepared to make a voluntary decision regarding the proposed intervention based on an accurate appreciation and understanding of the nature and risks of the interventions [6]. The informed consent process concludes with the patient providing voluntary authorization to proceed with a procedure. For surgical procedures, this takes place through a documentation process, a step that may serve two important purposes: (1) evidence of consent and (2) appreciation by the patient of the seriousness of what they are providing permission to undergo. When adequate informed consent has been achieved, then the patients' fundamental right of autonomy and self-determination is recognized in the therapeutic relationship and given a primary position in the care planning process.

As noted above, underlying legal standards provide minimum requirements and procedures that must be met, including obtaining written consent from the patient. Unfortunately, the legal underpinnings of the informed consent doctrine have led some clinicians to reduce the process to a perfunctory checklist of legal requirements culminating in the patient providing her signature on a legal consent document prior to undergoing a procedure [24]. While the legal aspects of the informed consent process are clearly important in the practice of medicine, they do not take precedence over the process of communication that is necessary for patients to make well-informed decisions about their healthcare. When viewed as a single event focused on completion of a legal document, the true purpose of the informed consent process is sacrificed. As a result, the patient is at risk for misunderstanding the indications, risks, and benefits of her medical options.

Table 3.1 Core components of the informed consent process

Ethical components
Medical decision-making capacity
Disclosure
Understanding
Voluntary choice
Authorization

One of the initial questions about the informed consent process is how to effectively facilitate it in a way that achieves its ethical and legal purposes. The following core components of the informed consent process serve as a guide for physicians about how to best empower patients to make well-informed, autonomous decisions. These core components include: (1) assessing competence or decision-making capacity, (2) disclosure of information, (3) ensuring understanding, (4) securing the voluntary choice of the patient, and (5) receiving patient authorization for the procedure (Table 3.1) [1]. Informed consent is only achieved when all of these components have been fulfilled.

Medical Decision-Making Capacity

Capacity is a threshold criterium for informed consent [1]. The informed consent process cannot take place unless the patient has the ability to make autonomous, cogent decisions about her healthcare. Traditionally, this has been most commonly described as competence, a concept with different definitions and criteria dependent upon the medical or legal context in which it is used. In the legal context, the competence of an individual is determined by a judge, who considers the evidence presented, including clinical assessments, and makes a global determination regarding an individual's ability to make decisions and to care for him- or herself. Generally, a patient deemed incompetent by a legal authority legally lacks medical decision-making capacity for all medical decisions. However, in the routine clinical setting, capacity is most often used interchangeably with the concept of decision-making capacity, a term that has a greater applicability in the clinical practice of outpatient gynecologic practice. This concept entails the ability for the patient to acquire and understand information about her condition and medical options, weigh the risks and benefits of different options in a rational fashion, communicate a preference for options, and provide authorization to initiate a plan of care [6].

In the clinical setting, decision-making capacity most often is determined by a clinical judgment rather than a formal psychiatric assessment and is assessed in the context of the specific decision at hand. In other words, a clinician may determine that a patient has the capacity to make medical decisions. A patient's decision-making capacity is presumed to be intact unless there is an evident reason to suspect otherwise by a member of the healthcare team. In some cases, there may be a transient impairment of decision-making abilities, such as an acute illness, the effects of a pharmaceutical agent, or substance abuse. While most patients with the former will rarely be undergoing an outpatient procedure, the latter may be more common in this setting, where the administration of medications for analgesia or anxiety may influence decision-making. In other cases, there may be a chronic condition affecting decision-making ability, such as in the case of severe psychiatric disease, impaired cognitive development, or dementia. If a physician has any reason to believe that a patient does not have full decision-making capacity, then the procedure should be deferred until a more complete assessment can be performed.

When a patient does not have adequate decision-making capacity, she cannot provide authorization for a procedure. In such cases, advanced directives can help care planning, driven by the underlying ethical principle of respecting and preserving the autonomy of the patient. Advanced directives can take the form of a document outlining treatment preferences, such as an advanced directive or a living will. Most often, in the outpatient gynecologic setting, decision-making would include an individual designated by the patient in a previously completed written healthcare power of attorney or other formal mechanism to make decisions on behalf of the patient [1]. This surrogate decision-maker is known as a healthcare proxy or an attorney-in-fact for healthcare. When this has not been formally established at the time a procedure is indicated, another individual is assigned this responsibility to make decisions on behalf of the patient, as based upon his or her knowledge of the patient's wishes. State laws and/or institutional policies may provide guidance as to who this individual may be. In most cases, this is a family member, such as a spouse or a member of the immediate family. In the case of surrogate decision-making, the authorizing agent must be familiar with the patient's wishes so that he or she can make decisions consistent with the patient's values and preferences. While the patient may not have decision-making capacity, the wishes of the individual should be included in the decision-making process, and care planning should reflect the values and preferences of the patient. Physicians should be aware of their institutional and state policies and procedures regarding surrogate decision-making, as these may vary in different practice settings.

Disclosure

As part of the informed component of the consent process, a patient must have adequate information pertinent to her medical condition and the proposed medical options in order to select a course of management that is consistent with her healthcare, personal needs, and values and belief system. The process of disclosure can present one of the greatest challenges to physicians in terms of determining the amount and detail of information to be conveyed, given that the process is individualized for each patient.

There are several different aspects of the treatment plan that should be presented to the patient as part of the consent process. Disclosure of information material to the procedure includes discussing the patient's medical condition and the procedure recommended to manage it. This

Table 3.2 Additional considerations for the informed consent process for office-based procedures

Benefits	Risks
• Avoidance of general anesthesia	• Inability to complete the expected procedure
	– Patient movement during the procedure
	– Patient intolerance of the procedure
	– Anatomical variation precluding adequate visualization or access
• Smaller time commitment on the part of the patient	• Management of complications
	– Staff and equipment available in the office setting
	– Distance to hospital or ambulatory center for additional management needs

begins with a discussion of the indication of the procedure and how it is performed. Once this has been established, then a discussion about the risks and benefits of the procedure can be initiated. In general, when discussing risks or benefits, a key aspect of a patient's decision-making is to be able to place these considerations in the context of her immediate and long-term health. This discussion includes not only the nature of those outcomes but also the likelihood of them occurring and the management of any adverse events. The patient should also be educated about the risk of procedure failure, including the chance that the procedure may not be able to take place as initially planned or that it may not resolve the clinical condition. Included in the disclosure process is a discussion of alternatives to the proposed intervention, including other medical options and courses of action if the patient elects against the recommended procedure or elects against any procedure at all. The risk of delay and/or not acting should also be discussed. Finally, she must also be aware of the fact that there is a choice to be made to accept or decline the procedure as part of the informed consent process.

The unique nature of office-based procedures requires additional considerations in structuring the informed consent process (Table 3.2). Specific to outpatient gynecologic procedures, physicians should also discuss aspects of the procedure that may be altered when performed in the clinical setting compared to the operating room. Some of the benefits of an office-based procedure include the avoidance of general anesthesia, and a reduction in the time required for the procedure. However, outpatient procedures are associated with risks that would not be encountered if the patient were under general anesthesia and in the operating room. As the patient will be awake, there are considerations specific to her response during the procedure. Patient discomfort, anxiety, or individual anatomical variation may play a role in the ability to safely and adequately perform the procedure. If complications are encountered, possible transfer for management to another facility may have an effect on the impact of those risks for the patient.

While there are several different approaches to the disclosure process, the physician should frame the counseling process in a way that enables the patient to make a meaningful and informed choice about her medical care. In general, a physician must disclose sufficient information that allows the patient to make a personalized, well-informed decision reflecting her beliefs and values. The disclosure process, however, does not consist merely of relaying a list of non-contextualized risks that could occur as part of the diagnostic or therapeutic procedure. Instead, to best enable a patient to make an informed choice, it is critical to present these risks in such a way that a patient can place the risks and benefits of a procedure within the contexts of her life, reproductive and sexual health, and overall well-being. An open dialog must exist between the physician and the patient to ensure that the patient obtains the quantity and detail of information she needs to qualify risks and benefits in relation to her health and interests, as well as the resources that will enable her to make a meaningful decision about treatment options.

Understanding

Understanding is an equally important component of the informed consent process. It is not sufficient merely to disclose information that is material to the procedure. Instead, the physician has an obligation to ensure the patient comprehends the information that has been communicated about her condition and recommended procedure. Without an understanding of the condition and options at hand, the patient will be unable to provide true informed consent for a procedure.

Understanding is a function of several different factors that can come together in the counseling process, including both health literacy and effective communication. The term health literacy denotes a patient's ability to acquire and process information to make meaningful and informed healthcare decisions [25]. This includes the patient's ability to comprehend the medical concepts used as part of care plan discussions. Some patients may not be familiar with the terminology used during the counseling process. For example, terms such as uterine perforation or hemorrhage, as well as the significance of these adverse events, may not be well understood by a patient who has not previously encountered them in her healthcare decisions. As a result, the meaning and significance of a proposed procedure may not be fully understood if such terms are not described in a meaningful way to the patient. Additionally, a patient's ability to individualize the advantages and disadvantages of a procedure requires understanding concepts of risk and numeracy. It is not uncommon for patients to struggle with comprehending risk as it is most often communicated in the physician–patient relationship, and thus they may have difficulty fully understanding key aspects of the procedure and how such aspects may apply to them [26].

For these reasons, it is important for physicians to lead the informed consent discussion using terms and concepts that their patients understand. It is equally critical that physicians take the time to assess patients' level of understanding at level stages of the consent process. There are several approaches to ensuring patients' comprehension, including methods in which physicians are actively engaged in assessing patient recall and understanding [27]. Such methods encourage patients to ask questions about their condition and about how the proposed procedure relates to it. Through a process of active listening and engagement in the informed consent process, physicians can pinpoint informational areas that could benefit from greater clarity and dispel misunderstanding before the procedure takes place.

Voluntariness

Valid informed consent can only be obtained through the voluntary authorization for a procedure by a patient. Coercion, manipulation, threat of force, harm, or access to treatment are all factors that are incongruous with the concept of informed consent. These are egregious behaviors that rarely emerge in their true form in the therapeutic relationship. However, there are other subtle influences that can affect the counseling process and have an unintentional impact on the patient's voluntary decision-making ability. For instance, a physician's bias toward a particular course of therapy may manifest during the informed consent process in the ways the advantages and disadvantages of a procedure are described. This can be driven by conflict of interest, increasingly recognized as a factor that can influence how physicians present and discuss medical options [28]. Conflict of interest can take several different forms, including influence from medical device manufacturers or the desire of the physician to learn and integrate a new procedure or surgical device into his or her practice. To avoid individual bias or placing undue pressure on the patient toward one treatment path or another, physicians should be aware of their own biases prior to counseling patients and have the interest and well-being of the patient as their primary goal in the informed consent process. This may include encouraging disclosure of an identified personal bias in regard to one path or another that may be appropriate given the circumstances, such as lack of familiarity or experience with the office-based procedure.

In the Office: Practical Clinical Challenges to Informed Consent for Outpatient Gynecologic Surgery

Sedation for Outpatient Procedures

One of the advantages to outpatient procedures is that they can be done without the use of general anesthesia. Despite the avoidance of general anesthesia, patients may still require a form of pain and symptom management, both for their own comfort and also to optimize safety during the procedure. Oftentimes, adequate analgesia can be achieved by using oral anti-inflammatory medications and/or a paracervical block. However, for some patients, narcotics or anxiolytics may be needed to provide more effective pain control or alleviate anxiety, respectively. To maximize effectiveness, these medications are usually recommended to be taken prior to the procedure. Based upon the dose of these medications and an individual's response to them, some patients will experience a degree of central nervous system depression. This, in turn, may affect their decision-making capacity, specifically limiting their ability to acquire information material to the procedure and/or postop period and process it in a way so as to provide informed consent.

If oral analgesics or anxiolytics are to be used during the procedure, steps should be taken to ensure the patient is able to participate in the informed consent procedure. For these situations, physician should consider obtaining informed consent prior to the administration of the medications, either during a separate clinical visit or earlier during the day of the procedure. In this way, the performing physician can be confident that the patient has the faculties to participate in the informed consent process prior to the outpatient procedure.

Limited Experience with a New Device or New Procedure

The integration of outpatient gynecologic procedures into clinical practice requires the physician to acquire new knowledge and skill sets. In some instances, this will include learning how to operate with a new instrument or surgical device for which the physician may not yet have experience with in either the outpatient or the operating room setting. In others, the physician may have experience with the equipment or device in the operating room but not yet in the unique circumstances of outpatient procedures. As the aim of the informed consent process is for the patient to provide informed and voluntary authorization for a specific procedure, both situations must be adequately addressed in the preoperative counseling period.

Physicians can optimize the patient's informed consent process by sharing their personal experience with the recommended outpatient procedure so that the patient can be best prepared to make an informed choice about the procedure and where it is performed. In terms of the utilization of new devices or instruments, counseling as part of the informed consent process should include some insight into individual experience with the device and reasons for selecting the recommended procedure over another, as such information is central to the patient's ability to weigh the risks, benefits, and alternatives of available medical options. This also requires the physician to be familiar with efficacy and safety data about the device and to be prepared to discuss their clinical opinions about how the recommended procedure is superior to other outpatient or operating room options.

Conclusion

The availability of office-based gynecologic procedures presents a new and important therapeutic option for patients. A key aspect to patients' decision-making regarding undergoing a procedure in the office is their ability to access a scientifically accurate and balanced representation about its use and applicability to their health. Physicians can ensure their patients have the ability to make informed choices by supporting an effective informed consent process. As physicians acquire new surgical skills to perform office-based procedures, it will also be important for them to become familiar with the informed consent process for the procedure in order to support the ability of patients to make meaningful and informed choices about their reproductive healthcare.

References

1. Beauchamp T, Childress J. Principles of biomedical ethics. 6th ed. New York: Oxford University Press; 2001.
2. AMA Code of Medical Ethics. [cited 2014 Mar 1]. Available from: http://www.ama-assn.org/ama/pub/physician-resources/medical-ethics/code-medical-ethics.page.
3. Gilligan C. Moral orientation and moral development. In: Kitty EE, Meyers PT, editors. Women and moral theory. Totowa: Rowman and Littlefield; 1987.
4. Pellegrino ED. Toward a virtue-based normative ethics for the health professions. Kennedy Inst Ethics J. 1995;5(3):253–77.
5. Tong R. Feminist approaches to bioethics. In: Wolf SM, editor. Feminism and bioethics: beyond reproduction. New York: Oxford University Press; 1996.
6. Berg JW, Appelbaum PS, Lidz CW, Parker LS. Informed consent: legal theory and clinical practice. 2nd ed. Fair Lawn: Oxford University Press; 2001.
7. Beauchamp T, Faden R. Informed consent: history of informed consent. In: Post S, editor. Encyclopedia of bioethics. 3rd ed. New York: Macmillan-Thomson; 2003.
8. Wu H, Nishimi R, Page-Lopez C, Kizer K. Improving patient safety through informed consent for patients with limited health literacy: an implementation report. Washington, DC: National Quality Forum; 2005.
9. President's Commission for the Study of Ethical Problems in Medicine and Biomedical and Behavioral Research. Making health care decisions: the ethical and legal implications of informed consent in the patient–practitioner relationship. Washington, DC: United States Government Printing Office; 1982.
10. ACOG committee opinion no. 390, December 2007. Ethical decision making in obstetrics and gynecology. American College of Obstetrics and Gynecology. Obstet Gynecol. 2;110(6):1479–87.
11. American College of Obstetricians and Gynecologists Committee on Ethics. Informed Consent. ACOG committee opinion no. 439; 2009.
12. Beauchamp T. Informed consent: its history, meaning, and present challenges. Camb Q Healthc Ethics. 2011;20(4):515–23.
13. American Medical Association. Code of medical ethics; 1847.
14. American Medical Association. Principles of medical ethics; 1903.
15. Mohr v. Williams, 104 N.W. 12 (Minn. 1905).
16. Pratt v. Davis, 118 Ill. App. 161 (1905).
17. Schloendorf v. Society of NY Hospital, 105 N.E. 92 (N.Y. Ct. App. 1914).
18. Salgo v. Leland Stanford Jr. Univ. Bd. of S et al., 317 P.2d 170 (Cal. Ct. App. 1957).
19. Canterbury v. Spence, 464 F.2d 772 (D.C. 1972).
20. Cobbs v. Grant, 502 P.2d 1 (Cal. 1972).
21. American Medical Association. Principles of medical ethics; 1957.
22. American Medical Association. Principles of medical ethics; 1980.
23. Katz J. Reflections on informed consent: 40 after its birth. J Am Coll Surg. 1998;186(4):466–74.
24. Lidz CW, Appelbaum PS, Meisel A. Two models of implementing informed consent. Arch Intern Med. 1988;148:1385–9.
25. National Research Council. Health literacy: a prescription to end confusion. Washington, DC: The National Academies Press; 2004.
26. Gates EA. Communicating risk in prenatal genetic testing. J Midwifery Womens Health. 2004;49:220–7.
27. Schillinger D, Piette J, Grumbach K, et al. Closing the loop: physician communication with diabetic patients who have low health literacy. Arch Intern Med. 2003;163(1):83–90.
28. American College of Obstetricians and Gynecologists Committee on Ethics. Committee opinion number 541: professional relationships with industry. Obstet Gynecol. 2012;120(5):1243–9.

4 Anesthesia and Analgesia for Office Gynecological Procedures

Nicholas Marcanthony, Sharon Marcanthony, and Englok Yap

Effective anesthetic coverage with regional anesthesia for any procedure involves a fundamental knowledge of several key ideas. The following key ideas will be addressed in this chapter as they pertain to common gynecological office procedure:

- Local anesthetics and the means to which they can be augmented
- Anatomy and innervation of the operative area
- Proper equipment and techniques for the procedure
- Familiarity with and availability of proper safety equipment and medications needed if complications arise

N. Marcanthony, M.D. (✉)
Department of Anesthesiology, Cleveland Clinic, 9500 Euclid Avenue, E30, Cleveland, OH 44195, USA

Anesthesiology Institute, Cleveland Clinic Wooster, 721 East Milltown Road, Cleveland, OH 44691, USA
e-mail: marcann@ccf.org

S. Marcanthony, M.D., F.A.C.O.G.
Department of Obstetrics/Gynecology, Women's Health Institute, Cleveland Clinic, 1739 Cleveland Road, Wooster, OH 44691, USA
e-mail: marcans@ccf.org

E. Yap, M.D., F.A.C.H.E., C.A.F.C.I.
Cleveland Pain Management and Acupuncture LLC, 24755 Chagrin Boulevard, Suite 135, Beachwood, OH 44122, USA
e-mail: englokyap@yahoo.com

Local Anesthetics

Local anesthetics' primary mechanism of action is via blockage of voltage-gated sodium channels on the internal side of a cell membrane. The major divide in local anesthetics is based on chemical structure; amide versus esters. All locals have a lipophilic end (usually a benzene ring) and a hydrophilic end (usually a tertiary amine). The intermediate chain between these is either an amide or ester [1]. All of the locals used in office practice for gynecology are amide locals. Whether amide or ester, their chemical structure is such that local anesthetics are weak bases [BH^+] [2].

The three primary properties of a local anesthetic are potency, onset, and duration. Potency of a local anesthetic is directly related to its lipid solubility. Both potency and lipid solubility increase with molecular size.

Onset of action is different from potency. The length of time it takes for a local anesthetic to start taking effect is based on the pK_a of the local. The greater the relative concentration of the nonionized form [B] compared to the ionized form [BH^+], the faster the onset, as only the non-charged particles can readily enter the cell through the cell membrane. As mentioned earlier, the receptor for the local anesthetic is on the interior side of the cell membrane. The clinical significance of this is that the anesthetic must enter the cell prior to any onset of action. Therefore, any hindrance to this will delay the effect.

J.D. Emery and M.F.R. Paraiso (eds.), *Office-Based Gynecologic Surgical Procedures*, DOI 10.1007/978-1-4939-1414-2_4, © Springer Science+Business Media New York 2015

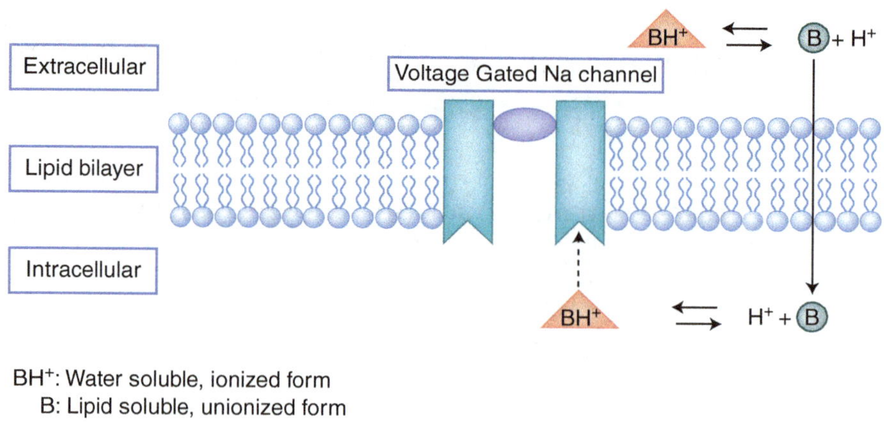

Fig. 4.1 Receptors for local anesthetics: only the nonionized form of the local can cross the cell membrane, but it is the ionized form that binds to the intracellular receptor

Table 4.1 Basic clinical properties of common local anesthetics

Generic (trade)	Potency/lipid solubility [2]	pK_a (onset) [1, 2]	Protein binding (duration of action) [1, 2]
Amides			
Bupivicaine (Marcaine)	High	8.1 (5 min)	High (~2–4 h)
Lidocaine (Xylocaine)	Moderate	7.8 (<2 min)	Moderate (0.5–1 h, 1.5–2 h with 1:200,000 epi)
Mepivacaine (Carbocaine)	Moderate	7.6 (3–5 min)	Moderate (0.5–1.5 h)
Ropivacaine	High	8.1 (5 min)	High (~2–4 h)
Esters			
Chloroprocaine (Nesacaine)	Low	9.0 (<2 min)	Low (0.5–0.75 h)
Tetracaine (Pontocaine)	High	8.2 (3–10 min)	Mod-high (2–3 h)

In short, the closer the pK_a is to the physiological pH, the faster the onset. It should also be noted that the addition of a buffered solution, like sodium bicarbonate, is advantageous in clinical practice because it will hasten the onset of action. As a secondary benefit, the patient may experience less pain with injection due to the more neutral nature of the solution (Fig. 4.1).

Duration of action is more multifactorial. The degree of protein binding of the local anesthetic involved is a main component. Lipid solubility and blood flow also play important roles (Table 4.1).

It is also important to understand that not all nerves are equally affected by local anesthetics. Several factors come into play when determining a nerve's sensitivity to locals. These include axonal diameter, degree of myelination, and classification of nerve (i.e., A_α, A_β, C, etc.). Clinically, this is manifested by a patient's loss of temperature and pain sensorium, while still maintaining proprioception, pressure awareness, and motor function [1].

The properties of local anesthetics can also be improved on and augmented. Vasoconstrictors, most commonly epinephrine, vasopressin, and phenylephrine, have been used in conjunction with locals to decrease vascular absorption and thereby increase the duration, improve overall quality, and decrease toxicity [1, 2]. Multiple other medications have been added as well, including clonidine, dexamethasone, and dexmedetomidine [2]. Specific adjunct will be discussed later with each particular regional block.

Use of local anesthetics necessitates that a provider be familiar with the complications that can arise with their use. These would include

Table 4.2 Maximum safe dosage of local anesthetics by weight

Local anesthetic	Maximum dose (mg/kg) [2]
Esters	
Chloroprocaine	12
Cocaine	3
Procaine	12
Tetracaine	3
Amides	
Lidocaine	4.5 (w/o epinephrine), 7 (w/ epinephrine)
Bupivacaine	3
Ropivacaine	3
Mepivacaine	4.5 (w/o epinephrine), 7 (w/ epinephrine)
Prilocaine	8

vasovagal response, toxicity, anaphylaxis, accidental intravascular injection, methemoglobinemia, and drug interactions.

Local anesthetic toxicity is a rare but serious complication of regional anesthesia. It is most often related to the local agents potency: the more potent the anesthetic, the greater the risk of toxicity [2]. There is a wide degree of toxicity from mild to severe to life threatening. Causes can include incorrect dosage (see Table 4.2), poor hepatic clearance, accidental intravenous injection, or worse, accidental intra-arterial injection. As with most procedural complications, early recognition of symptoms and rapid intervention are paramount (Table 4.2).

The central nervous and cardiovascular systems are particularly susceptible to the effects of local anesthetic toxicity [2]. The nervous system is usually the first to be affected. Classic symptoms include circumoral numbness, dizziness, and tinnitus. This is followed by an excitatory phase where the patient demonstrates restlessness, agitation, or a sense of impending doom. Finally, if the case is severe enough, an inhibitory phase can be seen where the patient becomes drowsy, unconscious, and may eventually produce tonic-clonic seizures.

As a rule, due to local anesthetics' nature as a sodium channel blocker, they all can have a profound effect on the cardiac muscle. In general, the more lipophilic a local is the greater the risk for cardiotoxicity [2]. Alterations in intrinsic cardiac electrical physiology can produce bradycardia. Increased dosages can lead to heart block and hypotension. Cardiovascular collapse can occur. However, it should be noted that the level of local anesthetic needed to produce a cardiovascular arrest is approximately three times the level needed to produce a seizure.

One additional benefit to regional anesthesia is that local anesthetics have relatively few drug interactions with other medications. However, it is important to note that local anesthetics do interact with each other, especially in terms of their toxicity. Local anesthetic toxicities are additive. For example, if a 50 % maximum dose of bupivicaine is used with a 50 % maximum dose of lidocaine, then the patient would be at 100 % the maximum allowed dose. Also, it is important to remember that amide locals are metabolized by the liver. Patients taking medications that alter the P450 system or with liver disease are at increased risk for toxicity and side effects [2]. The American Society of Regional Anesthesia and Pain Medicine (ASRA) has summarized all current literature in local anesthetic toxicity and produced guidelines for its treatment [3]. Some key points of the guidelines include:

- Call for help early
- Early airway management
- Seizure suppression with benzodiazepines if necessary
- Avoid vasopressin, calcium channel blockers, and beta blockers
- Reduce initial epinephrine doses to <1 μg/kg
- Treat with 20 % Lipid Emulsion Therapy (1.5 mL/kg bolus followed by 0.25 mL/kg/min infusion)

Drug allergies and anaphylactic reactions to local anesthetics are rare. They are more common with the ester locals. The esters are broken down in the blood by pseudocholinesterase. Para-aminobenzoic acid is a metabolite of this process and has been determined to be the true source of allergic reactions in most patients diagnosed with a local anesthetic allergy [1]. Because of this there is no cross-reactivity to amide in terms of anaphylaxis. True allergies to amide locals are exceedingly rare and have been associated with the preservative paraben, not the local itself.

Methemoglobinemia is a known possible effect of the use of prilocaine or benzocaine (common in anesthetic sprays). Symptoms include dyspnea, cyanosis, and altered mental status. Treatment of severe cases includes methylene blue 1–2 mg/kg [2].

Because of the possible complications, it is important that all necessary equipment be made available prior to any regional nerve block. In addition to the materials needed for the block itself, these items should always be present [4]:

- A thoroughly evaluated and consented patient
- A practitioner experienced with the technique to be used
- Appropriate monitoring of the patient, i.e., cardiac monitoring, blood pressure, pulse oximetry, and temperature
- Airway supplies including nasal cannulas, self-inflating bag-mask devices, and emergency airway equipment
- Suction equipment
- Intravenous cannulation equipment
- Resuscitation cart with appropriate medications and cardiac defibrillator

Paracervical Block

Anatomy

Cervical innervation is derived from T11 to T12. Pain from cervical dilation is carried through parasympathetic fibers running with the cardinal ligament and uterine vessels. Pain associated with uterine contractions is transmitted via sympathetic nerve fibers in the hypogastric nerve and superior hypogastric plexus into the posterior roots of the spinal cord at their respective levels [5].

A paracervical block is aimed at interrupting these pathways by blocking nerve transmission at the level of the inferior hypogastric plexus [5]. It is located in the uterosacral ligament on either side of the cervix in the lateral vaginal fornices. Because of this, paracervical blocks may be utilized in any procedure in which cervical manipulation, dilatation, biopsy, or ablation is planned.

Solution

As with any nerve block, choosing the correct local anesthetic is an important decision. For the purpose of office gynecological procedures, many combinations are possible. Lidocaine 1 % is a standard for most blocks that require anesthesia for less than 1 h. However, any of the longer acting locals previously discussed can be used for procedures that are expected to last longer or requiring continued post-procedural pain relief. A good office solution typical includes a local, a vasopressor, and a buffer (typically sodium bicarbonate). The following mixture can be used for paracervical blocks in office:

- 50 mL of lidocaine 1 % (mepivacaine 1 % is also a good choice if anesthesia is needed for long procedures)
- 0.25 mL of epinephrine 1:1,000 (final concentration of 1:200,000)
- 5 mL of 8.4 % sodium bicarbonate

Equipment

1. One 22 or 25 gauge Quincke spinal needle
2. One 20 mL syringe for injection (larger syringes are not recommended as more force is exerted during the block)
3. Sterile towels and sponges
4. Sterile prep of choice (Note: Items 2–4 usually will be found in a standard block tray)

Procedure [5, 6]

1. Internally and externally prep and drape your patient in your standard sterile fashion.
2. If a tenaculum will be used for cervical manipulation, the needle is inserted into the cervical stroma at the 12 o'clock position and a small amount (<2 mL) is superficially injected, prior to the tenaculum being applied to the cervix (Fig. 4.2).

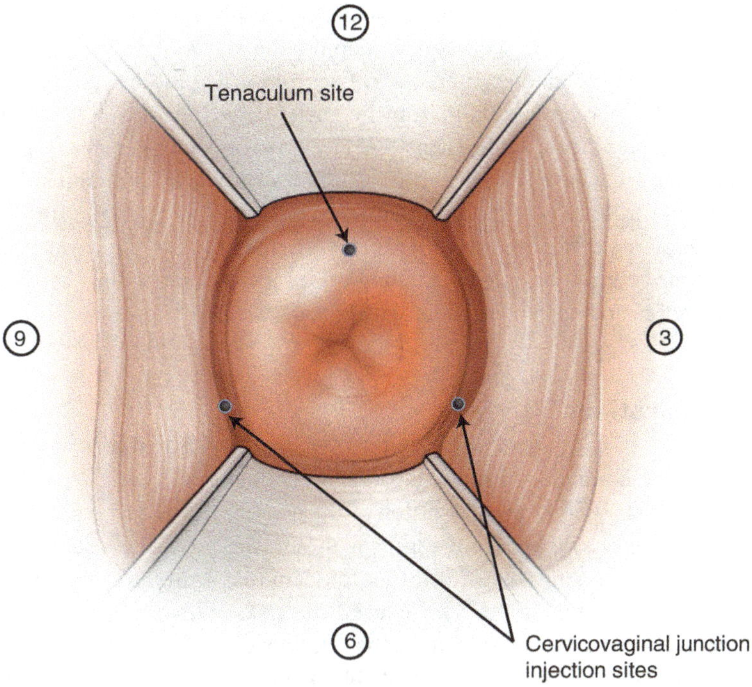

Fig. 4.2 Correct needle insertion sites for a paracervical block

3. Next the needle is inserted about 1 cm into the cervical stroma at the 4 o'clock position at the cervicovaginal junction.
4. Careful aspiration for blood on the syringe must be done prior to injection. If blood is obtained the needle should be withdrawn or advanced 1–2 mm until blood is no longer noted.
5. Inject 10–15 mL of local solution.
6. The needle should be removed and steps 3–6 should be repeated for an injection at the 8 o'clock position.
7. Wait an appropriate amount of time prior to beginning your procedure. Lidocaine with epinephrine will have an onset of action of less than 2 min (for other locals, refer to Table 4.1).

Tips

1. Depending on the amount of uterine descensus, a shorter needle rather than a spinal needle may be easier to administer the anesthetic.
2. Aspirate your syringe several times throughout the course of your injection, particularly at the onset, halfway, and conclusion of injection. This will confirm that your needle has not moved during the block.
3. Do not aspirate back on your plunger more than a couple mL's. Over-aggressive aspiration can produce negative pressure and collapse blood vessels to produce a false negative. This would lead to inadvertent intravascular injection.
4. Some physicians believe in divided doses on each side. This would lead to a total of four injections. Five milliliters each at 3, 5, 7, and 9 o'clock, or alternatively at 5 mL each 2, 4, 8, and 10 o'clock. Regardless of which approach is taken, the inferior hypogastric plexus and ganglia are blocked [5]. Technically, the 2, 4, 8, and 10 o'clock approach should be termed a uterosacral block. This, however, is purely semantics.
5. There is also dispute over the depth of which the needle should be advanced [5, 6]. The classical technique of 1–1.5 cm was described above. New techniques, particularly those with the divided dose technique, make their depth anywhere from 0.3 to 0.7 cm.

Several studies have tried to address these differences between techniques, depths, local anesthetic agent choice, and its concentration. Results have varied widely from no difference [7, 8] to significant difference [9–11]. Most of the studies that have shown no difference allowed relatively little to no time between injection and the beginning of the procedure. This fact reiterates the importance of understanding the local anesthetics and their pharmacological properties.

Complications

The most common complaint for paracervical blocks is pain upon initial insertion of the needle. This is simply a fact of doing regional anesthesia. For all but the simplest of in-office procedures, the benefits of the "pinch" far exceed the risks. However, complications can occur. Following a paracervical block, prolonged blockage or neuritis may occur. Prolonged blockage is usually a result of either too great a volume being injected or patient-specific pharmacokinetics. Neuritis is more often related to trauma to the nerves. Neuritis usually resolves in 1–2 weeks but has been known to linger for as long as 6 months [5].

Parametrial hematoma is another possible complication of a paracervical block. Usually, it requires no treatment. However, if neurological or vascular impairment is noted, incision and drainage may be needed [5].

Also, paracervical blocks done on the parturient have known associations with fetal bradycardia, fetal distress related uteroplacental insufficiency, inadvertent fetal injection, and death. For these reasons, paracervical blocks are not commonly used on pregnant patients anymore [2].

Intracervical Block

Anatomy

Intracervical blocks will block the same pain pathway as was described for the paracervical block. For this reason, intracervical blocks can be used for any procedure for which a paracervical block is indicated. Several studies have attempted to determine which block is superior for analgesia. While paracervical has been shown to provide good analgesic coverage [12], other blocks, such as the intracervical block, have been difficult for researchers to evaluate due to wide variations in techniques [13]. The anatomical differences in position for the block are noted in Fig. 4.3.

Solution

The same solutions used for paracervical blocks can be used with intracervical. Again, a good mixture for office procedures planned for less than 1 h is:

- 50 mL of lidocaine 1 %
- 0.25 mL of epinephrine 1:1,000 (final concentration of 1:200,000)
- 5 mL of 8.4 % sodium bicarbonate

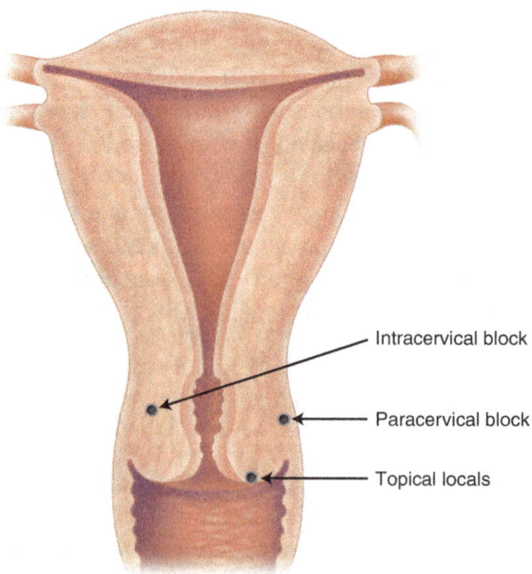

Fig. 4.3 Site comparison for paracervical, intracervical, and topical placement

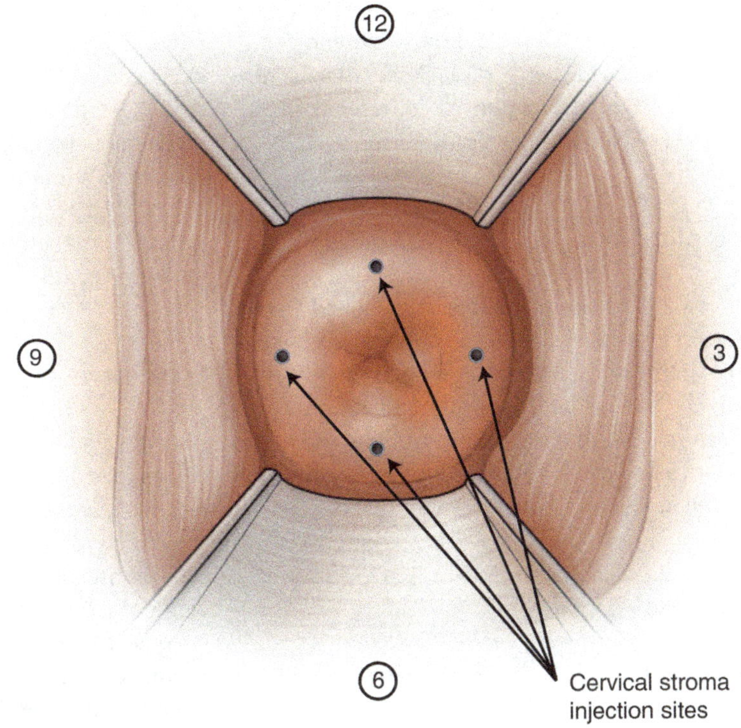

Fig. 4.4 Correct needle insertion sites for an intracervical block

Equipment

1. One 20-gauge needle (larger bore needle needled to compensate for the increased resistance of the cervical stroma)
2. One 20 mL syringe for injection (larger syringes are not recommended as more force is exerted during the block)
3. Sterile towels and sponges
4. Sterile prep of choice (Note: Items 2–4 usually will be found in a standard block tray)

Procedure [5, 6]

1. Internally and externally prep and drape your patient in your standard sterile fashion.
2. The needle is inserted about 1 cm into the cervical stroma at the 12 o'clock position (Fig. 4.4).
3. Careful aspiration for blood on the syringe must be done prior to injection. If blood is obtained the needle should be withdrawn or advanced 1–2 mm until blood is no longer noted.
4. Inject 5 mL of local solution.
5. The needle should be removed and steps 4–8 should be repeated for an injection at the 3, 6, and 9 o'clock positions around the cervix.
6. Wait an appropriate amount of time prior to beginning your procedure depending on the local anesthetic used.

Tips

1. Aspirate your syringe several times throughout the course of your injection, particularly at the onset, halfway, and conclusion of injection. This will confirm that your needle has not moved during the block.
2. Do not aspirate back on your plunger more than a couple mL's. Over-aggressive aspiration can produce negative pressure and collapse blood vessels to produce a false negative. This would lead to inadvertent intravascular injection.
3. Alternative techniques are also used in clinical practice. One such technique involves injections at the 4 and 8 o'clock positions as

described above. However, only 2 mL are injected at the 12 o'clock position and 5 mL are injected at the 6 o'clock position at the cervicovaginal junction (as described in the paracervical block section).

Complications

All of the complications associated with paracervical blocks have also been associated with intracervical blocks, including toxicity, prolonged blockade, neuritis, infection, and hematoma. All of the same precautions and monitoring should be applied when evaluating patients undergoing intracervical blocks.

Pudendal Block

Anatomy

Sacral nerve roots from S2, S3, and S4 are the origins of the pudendal nerves. Sensorium to the areas of the perineum, rectum, inner thighs, and female genitalia are covered by these nerves. They exit bilaterally via the greater sciatic foramen and traverse between the sacrospinous ligament and the sacrotuberous ligament [5]. While more commonly used during labor on parturient patients, pudendal nerve blocks are an option for patients with perineal pain, biopsies, or excisions. As with the other nerve blocks that have been discussed, there are several techniques, including the use of ultrasound [14] and nerve stimulators [15–17], for its placement exists. The technique for transvaginal administration and for transperineal will be described below (Fig. 4.5).

Solution

As always, the length of the procedure determines the appropriate anesthetic solution. For the purpose of an in-office procedure, the previously described solution of lidocaine 1 %, epinephrine, and bicarbonate is likely to be sufficient, so long as post-procedural pain relief is not needed. Mepivacaine 1 % is a good choice for prolonged office blockade. Another example would be the use of tetracaine 0.15 % with epinephrine 1:200,000 for a prolonged block for labor [5].

Equipment (Transvaginal)

1. Iowa trumpet (15 cm) (Fig. 4.6)
2. One 20-gauge 15 cm needle

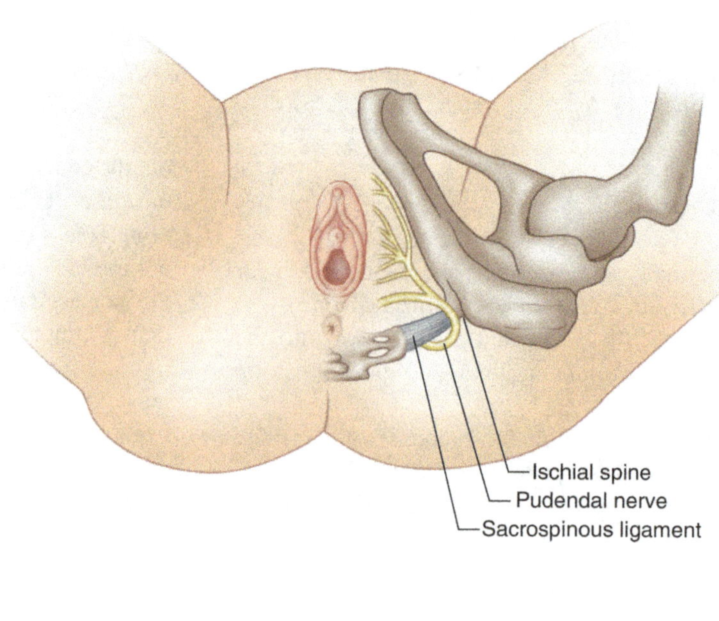

Fig. 4.5 Correct insertion sites for a pudendal block

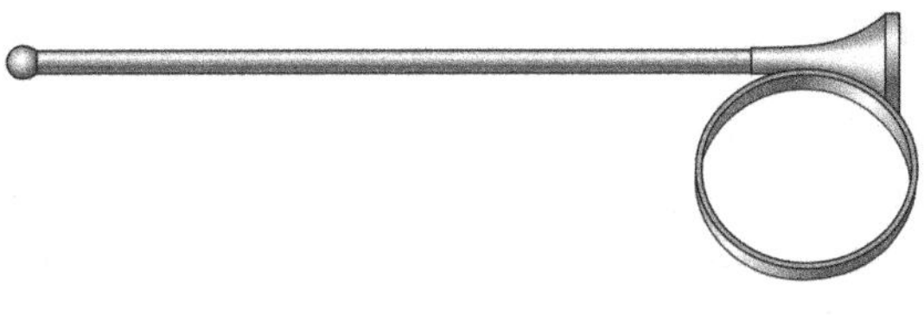

Fig. 4.6 Iowa trumpet

3. One 20 mL syringe for injection (larger syringes are not recommended as more force is exerted during the block)
4. Sterile towels and sponges
5. Sterile prep of choice (Note: Items 2–5 usually will be found in a standard block tray)

Procedure (Transvaginal) [5]

1. Internally and externally prep and drape your patient in your standard sterile fashion.
2. For a block performed on the patient's left side, the practitioner's left index and middle fingers are inserted vaginally and palpated the ischial spine.
3. Your needle guide of choice is directed 1 cm medial and posterior to the ischial spine.
4. The 20-gauge 15 cm needle is inserted through the guide and comes to rest on the vaginal mucosa.
5. The needle is slowly advanced through the mucosa until it passes through the sacrospinous ligament with a "pop" (total depth is 1.3–1.5 cm).
6. Careful aspiration for blood on the syringe must be done prior to injection. If blood is obtained the needle should be withdrawn or advanced 1–2 mm until blood is no longer noted.
7. Inject 10 mL of local solution.
8. Steps 4–7 should be repeated on the contralateral side if the procedure is bilateral.
9. The needle guide and needle should be removed.
10. Wait an appropriate amount of time prior to beginning your procedure depending on the local anesthetic used.

An optional way to perform this procedure is to infiltrate the area 1–2 cm lateral and parallel to the labia majora from the middle of the labia to the mons pubis. This will block the ilioinguinal, iliohypogastric and genitocrural nerves that innervate the superior half of the labia majora [5].

Tips

1. Aspirate your syringe several times throughout the course of your injection. Particularly at the onset, halfway, and conclusion of injection. This will confirm that your needle has not moved during the block.
2. Do not aspirate back on your plunger more than a couple mL's. Over-aggressive aspiration can produce negative pressure and collapse blood vessels to produce a false negative. This would lead to inadvertent intravascular injection.
3. The ischial spine, not the tuberosity, is the landmark that needs to be located. The spine lies posterior to the tuberosity.

Equipment (Transperineal)

1. Iowa trumpet or Kobak instrument (15 cm)
2. Two 22-gauge 10 cm needle
3. One 25-gauge needle (for skin infiltration)
4. One 20 mL syringe for injection (larger syringes are not recommended as more force is exerted during the block)
5. Sterile towels and sponges
6. Sterile prep of choice
7. Sterile marking pen (Note: Items 3–7 usually will be found in a standard block tray)

Procedure (Transperineal) [5]

1. Prep and drape your patient in your standard sterile fashion.
2. With your sterile marking pen, place bilateral "X's" over the inferior medial border of the ischial tuberosities.

3. Place a skin wheal at both "X's" with 1 % lidocaine.
4. The practitioner's non-dominate index finger is inserted rectally.
5. The 22-gauge 10 cm needle is inserted through one of the wheals and is guided by the non-dominate index finger to the ischial tuberosity (2.5–4.0 cm deep).
6. Careful aspiration for blood on the syringe must be done prior to injection. If blood is obtained the needle should be withdrawn or advanced 1–2 mm until blood is no longer noted.
7. Inject 5–10 mL of local solution on the lateral side of the tuberosity. This should anesthetize the inferior pudendal nerve.
8. With the non-dominate index finger again serving as a guide, the needle point is guided to the medial aspect of the tuberosity.
9. Careful aspiration is done again as described above.
10. Inject 5–10 mL of local solution on the lateral side of the tuberosity where branches of the pudendal nerve are often located.
11. Advance the needle point 2.5 cm past the tuberosity, aspirate, and inject 5–10 mL of local solution. Take care as the pudendal artery and vein travel here.
12. Guide the needle to the posterior spine of the ischium.
13. Palpate the sacrospinous ligament and insert the needle. It will give a "pop" when the needle is through. Advance 0.5 cm.
14. Aspirate and inject 5–10 mL of local solution.
15. Steps 5–14 are repeated for the opposite side if the procedure is bilateral.
16. Optional-infiltrate the area 1–2 cm lateral and parallel to the labia majora from the middle of the labia to the mons pubis. This will block the ilioinguinal, iliohypogastric, and genitocrural nerves that innervate the superior half of the labia majora.
17. Wait an appropriate amount of time prior to beginning your procedure depending on the local anesthetic used.

Tips

1. Aspirate your syringe several times throughout the course of your injection, particularly at the onset, halfway, and conclusion of injection. This will confirm that your needle has not moved during the block.
2. Do not aspirate back on your plunger more than a couple mL's. Over-aggressive aspiration can produce negative pressure and collapse blood vessels to produce a false negative. This would lead to inadvertent intravascular injection.
3. During Step 11, be careful to avoid intravascular injections, particularly into the pudendal artery and/or vein.
4. Double glove for the procedure. It will save time and reduce contamination between the parts of the procedure.

Complications

Pudendal neuritis is a rare, but known complication of pudendal nerve blocks. Similar to other types of neuritis, it is usually self-limiting and will resolve in less than 2 weeks. Hematomas of the parametrium are again possible as well. Sciatic nerve blockage may be noted after a pudendal block. Rectal puncture is possible using either transperineal or transvaginal. However it is more common with the transperineal. Because of the small gauge of the needle used, any sequela from the puncture, like fistula, is extremely rare [5]. Care should be taken to immediately change needles if rectal puncture is noted.

Topical Anesthetics

Topical anesthetics applied by way of sprays, gels, or creams have been studied with mixed results. Sprays on the ectocervix have proven to be ineffective for pain caused during biopsies [18]. However, they can lessen the pain caused by placement of the tenaculum [19]. The effectiveness of topical anesthetics for cervical canals has varied from study to study, some showing no difference [19] from placebo while others showed significant reductions [20, 21] in pain.

Conclusion

Regional blocks can improve patient satisfaction and decrease the pain associated with many gynecological procedures that are done in an office setting. However, for effective anesthesia to be administered many factors come into play.

An understanding of local anesthetics is needed for any regional technique to succeed. A practitioner must have a firm grasp on how the medications work, how they can be augmented, and how they will affect the patient.

The proper block needs to be chosen for an appropriate procedure. A working knowledge of the anatomy of the nerve or nerves needing to be blocked is a necessity, as well as an understanding on what to expect as a result of blocking those nerves.

For a regional block to be done safely in an office setting, the proper equipment and personnel must be readily available to manage any complications. While complications with the blocks discussed in this chapter are rare, preparation and vigilance will ensure safe and appropriate management of all patients.

Analgesia and Sedation for Office-Based Gynecologic Procedures

Sedation and analgesia for outpatient procedures in the Gynecology offices provide two main benefits. It allows patients to undergo potentially unpleasant procedures by relieving anxiety and pain. It also optimizes the technical aspect of the procedure for the gynecologist by minimizing patient movement and discomfort.

There is a well-defined continuum of sedation depth that has been developed by the American Society of Anesthesiologists. For office-based procedures, moderate sedation/analgesia or less will usually suffice. Moderate sedation, otherwise commonly known as "conscious sedation," is a drug-induced depression of consciousness during which patients respond purposefully to verbal commands, either alone or accompanied by light tactile stimulation. No interventions are required to maintain a patent airway and cardiovascular function is usually maintained [22].

Deep sedation/analgesia is a drug-induced depression of consciousness whereby patients cannot be easily aroused but respond purposefully after repeated or painful stimulation. These patients may need assistance in maintaining a patent airway as the ability to independently maintain ventilatory function may be impaired. Cardiovascular function is usually unaffected [22].

As it is not possible to always predict how a patient might respond to sedative medications, practitioners intending to attain a targeted level of sedation or analgesia have to be able to rescue patients whose sedation level has become deeper than intended. For moderate sedation, this translates to the ability to treat hypoventilation or manage a compromised airway in a patient who responds purposefully only after repeated stimulation. Deep sedation should therefore only be performed by practitioners qualified to conduct general anesthesia.

There are several components to office-based anesthesia that, if optimized, will increase the likelihood of satisfactory sedation and decrease the likelihood of adverse outcome. The process of sedation can be subdivided into three main parts: "pre-procedure," "intra-procedure" and "post-procedure." All three parts play an equally important role in patient safety.

Pre-procedure

Evaluation

A thorough pre-procedure evaluation is essential. Clinicians administering sedation should be familiar with the patient's medical history and how this might affect the patient's response to sedative medications. The evaluation should include: (1) a review of the major organ systems with particular attention to any abnormalities (2) prior experience with any anesthetic (3) drug allergies and medications currently taken with emphasis on potential interaction with sedation drugs (4) history of smoking, alcohol consumption, and illicit substance use (5) time and nature of last oral intake.

The clinician should perform a focused physical examination on the patient undergoing sedation. This should include a review of vital signs, ascultation of the heart and lungs as well as evaluation of the airway. Pre-procedure laboratory testing should be dictated by the patient's medical condition and the pertinence of the results to sedation.

Contraindications

Sedation in the office setting may be unsuitable for patients with the following:

- Lack of full mental capacity
- Inability to lie still for the time needed for the procedure
- Unstable medical condition
- A known or suspected difficult airway

Special Situations

Certain types of patients face an increased risk of complications related to sedation/analgesia unless precautions are taken. In patients with serious underlying medical conditions (ex. extreme elderly age; severe cardiac, pulmonary, hepatic or renal disease; drug or alcohol abuse), pre-procedural consultation with the appropriate medical specialist should be undertaken. Patients with significant sedation-related risk factors such as potentially difficult airway, sleep apnea, or morbid obesity should be referred to an anesthesiologist. In the face of any significant doubt or medical concern, the procedure should be performed with the assistance of an anesthesia provider in an ambulatory surgery center (ASC) or operating room (OR) setting.

Informed Consent

In addition to the procedural details, appropriate discussion of the benefits, risks, and alternatives to the proposed sedation should also be conducted with the patients. Patients should always be counseled that sedation or analgesia will usually relieve most but perhaps not all of their anxiety and pain. It would also not be unusual for them to sometimes "feel" parts of the procedure. A patient who is well-informed and who knows what to expect during the procedure will be a more satisfied patient. For appropriate patients, the option of undergoing the procedure without sedation should also be considered [23]. A full overview of Informed Consent may be found in Chap. 3.

Intra-procedure

Monitoring

The response of patients to verbal stimuli when they are sedated serves as a guide to their level of consciousness. Spoken responses also indicate that the sedated patients are breathing. Patients who only respond to painful stimuli are in a state of deep sedation that often approaches general anesthesia and should be treated accordingly.

The primary causes of morbidity associated with sedation/analgesia are drug-induced respiratory depression and airway obstruction. Monitoring of ventilation by direct observation or continuous ascultation reduces the risks of these adverse outcomes. Apnea monitoring by detection of exhaled carbon dioxide is a useful adjunct that is highly recommended. As ventilation and oxygenation are distinct physiologic processes, monitoring oxygenation with the use of pulse oximetry is not a substitute for monitoring ventilation.

Pulse oximetry, however, should be used in all patients undergoing sedation. Early detection of drug-induced hypoxemia through the use of oximetry decreases the likelihood of adverse outcomes such as cardiac arrest and death. In most instances, hypoxemia is more likely to be detected by oximetry than by clinical assessment alone.

Electrocardiographic monitoring should be used in all patients undergoing deep sedation. It should also be used for patients with significant cardiovascular disease who are undergoing moderate sedation. Since it is difficult to always be able to predict the precise depth of sedation or whether a patient might have cardiovascular disease, EKG monitoring should ideally be applied to every patient undergoing sedation. Blood pressure should be determined before the start of sedation/analgesia and at regular intervals thereafter during the procedure.

At a minimum, patients' level of consciousness, ventilation, oxygenation, and hemodynamic variables should be assessed and recorded at the following time periods: (1) before the start of the procedure (2) after administration of sedative/analgesic agents (3) at 5-min or less intervals during the procedure (4) during initial recovery (5) just before discharge from the office.

Personnel

A designated individual other than the practitioner performing the procedure should be present to monitor the patient throughout the procedure. During moderate sedation, the individual monitoring the patient may assist the practitioner with interruptible ancillary tasks of short duration. During deep sedation, the monitoring individual should not have any other responsibilities.

Since the primary complications of sedation are related to respiratory or cardiovascular compromise, the individual monitoring the patient needs to be trained to recognize these associated complications. Specifically, training should be focused towards the following concerns: (1) potentiation of respiratory depression by concomitantly administered sedatives and analgesics (2) insufficient time intervals between doses of sedative or analgesic medications possibly resulting in cumulative overdose (3) and lack of familiarity with the role of pharmacologic antagonists for sedative and analgesic agents.

At least one individual qualified in basic life support (bag-mask ventilation and cardiopulmonary resuscitation) should be present in the procedure room at all times for both moderate and deep sedation. For moderate sedation, an individual with advanced life support skills (including defibrillation, intubation, and use of resuscitation drugs) should be immediately available (not more than 5 min away). For deep sedation, this individual should be continually present in the procedure room.

Emergency Equipment

Resuscitative equipment should include a defibrillator, appropriately sized equipment of different sizes for establishing an airway and providing positive pressure ventilation, suction, resuscitation drugs as well as pharmacologic antagonists. These should always be present in the procedure room when sedation/analgesic is administered. Having a "sedation cart" in the procedure room available during these cases is advisable. It should contain all necessary emergency equipment and should be regularly assessed for medication expiration and adequacy of supplies.

Commonly Used Pharmacologic Agents

Midazolam

Midazolam is a water-soluble benzodiazepine that possesses anxiolytic, amnestic, and hypnotic properties. It does not have analgesic properties but is able to decrease analgesic requirements when used in combination with opioids. Midazolam elevates the seizure threshold; this is a safety advantage when local anesthetics are administered. It prevents nausea and vomiting, and seldom causes cardiovascular depression. However, significant respiratory depression and psychomotor impairment may occur, particularly when used in combination with opioids. Marked variability in dose-response is also common with the elderly being especially sensitive.

Midazolam has a quick onset and short duration of action. A single IV dose of 1–2 mg produces a peak effect in 2–3 min. Incremental doses of 0.5–1 mg can also be given every 3–5 min to attain the desired level of sedation. Midazolam can be given as a continuous infusion at 1–2 μg/kg/min. The elimination half-life is 1–4 h with overall duration dependent on the dose and age and/or condition of the patient (usually 15–80 min). Patients who take benzodiazepines on a regular basis may require a higher initial dose and more frequent redosing [23].

Flumazenil is a benzodiazepine antagonist that reverses Midzaolam's sedative effects. The initial dose is 0.2 mg IV with repeat dosing every 45–60 s to a maximum of 1 mg if desired effects are not attained. The duration of action is 45–90 min; as such, resedation can sometimes occur after this time period has elapsed.

Fentanyl

Fentanyl is an extremely lipid-soluble opioid that is approximately 100 times more potent than morphine. It has a very rapid onset, provides profound analgesia, and has a short duration of action. Analgesic doses of fentanyl usually do not affect the cardiovascular system. However, high doses can sometimes induce bradycardia which may lead to hypotension and a resultant decrease in cardiac output. Like all opioids, fentanyl can cause dose-related respiratory depression which is accentuated when used in combination with benzodiazepines. Unlike morphine, fentanyl is not associated with histamine release [23].

Fentanyl is usually given intravenously in doses of 1–2 μg/kg. It exerts a peak effect within 5 min and typically provides effective analgesic for approximately 30 min. Fentanyl may be redosed in increments of 25–50 μg if analgesia is insufficient. Although it quickly redistributes to inactive sites, frequent redosing of fentanyl can lead to saturation of fatty tissue which may significantly prolong its effects.

Naloxone is an opioid antagonist that reverses the effects of fentanyl. It is titrated in 0.04 mg doses intravenously every 2–3 min. Naloxone can reverse pruritis, nausea, and respiratory depression. However, it should be used with caution as it may acutely reverse analgesia and precipitate a withdrawal syndrome. It can also cause hypertension, pulmonary edema, and arrythmias. Renarcotization may occur, possibly requiring redosing of Naloxone every 30 min.

Morphine

Morphine has a delayed onset and prolonged duration of analgesic. It can cause histamine release which may lead to hypotension. These properties make morphine an inferior choice for sedation cases in which rapid titration to desired effect is needed. Morphine used in small doses towards the conclusion of the case may confer prolonged post-procedure analgesic if significant pain is expected after the procedure.

Propofol

Sedation with propofol is classified as deep sedation in most circumstances. Use of propofol may result in rapid and significant airway and cardiovascular compromise. As such, propofol should only be administered by clinicians qualified to rescue patients from any level of sedation up to and including general anesthesia [24].

Post-procedure Recovery Care

Patients may continue to be at significant risk for developing complications after the conclusion of their procedure. Respiratory or cardiac systems should be monitored as above but awareness of possible nausea and vomiting should be addressed and treated. Limiting post-procedural nausea and vomiting is a documented patient satisfier [25]. Decreased procedural stimulation, delayed drug absorption, and slow drug elimination may contribute to residual sedation and possibly cardiorespiratory depression in the recovery period. As such, following sedation/analgesia, patients should be recovered in an appropriately staffed and equipped area until they are near their baseline level of consciousness and are no longer at increased risk of cardiopulmonary depression. Appropriate discharge criteria should be established to address these concerns [24].

Medicolegal considerations mandate that physicians have evidence that the patient's discharge criteria have been met. All discharge instructions need to be signed by the patient and documented in the medical chart. Patients should be advised that discharge readiness does not imply the ability to drive or return to work and as such, office staff need to be certain that any patient who has undergone sedation have designated transportation post-procedure.

Conclusion

In-office gynecologic procedures can be safely accomplished with the assistance of regional anesthesia and sedation in the office setting. Following guidelines from the ASA will allow gynecologists to select patients who are appropriate for surgery in the office setting. A knowledge of both anesthetic properties and of sedatives is required in order to provide an optimal experience for the patient. Appropriate monitoring as well as pre- and post-procedure protocols are essential in order to provide a safe and successful procedure for your patients.

References

1. Strichartz GR, Berde CB. Local anesthetics. In: Miller RD, editor. Miller's anesthesia. 6th ed. Philadelphia: Elsevier; 2005. p. 573–99.
2. Morgan GE, Mikhail MS, Murray MJ. Clinical anesthesiology. 4th ed. New York: Lange; 2006.
3. Neal JM, Bernards CM, Butterworth 4th JF, Di Gregorio G, Drasner K, Hejtmanek MR, et al. ASRA practice advisory on local anesthetic systemic toxicity. Reg Anesth Pain Med. 2010;35(2):152–61.
4. Hausman LM, Rosenblatt MA. Office-based anesthesia. In: Barash PG, Cullen BF, Stoelting RK, editors. Clinical anesthesia. 5th ed. Philadelphia: Lippincott Williams & Wilkins; 2006. p. 1345–55.
5. Moore DC. Regional block: a handbook for use in the clinical practice of medicine and surgery. 4th ed. Springfield: Thomas Books; 1981.
6. Mankowski JL, Kingston J, Moran T, Nager CW, Lukacz ES. Paracervical compared with intracervical lidocaine for suction curettage: a randomized controlled trial. Obstet Gynecol. 2009;113(5):1052–7.
7. Vercellini P, Colombo A, Mauro F, Oldani S, Bramante T, Crosignani PG. Paracervical anesthesia for outpatient hysteroscopy. Fertil Steril. 1994;62 (5):1083–5.
8. Lau WC, Lo WK, Tam WH, Yuen PM. Paracervical anaesthesia in outpatient hysteroscopy: a randomised double-blind placebo-controlled trial. Br J Obstet Gynaecol. 1999;106(4):356–9.
9. Cicinelli E, Didonna T, Schonauer LM, Stragapede S, Falco N, Pansini N. Paracervical anesthesia for hysteroscopy and endometrial biopsy in postmenopausal women. A randomized, double-blind, placebo-controlled study. J Reprod Med. 1998;43(12):1014–8.
10. Titapant V, Chawanpaiboon S, Boonpektrakul K. Double-blind randomized comparison of xylocaine and saline in paracervical block for diagnostic fractional curettage. J Med Assoc Thai. 2003;86 (2):131–5.
11. Giorda G, Scarabelli C, Franceschi S, Campagnutta E. Feasibility and pain control in outpatient hysteroscopy in postmenopausal women: a randomized trial. Acta Obstet Gynecol Scand. 2000;79(7):593–7.
12. Cooper NAM, Clark TJ. Local anaesthesia for pain control during outpatient hysteroscopy: systematic review and meta-analysis. BMJ. 2010;340:c1130.
13. Munro MG, Brooks PG. Use of local anesthesia for office diagnostic and operative hysteroscopy. J Minim Invasive Gynecol. 2010;17(6):709–18.
14. Lean LL, Hegarty D, Harmon D. Analgesic effect of bilateral ultrasound-guided pudendal nerve blocks in management of interstitial cystitis. J Anesth. 2012;26:128–9.
15. Ismail MT, Nagat SE. Pre-emptive analgesia by nerve stimulator guided pudendal nerve block for posterior colpoperineorrhaphy. Eur J Obstet Gynecol Reprod Biol. 2012;163:200–3.
16. Naja Z, Ziade MF, Lönnqvist PA. Nerve stimulator guided pudendal nerve block decreases posthemorrhoidectomy pain. Can J Anaesth. 2005;52(1):62–8.
17. Imbelloni LE, Vieira EM, Gouveia MA, Netinho JG, Spirandelli LD, Cordeiro JA. Pudendal block with bupivacaine for postoperative pain relief. Dis Colon Rectum. 2007;50(10):1656–61.
18. Prefontaine M, Fung-Kee-Fung M, Moher D. Comparison of topical Xylocaine with placebo as a local anesthetic in colposcopic biopsies. Can J Surg. 1991;34(2):163–5.
19. Davies A, Richardson RE, O'Connor H, Baskett TF, Nagele F, Magos AL. Lignocaine aerosol spray in outpatient hysteroscopy: a randomized double-blind placebo-controlled trial. Fertil Steril. 1997;67 (6):1019–23.
20. Soriano D, Ajaj S, Chuong T, Deval B, Fauconnier A, Darai E. Lidocaine spray and outpatient hysteroscopy: randomized placebo-controlled trial. Obstet Gynecol. 2000;96(5 Pt 1):661–4.
21. Zullo F, Pellicano M, Stigliano CM, Di Carlo C, Fabrizio A, Nappi C. Topical anesthesia for office hysteroscopy. A prospective, randomized study comparing two modalities. J Reprod Med. 1999;44 (10):865–9.
22. Gross JB, et al. American Society of Anesthesiologists Practice Guidelines for sedation and analgesia by non-anesthesiologists. Anesthesiology. 2002;96:1004–17.
23. Toledano RD, Kodali BS, Camann WR. Anesthesia drugs in the obstetric and gynecologic practice. Rev Obstet Gynecol. 2009;2(2):93–100.
24. Abdemalak B, Riad I. Monitored anesthesia care and anesthesia outside the operating room. In: Longnecker DE, Brown DL, Newman MF, Zapol WM, editors. Anesthesiology. 2nd ed. New York, NY: The McGraw-Hill medical; 2012. p. 1260–74.
25. Perrott DH. Anesthesia outside the operating room in office based setting. Curr Opin Anaesthesiol. 2008;21:480–5.

Basic Gynecologic Procedures

5

M. Jean Uy-Kroh

Abbreviations

ACOG	American College of Obstetricians and Gynecologists
CDC	Centers for disease control
EMS/EMB	Endometrial sampling/endometrial biopsy
I&D	Incision and drainage
IUD	Intrauterine device
NSAIDs	Nonsteroidal anti-inflammatory drugs
PID	Pelvic inflammatory disease
STI	Sexually transmitted infections
US MEC	United States Medical Eligibility Criteria for contraceptive use
WHO MEC	World Health Organization Medical Eligibility Criteria

Introduction

Despite modern medical advances, the fundamental principles of gynecology procedures are remarkably resilient. Whether it is inserting an intrauterine device (IUD), obtaining a uterine biopsy, or draining a genital abscess, the tenets of these treatments endure with time, albeit with slight variations. This chapter will discuss basic gynecology office procedures offer clinical pearls for troubleshooting difficult situations, and review common procedure related complications.

Intrauterine Device

In 1909, the German physician, Dr. Richard Richter published the first account of IUDs used for human contraception. He described inserting a ring made of silkworm gut into the uterus. In the 1920s, Dr. Ernst Graefenberg of Berlin, made the silkworm ring "radio-opaque" by winding silver wire around the ring. Later, he replaced the silk with a spiral coil made of a copper, nickel, and zinc alloy. This device became known as the Graefenberg ring. The IUD ring was extensively used in England and the British territories but not in the United States or Europe [1].

Over the ensuing years, IUDs of various shapes and material modifications were created and widely used throughout the world. By 1959, 32 different IUD patterns were documented with 20 years of usage and in 20,000 women in Japan. Plastic IUDs were introduced and heralded for their ease of insertion, shape retention, and long-term efficacy and safety [2]. The popular Lippes Loop, was introduced by American obstetrician and gynecologist, Dr. Jack Lippes, in 1962. The Lippes Loop was known for its characteristic double S plastic loop with a monofilament nylon string that enabled its easy removal. But

M.J. Uy-Kroh, M.D., F.A.C.O.G. (✉)
Department of Obstetrics and Gynecology,
Women's Health Institute, Cleveland Clinic,
9500 Euclid Avenue, A81, Cleveland, OH 44195, USA
e-mail: uykrohm@ccf.org

J.D. Emery and M.F.R. Paraiso (eds.), *Office-Based Gynecologic Surgical Procedures*,
DOI 10.1007/978-1-4939-1414-2_5, © Springer Science+Business Media New York 2015

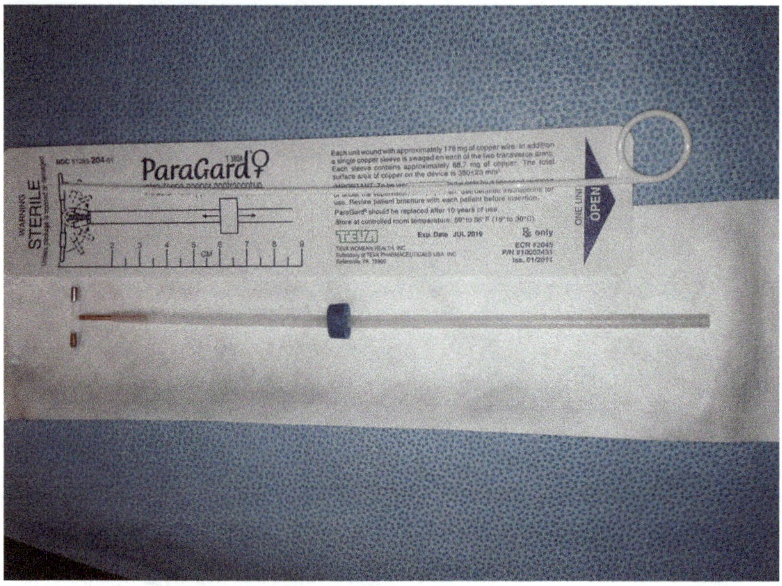

Fig. 5.1 ParaGard IUD—seen with sterile package contents which include device, loading instructions, ringed solid white insertion rod, and a measurement guide. Note the arms bend downward for loading

widespread American IUD acceptance and usage was hampered by IUD related deaths and bacterial infections from second generation devices, including the now infamous Dalkon Shield. Today, additional barriers that may hinder widespread usage include decreased patient access to IUDs and patient misconceptions regarding IUDs. Some common erroneous beliefs are that IUDs increase the risk of pelvic infections such as pelvic inflammatory disease (PID), IUDs act as abortifacients, and/or IUDs impair future fertility [3].

Currently, the IUD is the most commonly used form of reversible contraception in the world due to its excellent modern safety profile, outstanding efficacy, and ease of use. IUDs vary in size, composition, recommended duration, side effects, indicated usage, and insertion technique (Figs. 5.1, 5.2, and 5.3). As with initiating any contraceptive method, it is necessary to provide thorough patient counseling on alternative methods, the side effects, complications, benefits, and risks of initiating IUD usage versus the risk of accidental pregnancy to the patient's health and condition. As one considers IUD placement in the office, it is essential to remember that the financial, social, and medical access barriers to IUD placement are often far greater than the actual medical contraindications or relative restrictions of IUD usage for a patient. The policies regarding the initiation and continuation of IUDs and patient

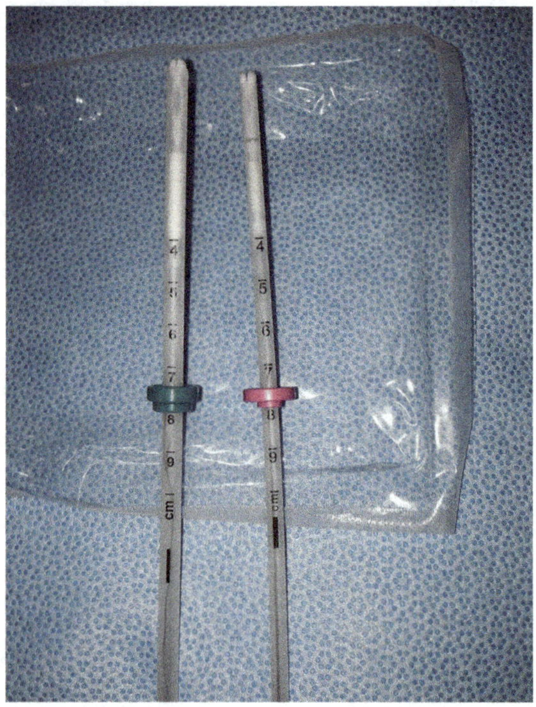

Fig. 5.2 Mirena and Skyla IUDs—a side by side comparison confirms the construction is very similar other than the distinguishing flange color, and the handle piece (not pictured)

recommendations are regularly detailed in the World Health Organization Medical Eligibility Criteria (WHO MEC) and the United States

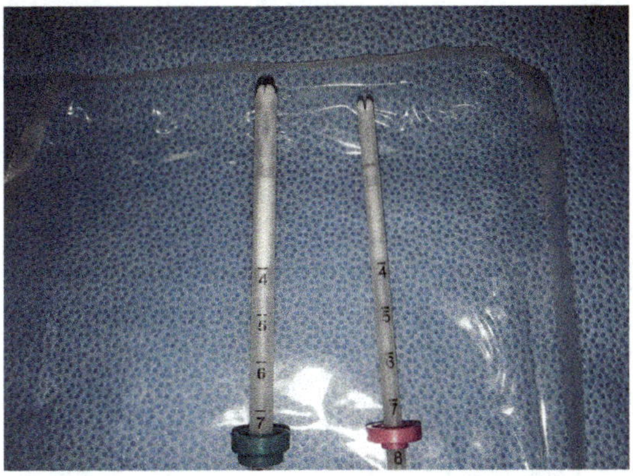

Fig. 5.3 Mirena and Skyla IUDs—close inspection of the two devices reveal the similarity that both devices have upward bending arms. But one can note, the variation in the outer insertion tube diameter (4.75 mm versus 3.8 mm), the device size discrepancy (32 × 32 mm versus 28 × 30 mm), and finally the identifying silver ring at the top of Skyla's vertical stem

Medical Eligibility Criteria for contraceptive use (US MEC) [4]. Absolute contraindications to IUD placement include: pregnancy, active known uterine infection, uterine or cervical malignancy, unexplained abnormal bleeding, adverse reaction to product ingredients, and the inability to place or retain the device [5].

IUD placement within the confines of the office is generally well tolerated. On a pain scale of 1–10, 46 % of women rated a pain score of 2 or below, and two thirds of the women had a pain score of 4 or lower. Although IUD insertion is "well tolerated" it is important to remember that it still produces pain. Pre-procedure treatment with nonsteroidal anti-inflammatory drugs (NSAIDs) is common and beneficial for reducing bleeding associated with IUD insertion, but only two treatments—tramadol (50 mg) and naproxen (550 mg) administered 40 min prior to insertion have been proven effective in decreasing pain [6–8]. Paracervical block was proven to decrease pain associated with cervical manipulation during hysteroscopy and may provide similar relief for IUD insertion [9] (Chap. 4). A paracervical block using 10–20 cc of 1 % lidocaine, is sometimes performed for patients who are prone to vasovagal reaction but the analgesic effect of this procedure must be weighed against the pain caused by the injection itself in relation to the pain produced by IUD insertion alone [10]. And finally, misoprostol may soften the cervix but its usefulness in decreasing pain and facilitating IUD insertion was not supported in four randomized control trials. Furthermore, some studies suggest the uterine activity promoted by misoprostol may worsen post-procedure cramping and increase the risk of device expulsion [11–14].

An IUD may be inserted at any time during the menstrual cycle but pregnancy should be excluded prior to insertion. In general, a pregnancy test is not necessary if the patient is: using a reliable form of contraception, in the late follicular phase (cycle day 5–10), or abstinent since her last menses. For patients with irregular menses, questionable compliance to contraception, or amenorrhea, a negative pregnancy test is recommended. Guidelines for recommended backup contraception, duration, and change from prior contraception is outlined by the Centers for Disease Control (CDC) and updated regularly [15].

Box 5.1: IUD Insertion Procedure Checklist

Signed informed consent

Patient counseling on procedure, side effects, post procedure contraception, and recovery instructions provided

Pregnancy has been excluded

STI screening (either prior to or at the time of IUD placement for higher risk patients)

Sterile speculum

Gloves (consider sterile gloves for Paragard IUD, dependent on provider loading preference)

Antiseptic cleansing solution and large applicator swabs

Single tooth tenaculum

Uterine sound

Scissors

IUD

± cervical dilator

Box 5.2: IUD Insertion Step by Step

Perform a pelvic exam to assess for cervical motion tenderness, uterine position, or uterine tenderness

Perform a sterile speculum exam and inspect the vagina and cervix

Cleanse the cervical portio with antiseptic solution

Perform paracervical block if necessary

Slowly and gently grasp the anterior lip of the cervix with a tenaculum (for anteverted or mid position uteri) and place gentle traction to align the cervical canal with the uterine cavity

Sound the uterus, for patency, noting the direction of the canal and the uterine length—gentle cervical dilation may be required

Load device for insertion (if necessary)

Using sterile technique, introduce the device through the endocervical canal with controlled, slow, and steady pressure

Be alert to sudden loss of resistance or increased uterine length

Deploy device per specific instructions (Table 5.2)

Remove insertion apparatus

Trim threads to 3 cm

Gently remove the tenaculum

Ensure hemostasis from the tenaculum site and os

Remove the speculum

Assess the patient's post-procedure condition

Schedule 4-week follow-up visit

Box 5.3: IUD Insertion Tips & Tricks

Place the tenaculum on the posterior lip of the cervix for retroverted uteri.

Slowly and gently close/open the tenaculum to reduce pain.

Quell patient anxiety: a calm and reassuring professional demeanor can significantly reduce patients' anxiety and fear. Patients are less likely to perceive increased pain if they are adequately counseled and emotionally supported.

If insertion is particularly painful or difficult due to extreme uterine flexion or fibroids, consider device insertion under ultrasound guidance or a post procedure ultrasound to confirm proper device placement.

Peri-procedural Complications

Vasovagal reaction—IUD insertion, removal, and transcervical procedures in general may provoke a vasovagal response. The patient may experience transient (pre)syncope, nausea, hypotension, diaphoresis, or bradycardia. Should this occur, terminate the procedure and provide supportive care to the patient. Place her in a supine position and if necessary, elevate her lower extremities. If her symptoms persist, consider placing a paracervical block or removing the IUD. For the truly refractive vasovagal episode, atropine (0.4 mg intramuscular injection) may be given to the patient while assessing for uterine perforation and intra-abdominal bleeding.

Infection—Active infection or symptoms suspicious for infection are clear contraindications to IUD insertion. For patients who are at low risk for sexually transmitted infections (STI), the use of prophylactic antibiotics at the time of insertion confers no benefit and is not recommended [16]. An international study did confirm a transient increased risk of PID due to bacterial contamination at the time of IUD insertion. The first 20 days after an IUD is inserted is the time of greatest infection risk [17]. This suggests that resultant PID is due to the introduction of pathogens during device insertion and underscores the importance of sterile technique. A retrospective cohort study of 57,000 IUD insertions revealed that the risk of PID after device insertion is only 0.54 %. As encouraged by device manufacturers, many clinicians screen for gonorrhea and chlamydia in patients based on their STI risk. According to the CDC, the prevalence of chlamydia is highest among women 14–25 years of age and is approximately 3 %. In addition, the American College of Obstetricians and Gynecologists defines women with multiple sexual partners and those younger than 25 years old as "high risk" for STI. Therefore, for this group of women, it is advised and reasonable to perform STI screening on the day of IUD insertion. Same day screening and insertion increases contraceptive access and decreases the chance of unintended pregnancy. If an infection is detected, the patient and her partner should be treated and the IUD may remain in place [18].

Perforation—This complication usually occurs at the time of insertion and is prone to involve the fundus, lower uterine segment, and midline posterior wall. Perforation may also occur remote from IUD insertion as a result of uterine contractions. These perforations are usually in a different plane or trajectory of insertion and more commonly involve the cervix. Perforation is a rare event occurring in 1 out of 1,000 insertions or less in experienced hands. The risk of perforation is dependent upon provider experience and increases with a stenotic cervix, immobile uterus, and a markedly flexed uterus. A sudden inappropriate, loss of resistance, severe patient pain, or a large discrepancy between uterine depth and anticipated uterine length should trigger an evaluation for perforation. The instrument should be removed gently and the patient should be observed for hemorrhage. If the patient's condition does not improve or there is a strong suspicion of intraperitoneal injury, swift surgical evaluation is necessary.

If uterine perforation occurs and the patient remains stable the clinician has two options: The procedure may be discontinued and the IUD inserted on a separate visit. Or, the IUD may still be inserted at the same visit, but care should be taken not to follow the previous tract. Although prophylactic antibiotics have been proven to be unnecessary for routine IUD insertion, when perforation occurs, the use of antibiotics is less clear since the procedure may have allowed passage of vaginal flora into the peritoneal cavity. In these instances, doxycycline (100 mg twice a day for 7 days) with or without metronidazole (500 mg twice a day for 7 days) may be considered [19, 20].

Expulsion—Expulsion of a device may occur even if the device was properly placed. Expulsion may be associated with pain and bleeding or the patient may be completely asymptomatic. Although it is a common practice to insert IUDs during a patient's menses, the expulsion risk during the first 5 days of a cycle is 5 % compared to 2 % if inserted during the luteal phase [21]. The risk of expulsion is also greater when IUD insertion is performed immediately after uterine evacuation and the uterus is still enlarged [22]. On the other hand, expulsion rates may also increase with smaller uteri, length less than 6 cm, and with anatomic uterine aberrations. If an IUD is expelled, consider performing the second IUD placement under ultrasound guidance. Or, sonographically confirm correct placement immediately afterward, since a patient with one previous expulsion has a 30 % chance of subsequent expulsion [23].

Malposition—Ideally, the IUD should be located in the uterine fundus. Occasionally, IUDs are malpositioned and are located in the lower uterine segment or endocervix (versus a partially expelled IUD that is visible at the external os and should be removed), embedded within the myometrium, or rotated out of the uterine plane. Prior to removing or replacing the device, the clinician should note several things including: the type of device, if the patient is symptomatic and warrants device removal, if the malpositioned device is still providing effective contraception, and if the risk of removing the device, particularly in an asymptomatic patient, will increase the chance of unintended pregnancy. Specifically, there is limited data that suggests that due to their different mechanisms of action, malpositioned Copper IUDs within the endocervix, unlike their levonorgestrol counterparts [24], do not provide adequate contraception. One study noted a malpositioned Copper IUD located in the cervix is almost 14 times as likely to be associated with concomitant pregnancy [25]. Therefore, before removing a malpositioned device and/or inserting a new

IUD, a clinician should assess for pregnancy and counsel the patient appropriately.

IUD Removal

Removal of an IUD is usually straightforward and swift. A sterile speculum is placed and using a ring forceps, the strings are grasped and used to gently remove the device from the uterus. Occasionally, removal is more involved. A sharply flexed uterus can be tricky and may decrease necessary visualization and access. In these instances, gentle traction applied with a tenaculum straightens the utero-cervical junction and aids in device retrieval. In addition, IUD strings are sometimes missing or retracted into the uterine cavity or endocervix. In this case, an ultrasound may be helpful to confirm that the device remains within the uterus. If the device is not seen within the uterus, a plain film X-ray of the abdomen and pelvis may confirm device perforation.

Endocervical speculums and endocervical brushes can be used to visualize the cervical canal and gently tease the threads outward. Furthermore, IUD hooks are also available and should be used by experienced clinicians to extricate the device threads. If the device is still unable to be retrieved flexible or rigid hysteroscopy can be performed to guide the threads outward.

Box 5.4: IUD Removal Tips & Tricks

Use a cytobrush or endocervical speculum to locate "lost" threads.

Ultrasound and pelvic radiographs are helpful in locating the device position and location.

Exercise caution when utilizing IUD hooks.

Flexible hysteroscopy can decrease time and patient discomfort, and can be used to produce a portion of the device or the threads at the external os.

Box 5.5: IUD Removal Procedure Checklist

Signed informed consent

Patient counseling on procedure, side effects including return to fertility, post procedure contraception, and recovery instructions provided

In the event of a partially expelled or a malpositioned device, confirm that the patient is not pregnant

Sterile speculum

Ring forceps

Gloves

As needed

- Single tooth tenaculum
- Cytobrush
- Endocervical speculum
- IUD hook
- Ultrasound
- Flexible or rigid hysteroscopy

Endometrial Sampling

Endometrial sampling (ES) in the office is a simple, safe, well tolerated, and cost-efficient method to obtain uterine tissue for histology diagnosis. As early as the 1920s, in-office endometrial biopsy (EMB) was lauded for the advantages of avoiding general anesthesia and allowing the patient to quickly resume her normal daily function.

The original Novak and Randall curettes are rigid, metal sheaths with an outer diameter of 4.2–3 mm respectively. The most distal end contains a small serrated or beveled lateral opening and the most proximal end attaches to an aspirator that provides suction. In 1968, Jensen described a modification. Using a rigid 3 mm cannula attached to 600 mmHg of vacuum suction, an in-office vacuum-abrasion technique, or Vabra, aspirator was introduced. Despite the small outer diameter and apparent effectiveness, the Vabra device and technique did not gain widespread office adoption. Significant patient discomfort and the reliance upon a machine to produce sufficient vacuum suction caused many clinicians to return to the operating room to perform a standard dilation and curettage until a superior in-office device came to market. Additional electronic and vacuum syringe devices were trialed but they too had limited clinical acceptance [26].

Today, the original curettes and aspirators have mostly been replaced with flexible, 2–4 mm, plastic pipelles that are very well tolerated by patients. The newer pipelle biopsy device is disposable and does not require an aspirator. Instead, a vacuum is created by withdrawing the inner piston from the pipelle cannula. This creates a negative pressure that draws the endometrial tissue into the pipelle channel. No additional personnel or equipment is necessary to perform the simple procedure. There are a number of pipelle kits available today—all with varying accessories such as additional suction syringes, multi-perforated channels, and even cytology abrasion brushes.

Given the numerous and varied indications for endometrial sampling, EMB is one of the most common procedures encountered in a gynecology office. The procedure's efficacy for detecting malignancy has been investigated numerous times. Two separately conducted, large reviews—revealed that EMB has high accuracy in diagnosing endometrial cancer especially if the endometrial process is global and if an adequate specimen is obtained. If the malignancy occupies less than half of the endometrial surface, however, the cancer may not be detected by a blind, random, cavity sampling. Therefore, the procedure is more accurate at confirming a uterine cancer diagnosis than excluding an intrauterine malignancy [27, 28]. In summary, if a patient has a negative EMB result but continues to have symptoms, further clinical evaluation is warranted with either saline infusion sonography or office diagnostic hysteroscopy (Chaps. 6 and 7).

EMB should not be performed in cases of pregnancy, coagulopathy, or known pelvic infection. If possible, avoid scheduling a biopsy when the patient is having heavy uterine bleeding as this may increase the risk of insufficient tissue sampling. In addition, EMB can interfere with an early, undiagnosed pregnancy. Therefore, it should not be performed more than 14–16 days after ovulation.

Box 5.6: ES/EMB Procedure Checklist

Signed informed consent

Patient counseling on procedure, side effects, and post-procedure recovery instructions provided

Pregnancy has been excluded

STI screening (if needed)

Sterile speculum

Gloves

Antiseptic cleansing solution and large applicator swabs

± single tooth tenaculum

± cervical dilator

± paracervical anesthetic equipment

EMB pipelle or sampling device

Labeled, sterile pathology container

Box 5.7: ES/EMB Step by Step

Perform a pelvic exam to assess for cervical motion tenderness, uterine position, or uterine tenderness

Perform a sterile speculum exam and inspect the vagina and cervix

Cleanse the cervical portio with antiseptic solution

Perform a paracervical block if necessary

If the uterus is highly mobile, slowly and gently grasp the cervix with a tenaculum and place gentle traction to align the cervical canal with the uterine cavity

Using sterile technique, introduce the pipelle/sampling device through the endocervical canal with controlled, slow, and steady pressure—cervical dilation may be necessary, especially in postmenopausal patients

Be alert to sudden loss of resistance or increased uterine length

(continued)

Box 5.7 (continued)

Gently advance the sampling device until resistance is met

Steady the device in one hand, while the other hand withdraws the inner piston from the outer cannula. Move the piston to its maximally extended position—it will remain attached to the cannula

Rotate the pipelle in a continuous 360° fashion and observe for tissue or blood to draw up into the plastic cannula

Continue a rotary motion while slowly removing the device

Maintain sterile technique and remove the entire device from the uterus

Expel the biopsy into a sterile formalin or saline specimen cup by replacing the inner piston into the cannula, avoid contaminating the pipelle

Assess tissue sample adequacy and if necessary repeat the procedure

Gently remove the tenaculum and ensure hemostasis from the tenaculum site and os

Remove the speculum

Assess the patient's post procedure condition

Schedule 4-week follow-up visit

Box 5.8: ES/EMB Tips & Tricks

Challenging exams

As with most gynecologic procedures, supportive, patient positioning is key to any successful procedure. Updated or specialized examination tables and stirrups that accommodate patients with large habitus are increasingly necessary and their value in ensuring patient safety and comfort cannot be understated. In addition, adequate lighting, protective gowning, and extra-long gloves are sometimes necessary for clinician safety and comfort.

If vaginal tissue dystocia hinders cervical visualization consider "gloving" a speculum to create a modified tissue retractor. Cut the thumb of a sterile glove and slide it over the arms of the speculum, allowing the most distal ends of the arm to be uncovered by the glove. Together, these techniques usually improve access and visualization of the cervix.

Avoid moving the pipelle in an in/out motion as this increases the risk of uterine perforation.

Instead, rely on the rotational movement of the pipelle and the vacuum generated by the internal piston.

Provide emotional assurance to the patient when/if she expresses discomfort.

If cramping is severe, expeditiously complete the procedure

Assess the specimen for adequacy before removing all instruments by transilluminating clear specimen cups—mucus and organized blood can be identified from tissue and can indicate the need for a second or third pass.

Sometimes less is more

Some patients do not tolerate even a small speculum or may have anatomy that makes prolonged speculum positioning difficult (i.e., an anterior cervix located behind the pubic symphysis) Once the cervix has been adequately inspected and cleansed with antiseptic, remove the speculum, don sterile gloves, and perform an EMB by tactile sensation. This technique significantly limits patient discomfort.

Peri-procedural Complications

Vasovagal reaction, infection, and uterine perforation are all known complications of EMB. Vasovagal reaction is treated mostly with supportive care and rarely requires further intervention. Infection following EMB may be associated with marked uterine tenderness, foul discharge, and/or fever. The patient should be treated for endometritis with doxycycline (100 mg twice a day for 7 days) with or without metronidazole (500 mg twice a day for 7 days.) Uterine perforation is rare and has been reported to have an incidence of 1 or 2 cases per 1,000. Unless the patient is unstable, supportive therapy is advocated [29]. Finally, insufficient tissue for histologic diagnosis can be encountered regardless of the type of sampling device employed. In these instances, further clinical evaluation is advised.

Bartholin Gland Cyst & Abscess Treatment

Normally, the Bartholin glands are pea-sized, non-palpable glands located bilaterally at the 5 and 7 o'clock position of the posterolateral aspect of the vaginal orifice. The gland drains into a 2.5 cm long duct and the duct drains into the space between the hymen and the labia minora (see Fig. 5.4). Occasionally, trauma, inflammation, or obstruction of the orifice causes the ducts to dilate. Many of these dilations range from 1 to 3 cm in diameter and are commonly referred to as a Bartholin cyst, although it is actually an obstructed and dilated duct. An asymptomatic Bartholin cyst does not require treatment and is not an infection. One exception to this is a Bartholin cyst in a 40-year-old, or older, woman or a woman with Paget's disease of the vulva. For these patients, incision, drainage, and additional biopsy of the gland is recommended to exclude carcinomas such as adenocarcinoma and squamous cell carcinoma [30, 31].

Sometimes, the duct rapidly enlarges over just a few days and causes significant pain. In addition, the dilated duct may become infected and progress to a polymicrobial abscess characterized by a fluctuant vulvar mass (that may extend past the vestibular area), severe pain, warmth, tenderness, edema and/ or cellulitis (see Fig. 5.5). A symptomatic Bartholin cyst or an overt Bartholin abscess requires intervention and this can be safely performed in the office. Definitive treatment for recurrent duct dilation or abscess formation is excision of the gland but given the risk of bleeding and need for adequate anesthesia, this procedure is usually performed in the operating room. It is also important to note that unusual or unremitting Bartholin gland infections warrant

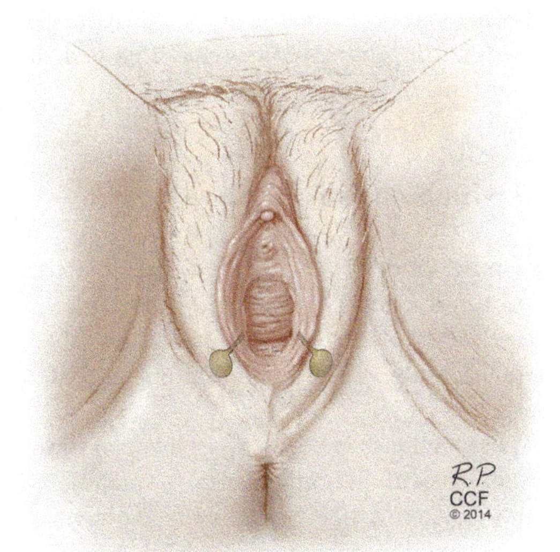

Fig. 5.4 Bartholin gland and duct—the bilateral glands and ducts are seen in normal anatomic relationship to the ductal orifice and hymen. The duct is approximately 2–2.5 cm in length and empties into a groove within the hymen and the labia minora

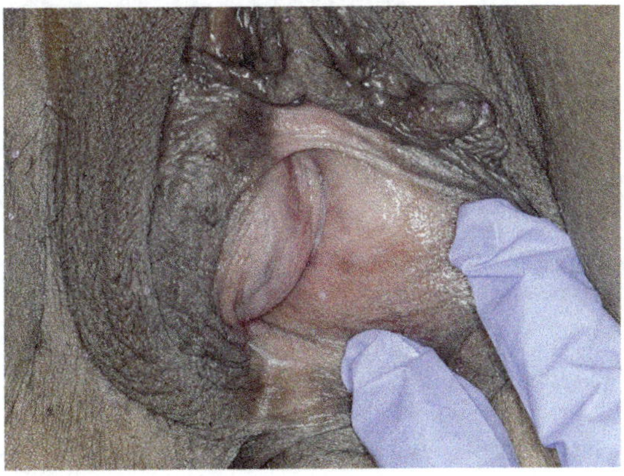

Fig. 5.5 Bartholin abscess—this 46-year-old patient had a recurrent, symptomatic right Bartholin abscess and was seen in the office for intense pain and swelling. Note the edema, erythema, and distortion of normal anatomy

Table 5.1 Differential diagnosis of vulvar masses in the Bartholin gland region

Inclusion cyst[a]
Gartner duct cyst[b]
Sebaceous cyst
Fibroma
Leiomyoma
Lipoma
Hidradenoma[c]
Peri-rectal abscess
Skene's duct cyst
Endometriosis
Canal of Nuck cyst
Necrotizing fasciitis
Malignancy

Droegmemueller W. Benign Gynecologic Lesions. In: Stenchever M, Droegemueller W, Herbst A, Mishell D, editors. Comprehensive gynecology. St Louis: Mosby; 2001. p. 233

[a]The most common cystic structures of the vagina, usually located in the posterior or lateral walls of the lower third of the vagina. They are more common in parous women as they usually result from birth trauma or gynecologic procedures and occur when a small island of epithelium is buried beneath the surface after a procedure. Histologically, they are lined by stratified squamous epithelium and contain a thick pale yellow substance formed by degenerating epithelial cells. Due to their contents they are often erroneously referred to as sebaceous cysts

[b]Mesonephric in origin, they are usually found in the lateral vagina

[c]Originate from the apocrine sweat glands, they are usually small, benign, vulvar tumors

further evaluation. Immunocompromised and diabetic patients are more susceptible to rare, but life threatening, necrotizing subcutaneous infections which require immediate surgical excision and debridement.

In addition to malignancy, other benign vulvar masses can be found in the area of the Bartholin gland and should be considered prior to treatment. The differential diagnosis of these lesions is listed in Table 5.1. Simple Bartholin gland cysts do not require antibiotic treatment. For a cyst that is already draining, warm compresses and Sitz baths alone can be therapeutic. For patients affected by recurrent ductal dilation, abscess, extensive cellulitis, concomitant STI, pregnancy, immunosuppression, hospitalization, or increased risk of methicillin-resistant staphylococcus aureus infection, administer dual treatment with clindamycin (300 mg by mouth four times a day for 7 days) and amoxicillin–clavulanate (875 mg by mouth two times a day for 7 days) [32]. Antibiotic treatment should be reevaluated and tailored based on microbiology findings and correlation with the patient's clinical condition.

Possible office treatments include: Simple incision and drainage (I&D) of the symptomatic cyst, I&D with fistulizing device placement (such as a Word catheter), for 40-year-old and older women I&D and gland biopsy, and finally, marsupialization of the Bartholin duct.

The patient should be re-evaluated if she experiences persistent bleeding, fever, discomfort, or if her cellulitis worsens as these are all concerning signs and symptoms that require investigation.

Simple I&D

This procedure may be performed for symptomatic Bartholin duct enlargement. It is the fastest and simplest of all of the options. It provides immediate decompression of the enlarged duct but reoccurrence is common.

I&D with Fistula Formation

This procedure is the preferred first line treatment for a painfully enlarged Bartholin duct since it attempts to not only create, but also to maintain, a new orifice for the entrapped contents to drain.

Word catheter placement is the classic and most extensively reported fistula formation treatment (see Box 5.10). Newer methods have also been invented that similarly establish a fistulized tract. The Jacobi ring and dual exit plastic tubing have been reported to successfully treat Bartholin pathology [33]. The Jacobi ring was described in 2005 by Gennis et al. and involves fistulizing an entry and exit orifice from the abscess.

Table 5.2 Comparing IUDs[a]

	ParaGard	Mirena	Skyla
IUD	Copper TCu380A (see Fig. 5.1)	LNg-20 (see Fig. 5.2)	LNg-14 (see Fig. 5.3)
Hormone	None Contains 176 mg of copper wire with exposed copper surface of 380 ± 23 mm	Levonorgestrol 52 mg 20 μg/day	Levonorgestrol 13.5 mg 14 μg/day declines to 5 μg/day after 3 years
Device duration	10 years, may be effective up to 12–20 years[b]	5 years, may be effective up to 7 years[b]	3 years
Dimensions	32 × 36 mm Outer diameter of insertion tube 4.4 ± 0.1 mm	32 × 32 mm Outer diameter of insertion tube 4.75 mm	28 × 30 mm Outer diameter of insertion tube 3.8 mm
Radio-opaque	T body barium infused	T body barium infused	T body barium infused + silver ring located at the top of vertical stem is visible by ultrasound
Mechanism of action	Sterile inflammatory reaction Copper spermicidal action	Sterile inflammatory reaction Thickens cervical mucous Thins endometrium Reduces sperm capacitation	Sterile inflammatory reaction Thickens cervical mucous Thins endometrium Reduces sperm capacitation
Recommended uterine cavity length	6–9 cm[c]	6–10 cm[c]	No recommendation
Additional information	Contraindicated (theoretical) for patients with Wilson's disease	Contraindicated in patients with hormone-sensitive malignancy and some liver diseases Ovulation is inhibited in a minority of women. 45 % of menstrual cycles were ovulatory in a 1 year study. In another study, 75 % of cycles were ovulatory after 4 years.[d]	Contraindicated in patients with hormone-sensitive malignancy and some liver diseases
Common uses other than contraception	Emergency contraception within 5 days of unprotected intercourse[e]	Heavy uterine bleeding that has been evaluated (FDA approval 2009) Endometriosis Medical management for poor surgical candidates with endometrial hyperplasia	None
Device loading	Don sterile gloves or load the IUD using the sterile, transparent, plastic packaging as a barrier The thread should be preloaded into the tube *Bend the arms of the device downward* and secure the tips into the clear, inserter tube (for no more than 5 min)	Free the ends of the IUD strings from the base of the handle so they move freely and the numbers on the inserter are facing upward Lift the handle while resting the device arms against the sterile package Align the arms in a horizontal position	*~Do not move the slider to a reverse position since the strings are pre-contained and this movement will release them prematurely.*

(continued)

Table 5.2 (continued)

	ParaGard	Mirena	Skyla
IUD	Copper TCu380A (see Fig. 5.1)	LNg-20 (see Fig. 5.2)	LNg-14 (see Fig. 5.3)
	Ensure the elliptical flange is in the same horizontal plane as the arms and slide it to the sounded uterine length	*Advance and hold the green slider* in the most forward "up" position	*Advance and hold the pink slider* in the direction of the arrow in the most forward "up" position to draw the insertion tube over the IUD *folding the arms upward*
	Thread the solid white rod into the free end of the tube until it just touches the base of the loaded IUD and the ringed end protrudes Both the device and solid rod should be partially contained within the inserter tube	Firmly pull the threads downward to draw the IUD into the insertor tube, *folding the arms upward*, and secure the threads in the handle cleft Adjust the flange to the sounded uterine length	Adjust the flange to the sounded uterine length
Device insertion	Grasp the tenaculum with the non-dominant hand and apply traction Using the dominant hand, insert the loaded device through the cervix and gently advance until the flange abuts the cervix This places the device at the fundus Do not advance the solid rod or perforation may occur	Grasp the tenaculum with the non-dominant hand and apply traction Using the dominant hand, insert the device through the cervix until the flange is 1.5–2 cm from the cervix	Grasp the tenaculum with the non-dominant hand and apply traction Using the dominant hand, insert the device through the cervix until the flange is 1.5–2 cm from the cervix
	Hold the solid white rod steady to stabilize the IUD at the fundus and retract the clear tube less than 1 cm to allow the arms to expand	*Hold the entire inserter steady and move only the slider* toward the raised linear notch and wait 10 s for the arms to expand	*Hold the entire inserter steady and move only the slider* to the raised linear notch and wait 10 s for the arms to expand
	Then, advance the clear insertion tube forward until slight fundal resistance is met	Then, advance the entire inserter until the flange abuts the cervix and fundal resistance is met This places the device at the fundus	Then, advance the entire inserter until the flange abuts the cervix and fundal resistance is met This places the device at the fundus
	Hold the insertion tube steady while completely removing the solid white rod	*Hold the entire inserter steady and move only the slider* completely in the most "downward" position to release the IUD	*Hold the entire inserter steady and move only the slider* completely in the most "downward" position to release the IUD and strings
	Take care not to pull on the threads and remove the clear insertion tube	Take care not to pull on the threads, and remove the inserter	Remove the inserter

Sivin I: Utility and drawbacks of continuous use of a copper T IUD for 20 years. Contraception. 2007;75(6 Suppl): S70–5. Epub 2007 Apr 16

ACOG Practice Bulletin No. 121: Long-acting reversible contraception: Implants and intrauterine devices. Obstet Gynecol. 2011;118(1):184–96

[a]The three IUDs compared in this chart are notably all T shaped. An Intrauterine Ball (IUB) has a promising new design that consists of copper spheres that are threaded over a flexible nitinol wire. When deployed through its 3.2 mm outer diameter insertion tube, the IUB claims to conform to a woman's uterine cavity in the form of a three-dimensional ball. An additional hormone eluting IUB of similar design is also being developed. Further trials and testing of the IUB's efficacy and safety will determine its place amongst IUDs. Baram I, Weinstein A, Trussell J. The IUB, a newly invented IUD: a brief report. Contraception. 2014;89(2):139–41

[b]Long-term reversible contraception: twelve years of experience with the TCu380A and TCu220C. Contraception. 1997;56(6):341–52

[c]Per Mirena and Paragard prescribing information package insert. *Note*: expulsion rates are higher when the uterus sounds to less than 6 cm but is not considered an absolute contraindication. Additionally, on the other end of the spectrum an IUD may also be inserted postpartum or post termination, or in enlarged uteri

[d]Mirena prescribing information package insert 2/2013

[e]Trussell J, Ellertson C. Efficacy of emergency contraception. Fertil Control Rev. 1995;4:8–11

A simple I&D is performed in the most gravity-dependent portion of the enlarged duct. Then, a thin plastic tubing thread through a long piece of free suture is introduced through a separate, more cephalad puncture site. The entire apparatus is threaded through the duct cavity and exits via the original I&D site. The tails of the free suture are then tied together and effectively form a closed "ring" of tubing. In a small prospective trial the Jacobi ring was well tolerated and appeared to have at least equal if not better results than the standard Word catheter technique [34]. The simplicity of the procedure and the concept of securing the fistulizing device with a closed ring to prevent premature expulsion is attractive but a larger, randomized prospective trial is needed to adequately assess its efficacy.

Both Word catheter and Jacobi ring removal at the follow-up visit is easily accomplished by either deflating the catheter or cutting the free suture and removing the apparatus from the ductal cavity. Only gloves and a syringe to decompress the catheter, or scissors to cut the ring suture are needed.

There are many advantages to this type of procedure. Mostly, it provides almost immediate symptomatic relief for the patient. It also allows for prophylactic therapeutic intervention. And finally, it is a quick, efficient office alternative to other invasive treatments such as marsupialization.

There are two main disadvantages to simple I&D and fistula formation. The first disadvantage is irritation and discomfort caused by the continued drainage and by the catheter or ring apparatus itself. The procedure also requires the patient to wear absorbant mini-pads for a prolonged period to allow epithelialization of the tract. Second, premature word catheter displacement prior to 4 weeks may occur and may not allow the tract to adequately form and thus, increases the risk of cystic recurrence. Similarly, overzealous re-approximation of the free suture ends of the Jacobi ring, can cause pressure necrosis that prevents adequate tract formation and hinders healing.

For Women over 40 Years of Age I&D and Biopsy

Although the incidence of Bartholin gland carcinoma is low [35], a firm or fixed vulvar mass in the Bartholin gland vicinity, should be biopsied and is suspicious for malignancy. Vulvar carcinoma typically presents as a painless vulvar mass. It is recommended that women with Paget's disease or those who are 40 years old or greater undergo this evaluation.

The Bartholin glands, also known as the greater vestibular glands, are usually 0.5 cm in size and lie 15 mm below the surface of the vestibule. To provide anatomic relationship reference points, at the 6 o'clock position, the rectum is 3–4 mm below the vagina and at the 12 o'clock position the urethra is 2–3 mm anterior to the vagina [36]. The duct is approximately 2 cm in length and empties into a groove between the hymen and the labia minorum [37].

Knowledge of the gland and duct anatomy is useful when performing the biopsy. Excisional biopsy provides histologic assessment with the additional benefit of decreased morbidity, decreased discomfort, and increased convenience of an in-office treatment for the patient. During the acute inflammatory stage, the difference between ductal and glandular tissue is difficult to distinguish. Prior to Word catheter placement, grasp the glandular tissue with a forceps and excise a small amount of tissue. If in doubt, measure the depth (it should be at least 1.5 cm) of the duct cavity, with a pre-measured sterile guide to ensure you are in the correct glandular vicinity prior to any excisional biopsy. Place the biopsy in a labeled surgical pathology container. Ensure hemostasis by either applying pressure, or if necessary, place a small hemostatic suture or sparingly apply silver nitrate. Then, place the word catheter as described above.

The main disadvantage to this procedure is that a secondary excisional procedure may be necessary and the patient may still be at risk for post-procedural complications.

Box 5.9: Bartholin Duct Procedure Checklist (Fig. 5.6)

Signed informed consent

Patient counseling on procedure, side effects, and post-procedure recovery instructions provided

Sterile draping

Sterile gloves

Antiseptic cleansing solution to prepare the procedure site and large applicator swabs

1 % lidocaine in a 5 cc syringe with 25 gauge needle

Microbiology culturette, nucleic acid amplification swabs

Sterile instruments:

Scalpel, number 11 or number 15 blade

Forceps

Hemostat

Word catheter with 3 cc saline syringe to inflate catheter

Sterile gauze

Sterile, nonpermanent, marking pen with measuring guide

± sterile scissors

± needle driver

± 2–0 delayed absorbable suture

Labeled, sterile pathology container

For marsupialization also include:

Pre-drawn sterile saline syringes for irrigation

± sterile angiocatheter tips

Box 5.10: Bartholin Cyst I&D with Word Catheter Placement (and Additional Biopsy) Step by Step

Test the Word catheter by inflating and deflating the bulb

Prepare the affected area with the cleansing solution

Identify a gravity-dependent area at or within the hymenal ring

Infiltrate this site with local anesthetic (Fig. 5.7)

Incise the cyst while preventing wall collapse with forceps

A small incision less than 1 cm is necessary for word catheter retention

Lyse loculations with a hemostat (Figs. 5.8 and 5.9)

Culture any effluent

(Excise a small portion of tissue and ensure hemostasis, see Fig. 5.10)

Place the Word catheter into the cystic duct as deep as possible, and inflate the catheter

The tail of the catheter may be tucked into the vagina to decrease discomfort

Assess the patient's post-procedure condition

Schedule 4-week follow-up visit

**Tip*—The overwhelming tendency is to create a larger than needed incision to facilitate spontaneous drainage of the duct.

In addition, the mechanical lysis of loculations may further enlarge the initial stab incision.

Therefore, always aim the initial point of entry *perpendicular* to the vertical vulvar plane and exceedingly limit the size.

Ensure the cavity is entered at least 1.5 cm deep (remember most ducts range from 2 to 2.5 cm in length prior to reaching the Bartholin gland)

If a hemostat is needed to break up septations, do not spread the hemostat tips until the depth of the ductal cavity has been reached or the dissatisfying result will be over dilation of the epidermal layer only.

Prior to incision, a sterile marking pen (that has pre-made measurements on the implement) can assist in two ways.

First, mark the point of entry and measure the incision by creating a *5 mm wide dot*. This dot will expand slightly with manipulation but should remain less than 1 cm.

Second, use the marking pen to measure cavity depth prior to lysing loculations or inserting the word catheter to ensure adequate duct access has been achieved.

These simple pre-procedure planning tips can avoid the frustrating scenario of an inexplicably expanded, bleeding incision and an unruly Word catheter that dislodges with each inflation attempt.

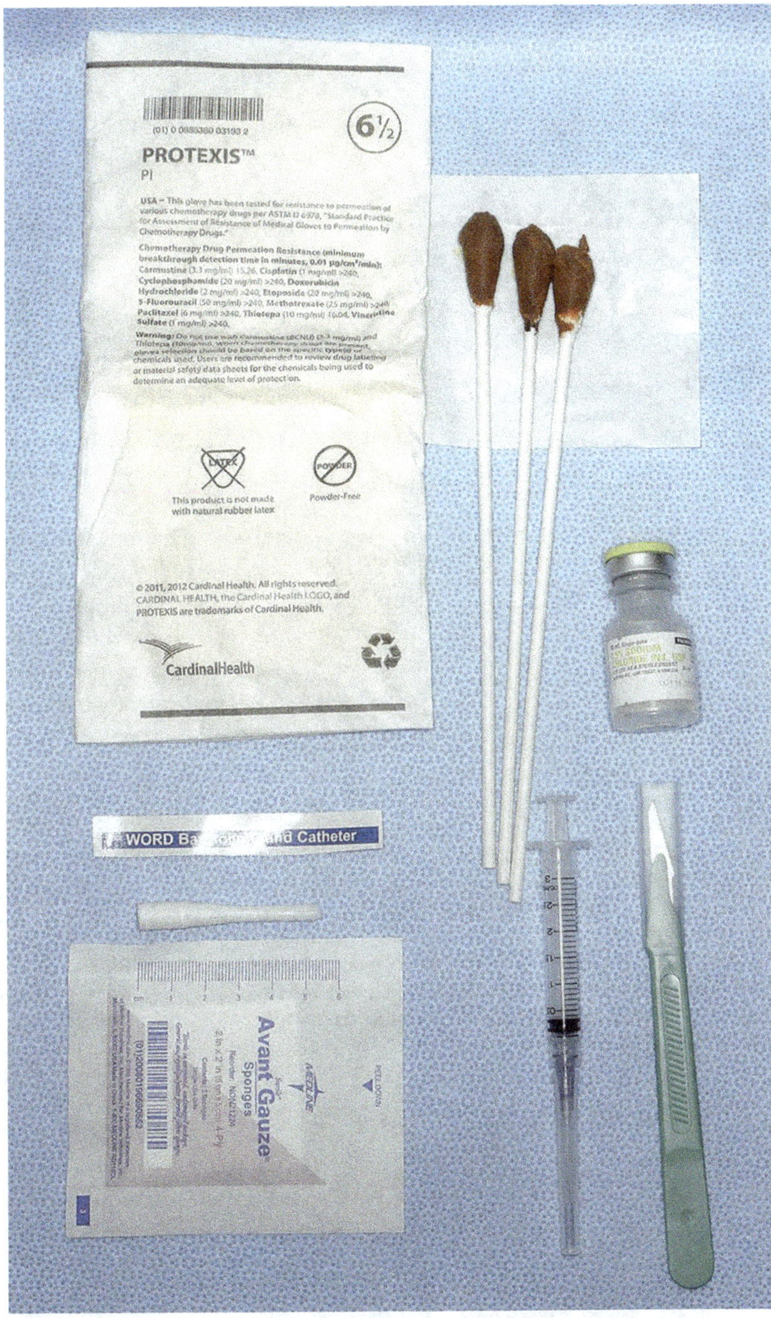

Fig. 5.6 Bartholin procedure supplies—cleansing solution, sterile instruments, local anesthetic, gauze, and word catheter

Marsupialization of the Bartholin Duct

This procedure is reserved for women who despite previous Word catheter placement, continue to suffer from recurrent, symptomatic Bartholin cysts or for women who refuse a catheter/ring placement. This procedure creates a new, larger and permanent egress to allow improved drainage from the duct. This fenestration is achieved by tacking the edges of the cystic duct "open" to the adjacent vulvo-vaginal epithelium. Marsupialization is usually performed once the acute inflammatory stage has resolved.

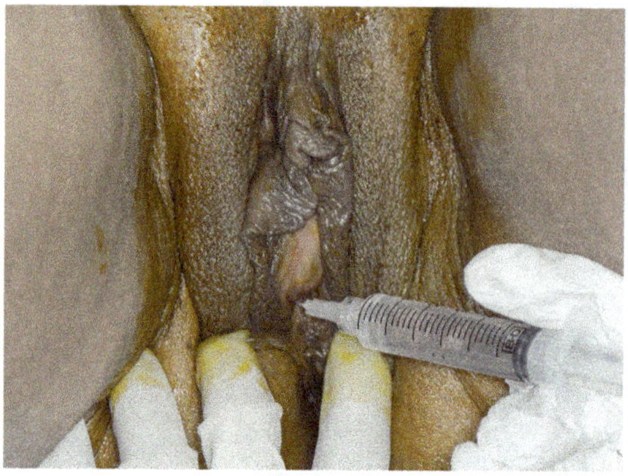

Fig. 5.7 Bartholin procedure—preparing the affected area and injecting local anesthetic

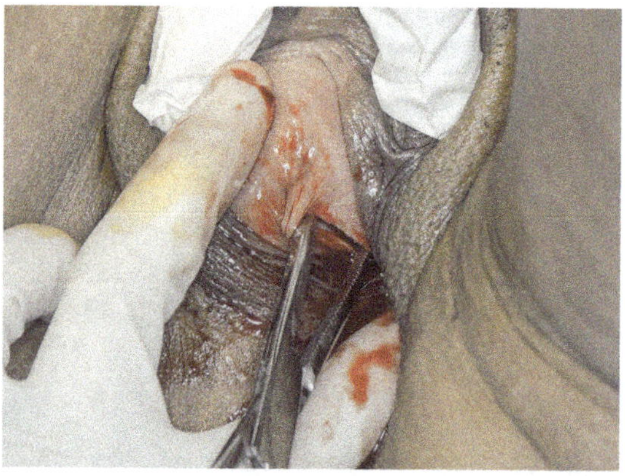

Fig. 5.8 Bartholin abscess—an incision is made and the abscess entered with immediate bloody effluent return. The cavity was cultured. Note, the smooth duct walls held open by the hemostat

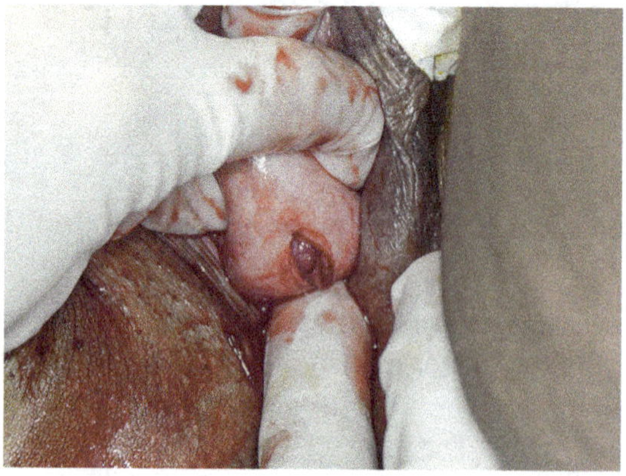

Fig. 5.9 Bartholin duct with debris—the duct was measured and confirmed to be approximately 2 cm in length. A large amount of debris and inspissated material was irrigated from the cavity

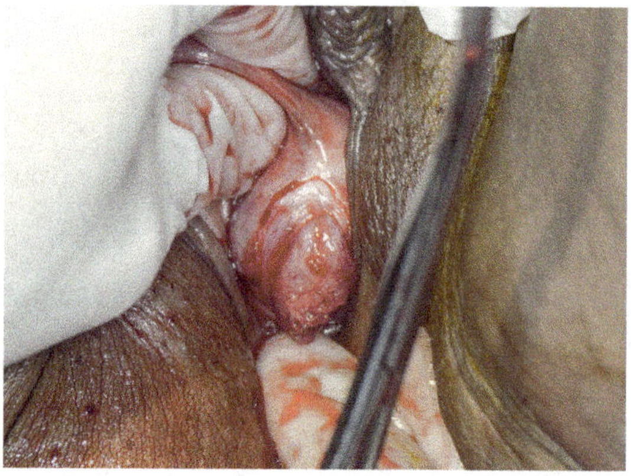

Fig. 5.10 Bartholin gland—after the cavity was irrigated the enlarged palpable gland was exposed and biopsied

The advantage of this procedure is that a larger orifice is created to allow the duct to drain without a catheter and it may have less post-procedure discomfort. The disadvantages are that it takes more time to perform, is more invasive to the patient, and may be associated with more post-procedure complications.

Box 5.11: Marsupialization of the Bartholin Cyst Step by Step

Prepare the affected area with the cleansing solution

Infiltrate this site with local anesthetic

Use the scalpel to incise a vertical, wedge-shaped ellipse of tissue overlying the center of the protrusion, just outside of the hymenal ring.

Lyse loculations with a hemostat

Culture any effluent

Evacuate the inspissated material

Irrigate the cavity with sterile saline

Identify the edges of the dilated ductal walls

Evert the duct lining and approximate the cavity wall to the vulvo-vaginal epithelium using interrupted sutures.

Assess the patient's post-procedure condition

Schedule 4-week follow-up visit and instruct the patient on post-procedure hygiene and sitz baths

(continued)

Box 5.11 (continued)

Tip—For large dilated ducts, a flexible, sterile angiocatheter attached to a saline syringe may be useful to irrigate and reach the depths of the cavity without overly enlarging the orifice.

Tip—Place sutures at least 5 mm away from the everted wall edge. The tissue can be friable and the success of the marsupialization lies in solidly affixing the glandular tissue to the adjacent epithelial tissue.

Tip—Meticulous and efficient suture placement dictates post-procedure discomfort. Secure sutures firmly but avoid tight knots that can cause tissue necrosis.

Additional Bartholin Treatments

Two other less commonly used treatments include silver nitrate ablation and carbon dioxide laser vaporization. Neither method creates a new permanent egress from the walled off duct.

Silver nitrate ablation involves simple I&D followed by placing 0.5 cm silver nitrate sticks into the duct cavity. Gauze dressing is then used to occlude the wound and the patient returns in 48 h for debridement of the cavity. Despite two studies that have shown promising results, this method has not been universally adopted [38, 39]. The disadvantages to this method include a close interval office follow-up and possible, additional painful side effects such as inadvertent chemical burn of adjacent tissue, ecchymosis, and labial edema. One prospective randomized trial of marsupialization versus silver nitrate application included 212 women and found similar recurrence rates but a statistically significant decrease in less scar formation with the silver nitrate group [40].

Carbon dioxide laser vaporization is another office alternative. The carbon dioxide laser is not a staple in most gynecology offices and the cost of procuring and maintaining equipment may be prohibitive but at least two different studies that included 219 women resulted in encouraging outcomes that once again offer a viable alternate treatment. Independently, Panici and Fambrini describe using the laser via a colposcope at 25 W continuous mode with a laser diameter between 0.5 and 1 mm, and power density ranging from 600 to 1,200 W/cm^2 to incise the enlarged duct. The duct is then irrigated and then vaporized with the laser [41].

In the larger study it was noted that a single laser treatment was curative for 95.7 % of the patients. Of note, three cases were complicated by bleeding and required diathermy and nine patients had recurrence that was later cured with additional laser treatment(s) [42]. The main advantage to this is similar to marsupialization: single visit treatment. Disadvantages again are the cost, training, and access to laser equipment.

Peri-procedural Complications

Like any vulvar procedure, complications from all of these procedures may include pain, infection, bleeding, hematoma, scarring, dyspareunia, and premature displacement of any fistula promoting device. In addition, up to 4–17 % of patients who undergo Word catheter or marsupialization procedure experience a recurrence [43]. This risk of recurrence is especially important when counseling patients.

Robust, prospective comparative trials of traditional I&D, catheter, and marsupialization techniques versus newer fistula methods, silver nitrate application, and laser vaporization are needed to better guide future office management of Bartholin pathology.

Conclusion

Necessity and innovation led to the most rudimentary office procedures. As we refine our understanding of human biology and improve our practice of medicine the boundary between the operating theater and the office procedure suite lessens. Despite changing times, one thing remains steadfast: the desire and ability to provide safe, effective, and efficient diagnostic therapies and treatments to our patients. Who knows what form the next generation of IUDs will embody. Or, if painless endometrial sampling and singular Bartholin abscess treatment can become a new gold standard. Either way, with advanced technologies and the need for expedited recoveries our quest to improve even the most basic of office gynecologic procedures will, and should, improve the lives of our patients.

References

1. Margulies L. History of intrauterine devices. Bull N Y Acad Med. 1975;51(5):662–7.
2. Ishihama A. Clinical studies on intrauterine contraception, especially the present state of contraception in Japan and the experience in the use of intrauterine rings. Yokohama Med J. 1959;10:89.
3. American College of Obstetricians and Gynecologists. ACOG Committee opinion no. 539: adolescents and long-acting reversible contraception: implants and intrauterine devices. Obstet Gynecol. 2012;120(4):983–8.
4. The WHO states that the WHO MEC are, "Intended to be used by policy-makers, programme managers, and the scientific community, to support national programmes in the preparation of service delivery guideline." The United States Medical Eligibility Criteria for contraceptive use (USMEC) is a formal adaption of the WHO MEC and also has a companion document, U.S. Selected Practice Recommendations for Contraceptive Use, (US SPR), intended for health care providers.
5. Nelson AL. Contraindications to IUD and IUS use. Contraception. 2007;75(6 Suppl):S76–81. Epub 2007 Mar 2.
6. Nelson AL, Fong JK. Intrauterine infusion of lidocaine does not reduce pain scores during IUD insertion. Contraception. 2013;88(1):37–40.
7. Karabayirli S, Ayrim AA, Muslu B. Comparison of the analgesic effects of oral tramadol and naproxen sodium on pain relief during IUD insertion. J Minim Invasive Gynecol. 2012;19(5):581–4.
8. Allen RH, Bartz D, Grimes DA, Hubacher D, O'Brien P. Interventions for pain with intrauterine device insertion. Cochrane Database Syst Rev. 2009;(3): CD007373.
9. Chudnoff S, Einstein M, Levie M. Paracervical block efficacy in office hysteroscopic sterilization: a randomized controlled trial. Obstet Gynecol. 2010;115:26.
10. Mody SK, Kiley J, Rademaker A, et al. Pain control for intrauterine device insertion: a randomized trial of 1% lidocaine paracervical block. Contraception. 2012;86:704.
11. Lathrop E, Haddad L, McWhorter CP, Goedken P. Self-administration of misoprostol prior to intrauterine device insertion among nulliparous women: a randomized controlled trial. Contraception. 2013;88 (6):725–9.
12. Espey E, Singh RH, Leeman L, Ogburn T, Fowler K, Greene H. Misoprostol for intrauterine device insertion in nulliparous women: a randomized controlled trial. Am J Obstet Gynecol. 2014;210(3):208e.1–5. pii: S0002-9378(13)02017-6.
13. Ibrahim ZM, Sayed Ahmed WA. Sublingual misoprostol prior to insertion of a T380A intrauterine device in women with no previous vaginal delivery. Eur J Contracept Reprod Health Care. 2013;18 (4):300–8.
14. Scavuzzi A, Souza AS, Costa AA, Amorim MM. Misoprostol prior to inserting an intrauterine device in nulligravidas: a randomized clinical trial. Hum Reprod. 2013;28(8):2118–25.
15. Centers for disease control and prevention, morbidity and mortality weekly report, vol. 62, June 14, 2013. U. S. Selected Practice Recommendations for Contraceptive Use, 2013. Adapted from the World Health Organization Selected Practice Recommendations for Contraceptive Use, 2nd ed.
16. American College of Obstetricians and Gynecologists. ACOG practice bulletin no. 121: long-acting reversible contraception: implants and intrauterine devices. Obstet Gynecol. 2011;118:184.
17. Farley TM, Rosenberg MJ, Rowe PJ, et al. Intrauterine devices and pelvic inflammatory disease: an international perspective. Lancet. 1992;339:785.
18. Sufrin CB, Postlethwaite D, Armstrong MA, et al. Neisseria gonorrhea and Chlamydia trachomatis screening at intrauterine device insertion and pelvic inflammatory disease. Obstet Gynecol. 2012;120:1314.
19. Grimes DA. Intrauterine devices (IUDs). In: Hatcher RA, Trussell J, Nelson AL, et al., editors. Contraceptive technology. New York: Ardent Media; 2007. p. 117–43.
20. Grimes DA, Lopez LM, Schulz KF. Antibiotic prophylaxis for intrauterine contraceptive device insertion. Cochrane Database Syst Rev. 2012.
21. White MK, Ory HW, Rooks JB, Rochat RW. Intrauterine device termination rates and the menstrual cycle day of insertion. Obstet Gynecol. 1980;55:220.
22. Bednarek PH, Creinin MD, Reeves MF, Cwiak C, Espey E, Jensen JT, Post-Aspiration IUD Randomization (PAIR) Study Trial Group. Immediate versus delayed IUD insertion after uterine aspiration. N Engl J Med. 2011;364(23):2208–17.
23. Bahamondes L, Diaz J, Marchi NM, Petta CA, Cristofoletti ML, Gomez G. Performance of copper intrauterine devices when inserted after an expulsion. Hum Reprod. 1995;10(11):2917–8.

24. Pakarinen P, Luukkainen T. Five years' experience with a small intracervical/intrauterine levonorgestrel-releasing device. Contraception. 2005;72(5):342–5.
25. Inal MM, Ertopçu K, Ozelmas I. The evaluation of 318 intrauterine pregnancy cases with an intrauterine device. Eur J Contracept Reprod Health Care. 2005;10 (4):266–71.
26. Jimenez-Ayala M, Jimenez-Ayala Portillo B. Endometrial adenocarcinoma: prevention and early diagnosis. Basel: Karger Medical and Scientific; 2008. p. 22–4.
27. Guido RS, Kanbour-Shakir A, Rulin MC, Christopherson WA. Pipelle endometrial sampling. Sensitivity in the detection of endometrial cancer. J Reprod Med. 1995;40:553–5.
28. Clark TJ, Mann CH, Shah N, Khan KS, Song F, Gupta JK. Accuracy of outpatient endometrial biopsy in the diagnosis of endometrial cancer: a systematic quantitative review. BJOG. 2002;109:313–21.
29. Droegemueller W, Katz V. Diagnostic procedures. In: Stenchever M, Droegemueller W, Herbst A, Mishell D, editors. Comprehensive gynecology. St. Louis: Mosby; 2001. p. 232–3.
30. Marzano DA, Haefner HK. The bartholin gland cyst: past, present, and future. J Low Genit Tract Dis. 2004;8:195.
31. Visco AG, Del Priore G. Postmenopausal bartholin gland enlargement: a hospital-based cancer risk assessment. Obstet Gynecol. 1996;87:286.
32. Stevens DL, Bisno AL, Chambers HF, et al. Practice guidelines for the diagnosis and management of skin and soft-tissue infections. Clin Infect Dis. 2005;41:1373.
33. Kushnir VA, Mosquera C. Novel technique for management of Bartholin gland cysts and abscesses. J Emerg Med. 2009;36(4):388–90.
34. Gennis P, Li SF, Provataris J, Shahabuddin S, Schachtel A, Lee E, Bobby P. Jacobi ring catheter treatment of Bartholin's abscesses. Am J Emerg Med. 2005;23(3):414–5.
35. "Based on local New York State Department of Health census data, the incidence of Bartholin gland carcinoma was 0.023 per 100,000 woman-years in premenopausal women and 0.114 per 100,000 woman-years in postmenopausal women (incidence rate ratio 5.01, 95% confidence interval [CI] 0.67-25.1). The overall incidence rate of squamous cell vulvar carcinoma was 0.42 per 100,000 woman-years in premenopausal and 4.72 per 100,000 woman-years in postmenopausal women (odds ratio [OR] 11.55, 95% CI 7.82-17.14)" from Visco AG, Del Priore G. Postmenopausal bartholin gland enlargement: a hospital-based cancer risk assessment. Obstet Gynecol 1996;87:286.
36. Baggish M, Karram M. Anatomy of the vagina in Atlas of pelvic anatomy and gynecologic surgery. Philadelphia: Saunders; 2006. p. 529.
37. Droegmemueller W. Infections of the lower genital tract. In: Stenchever M, Droegemueller W, Herbst A, Mishell D, editors. Comprehensive gynecology. St Louis: Mosby; 2001. p. 233.
38. Yüce K, Zeyneloglu HB, Bükülmez O, Kisnisci HA. Outpatient management of Bartholin gland abscesses and cysts with silver nitrate. Aust N Z J Obstet Gynaecol. 1994;34:93.
39. Mungan T, Uğur M, Yalçin H, et al. Treatment of Bartholin's cyst and abscess: excision versus silver nitrate insertion. Eur J Obstet Gynecol Reprod Biol. 1995;63:61.
40. Ozdegirmenci O, Kayikcioglu F, Haberal A. Prospective randomized study of marsupialization versus silver nitrate application in the management of Bartholin gland cysts and abscesses. J Minim Invasive Gynecol. 2009;16:149.
41. Panici P, Manci N, Bellati F, et al. CO2 laser therapy of the Bartholin's gland cyst: surgical data and functional short- and long-term results. J Minim Invasive Gynecol. 2007;14:348.
42. Fambrini M, Penna C, Pieralli A, et al. Carbon-dioxide laser vaporization of the Bartholin gland cyst: a retrospective analysis on 200 cases. J Minim Invasive Gynecol. 2008;15:327.
43. Wechter ME, Wu JM, Marzano D, et al. Management of Bartholin duct cysts and abscesses: a systematic review. Obstet Gynecol Surv. 2009;64(6):395–404.

Saline Infusion Sonohysterography

6

Jamie Stanhiser and Rebecca Flyckt

Introduction

Saline infusion sonohysterography (SIS) is a procedure in which sterile saline is infused transcervically into the uterus to improve visualization of the endometrium during endovaginal ultrasonography [1]. This procedure augments the clinician's ability to detect endometrial pathology including hyperplasia, polyps, leiomyomata, adhesions, and even cancer [2]. It is easily and quickly performed in the office with minimal cost, has very few complications, and is well tolerated by patients [3]. SIS is therefore an excellent screening technique to triage patients with suspected endometrial pathology, and it can often avert more invasive diagnostic procedures when used appropriately [4].

History and Background

Transvaginal ultrasonography (TVUS) is an essential tool of the gynecologist to evaluate the pelvic cavity with high accuracy. However, the uterine cavity and the endometrial lining are often not clearly delineated using conventional TVUS. In cases where endometrial sonographic images are not clear, infusing saline through a transcervical catheter to expand the uterine cavity creates visual contrast and thereby enhances the clinician's ability to distinguish and diagnose uterine pathology. The term "sonohysterography" was coined by Parsons et al. [1]; however, the technique was described a decade prior following clearer observations of intrauterine pathology in postmenopausal women with cervical stenosis and fluid-filled cavities [5]. It has also been referred to as saline ultrasonography or SIS. Images of a normal uterine cavity during SIS are shown in Fig. 6.1. Soon after its implementation, SIS became not only a tool to enhance transvaginal ultrasound, but an attractive alternative to more invasive procedures that can be used to evaluate the uterine cavity, specifically hysterosalpingography (HSG) and hysteroscopy [6].

Supporting Data

When compared to traditional two-dimensional (2D) transvaginal sonography, SIS has been found in numerous studies to be superior in the detection of endometrial abnormalities. For example, a prospective study comparing the accuracy of TVUS and SIS in pre and postmenopausal women with abnormal uterine bleeding reported that the sensitivity and specificity of

J. Stanhiser, M.D.
Department of Obstetrics and Gynecology, Cleveland Clinic Foundation, 9500 Euclid Avenue, Desk A81, Cleveland, OH 44195, USA
e-mail: jamiestanhiser@gmail.com

R. Flyckt, M.D. (✉)
Department of Obstetrics and Gynecology & Women's Health Institute, Cleveland Clinic, 8500 Euclid Avenue, A81, Cleveland, OH 44195, USA
e-mail: flycktr@ccf.org

J.D. Emery and M.F.R. Paraiso (eds.), *Office-Based Gynecologic Surgical Procedures*, DOI 10.1007/978-1-4939-1414-2_6,

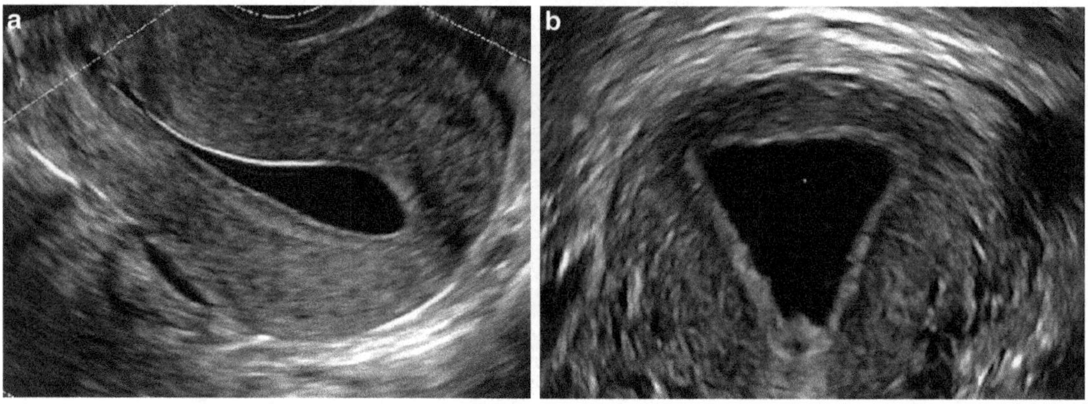

Fig. 6.1 Normal saline infusion sonohysterography (SIS). (**a**) Sagittal view. (**b**) 3D rendering

SIS for the detection of endometrial pathologies were significantly higher than that of transvaginal ultrasound (98 % and 93 %, respectively, for SIS versus 83 % and 71 % for TVUS) [7]. SIS is particularly useful in diagnosing focal endometrial abnormalities and intracavitary masses such as endometrial polyps and fibroids. In the above mentioned study, the sensitivity and specificity of SIS in the detection of endometrial polyps were 100 % and 92 %, and in the case of fibroids were 95 % and 100 %, respectively. Another prospective study of a similar patient population compared the detection of polyps and fibroids using these two techniques. This study found that the sensitivity and specificity of SIS for polyps were significantly higher than TVUS (91 and 93 % for SIS versus 65 and 88 % for TVUS) [8]. The sensitivity and specificity for the detection of fibroids between the two techniques were similar in this study (92 % and 99 % for SIS versus 96 % and 95 % for TVUS), although other studies have demonstrated a small advantage of SIS over TVUS for the detection of myomas [6, 9]. The clear visual advantage of SIS for the detection of polyps and fibroids can be seen in Figs. 6.2, 6.3, and 6.4. Figure 6.2 illustrates the typical appearance of a polyp during SIS, while Figs. 6.3 and 6.4 demonstrate leiomyomas. Numerous studies confirm that SIS improves the diagnostic utility of standard 2D transvaginal sonography [2, 6–8, 10].

It has been suggested that SIS may also serve as an alternative to HSG. HSG is often used to simultaneously evaluate the uterus and fallopian tubes. HSG is superior to SIS in the detection of tubal abnormalities, as nonpathologic fallopian tubes are not visualized ultrasonographically. While SIS can reliably identify tubal spill, all that can be concluded from the finding of free fluid on endovaginal ultrasound after SIS is that at least one of the fallopian tubes is patent. Recent adaptations to improve tubal evaluation during ultrasound include the instillation of either air bubbles or echogenic contrast media rather than saline (hysterosalpingo-contrast sonography [HyCoSy]) [11]. Although HSG remains the gold standard for evaluation of tubal pathology, SIS has higher accuracy than HSG in the detection of uterine anomalies, in particular septate and bicornuate uteri (100 % versus 81 % for HSG) [12]. The ability to assess fundal contour in the evaluation of uterine anomalies is a valuable addition provided by sonography as compared to HSG, especially when combined with 3D ultrasound images. SIS is also superior to HSG in the diagnosis of polyps and endometrial hyperplasia [13]. Both HSG and SIS have limited accuracy in diagnosing intrauterine adhesions, with high false positive rates from blood clots, shearing of normal endometrium, and mucus plugs [14]. Such uterine synechiae as visualized on SIS in a patient with Asherman's Syndrome are shown in Fig. 6.5.

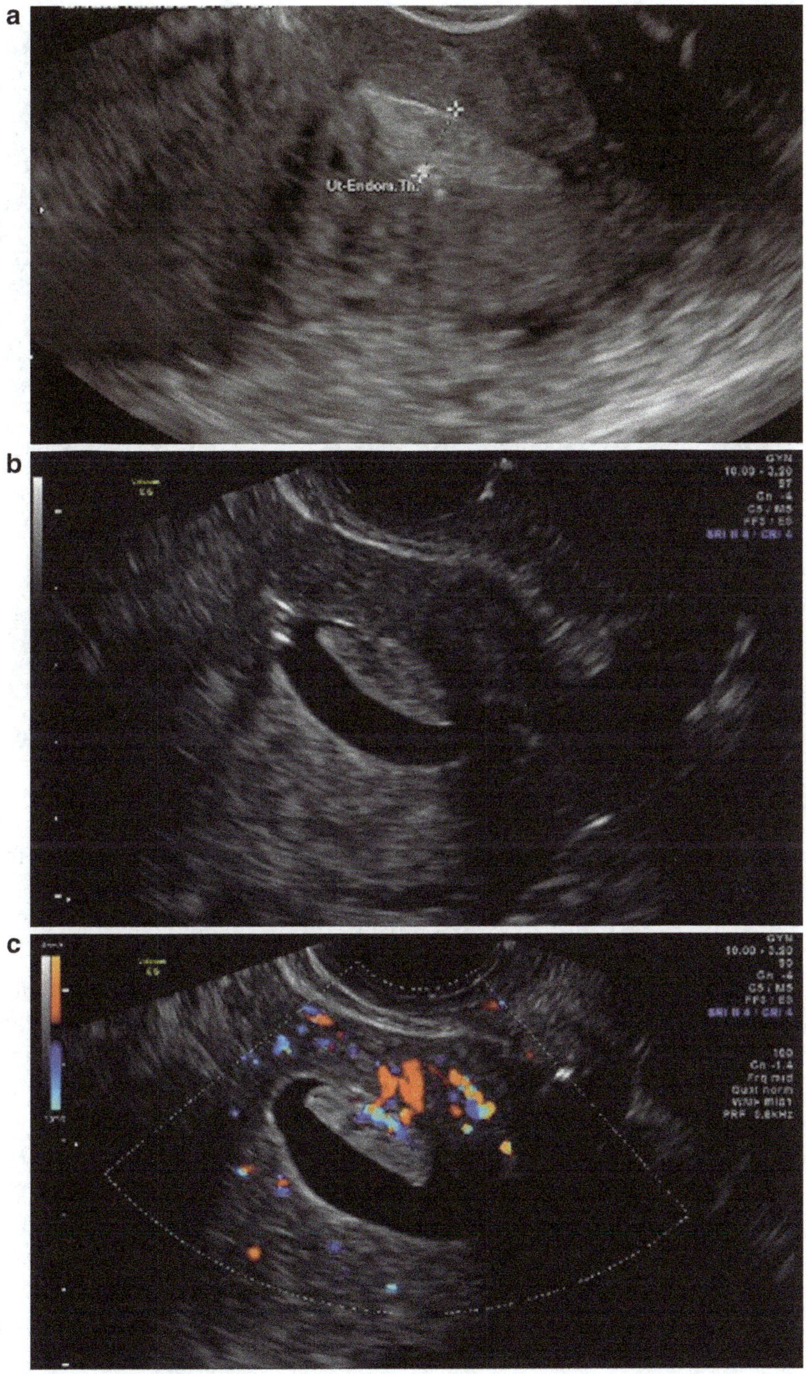

Fig. 6.2 Polyp in a perimenopausal woman with menorrhagia. (**a**) Standard 2D transvaginal imaging shows a thickened endometrial stripe. (**b**) SIS shows a 2 × 2 cm lesion of the anterior endometrium. (**c**) Color Doppler imaging shows flow within the lesion that is typical of a polyp. (**d**) 3D imaging of the endometrial cavity demonstrate two polyps on transverse view that were not apparent on original longitudinal view

Some authors have reported additional advantages of SIS which make it an appealing choice over HSG, including decreased patient discomfort, less expense, the absence of radiation exposure, and its availability in an office setting [12, 13].

Diagnostic hysteroscopy with endometrial biopsy is the gold standard to evaluate uterine

d

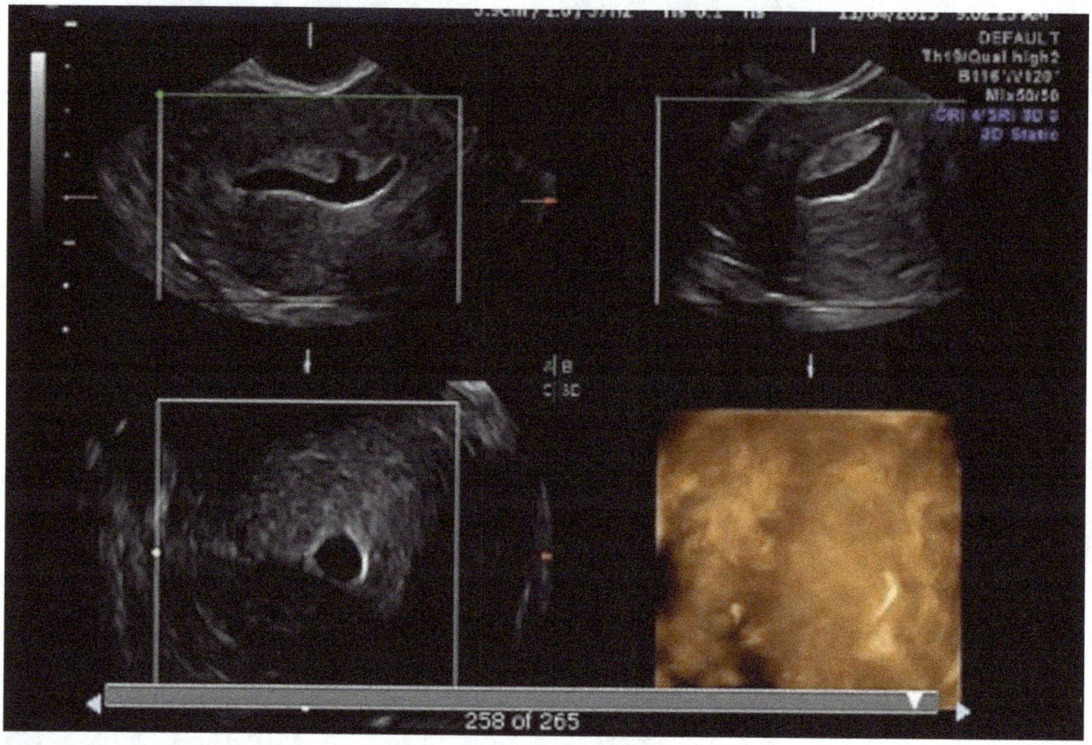

Fig. 6.2 (continued)

cavity abnormalities [6]. However, office hysteroscopy is expensive, invasive, and causes more discomfort to the patient than SIS [15, 16]. Additionally, hysteroscopy cannot visualize the myometrium and therefore cannot classify the depth of myometrial invasion of leiomyomas or carcinoma as SIS can [17]. In direct comparisons, the diagnostic accuracy for polyps, endometrial hyperplasia, and submucosal myomas with SIS has been found to be equivalent to hysteroscopy [6]. Several studies have reported that in patients with abnormalities on transvaginal ultrasound, SIS use, first-line was preferable to proceeding directly to hysteroscopy, as the latter could be avoided in 72–88 % of patients who could then be managed conservatively [4, 17, 18]. More support for this triaging method is reported in a study on cost-effectiveness which indicates that SIS as an initial screening procedure is superior to first-line diagnostic hysteroscopy [19]. Another set of authors stated that diagnostic hysteroscopy should be reserved for situations where SIS is either inconclusive or not feasible [20].

In conclusion, SIS is a safe, simple, inexpensive procedure with few side effects. It is well tolerated by patients, and it can easily be performed in the office setting [21] without the need for an operating room, extra personnel, anesthesia, or exposure to radiation. Distention of the uterine cavity with saline clearly improves upon traditional 2D transvaginal sonographic imaging of the uterine cavity, endowing SIS with greater sensitivity and specificity for the detection of endometrial pathologies. SIS is superior to HSG for the detection of uterine anomalies, and new adaptions may help SIS to overcome its longstanding inferiority to HSG in tubal evaluation. SIS is less invasive than hysteroscopy, and is cost-effective as a screening test prior to more invasive methods in investigating patients with abnormal or inconclusive transvaginal sonographic results [3, 8, 22].

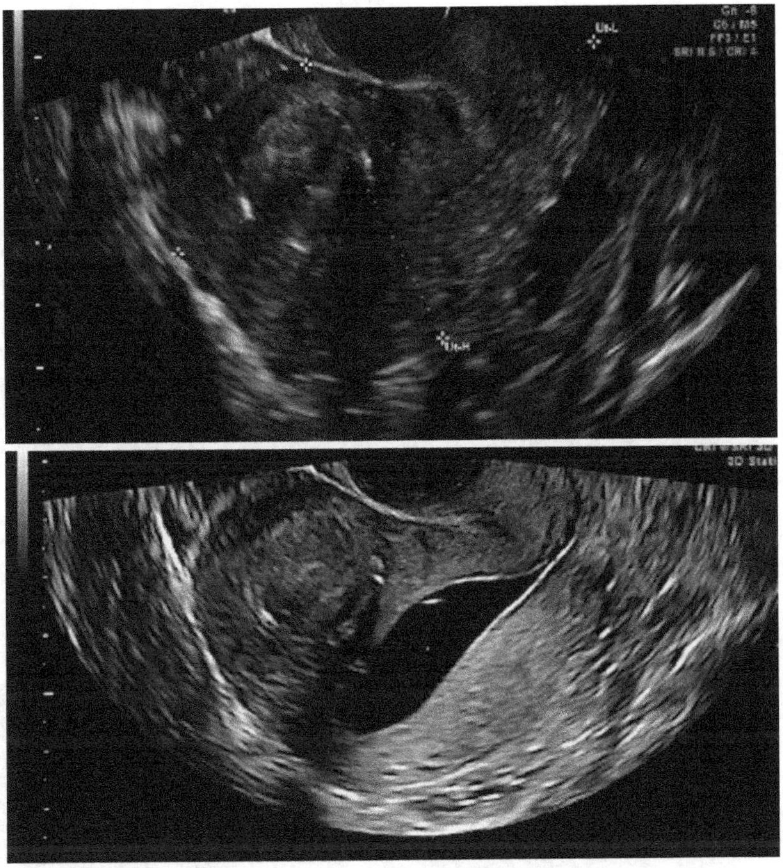

Fig. 6.3 Fibroid in a 38-year-old woman with infertility. (**a**) Gray scale images demonstrate a fibroid of the anterior uterus. (**b**) Instillation of saline demonstrates that the fibroid is intramural without distortion of the endometrial cavity. This fibroid is unlikely to interfere with implantation or pregnancy

Indications and Contraindications

SIS is indicated when the etiology of a woman's symptoms is suspected to arise from an abnormality of her endometrium or uterine cavity, and it can be useful in other situations when transvaginal ultrasound is inadequate [23, 24]. Specifically, indications for SIS include, but are not limited to, evaluation of the following:

- Abnormal uterine bleeding
- Infertility
- Recurrent pregnancy loss
- Congenital abnormalities of the uterus
- Evaluation of uterine cavity polyps, myomas, and synechiae
- Abnormalities on transvaginal ultrasound, including focal or diffuse endometrial or intracavitary abnormalities

Absolute contraindications to SIS include pregnancy, pelvic infection, and unexplained pelvic tenderness [23, 24]. SIS can be performed during menses as active bleeding is not a contraindication. However, heavy menstrual bleeding may make interpretation of the study more difficult, as blood clots are known to cause false positive examinations [23].

Although not a contraindication, a concern exists regarding sonohysterography for the patient in whom there is high suspicion of endometrial carcinoma. In this situation, there is the potential risk of disseminating malignant cells into the pelvic cavity via transtubal spill of saline. Two prospective studies performed in women with endometrial cancer found malignant or suspicious cells from SIS in 25 % of cases [25, 26]. During surgical staging for endometrial cancers, the presence of malignant cells in

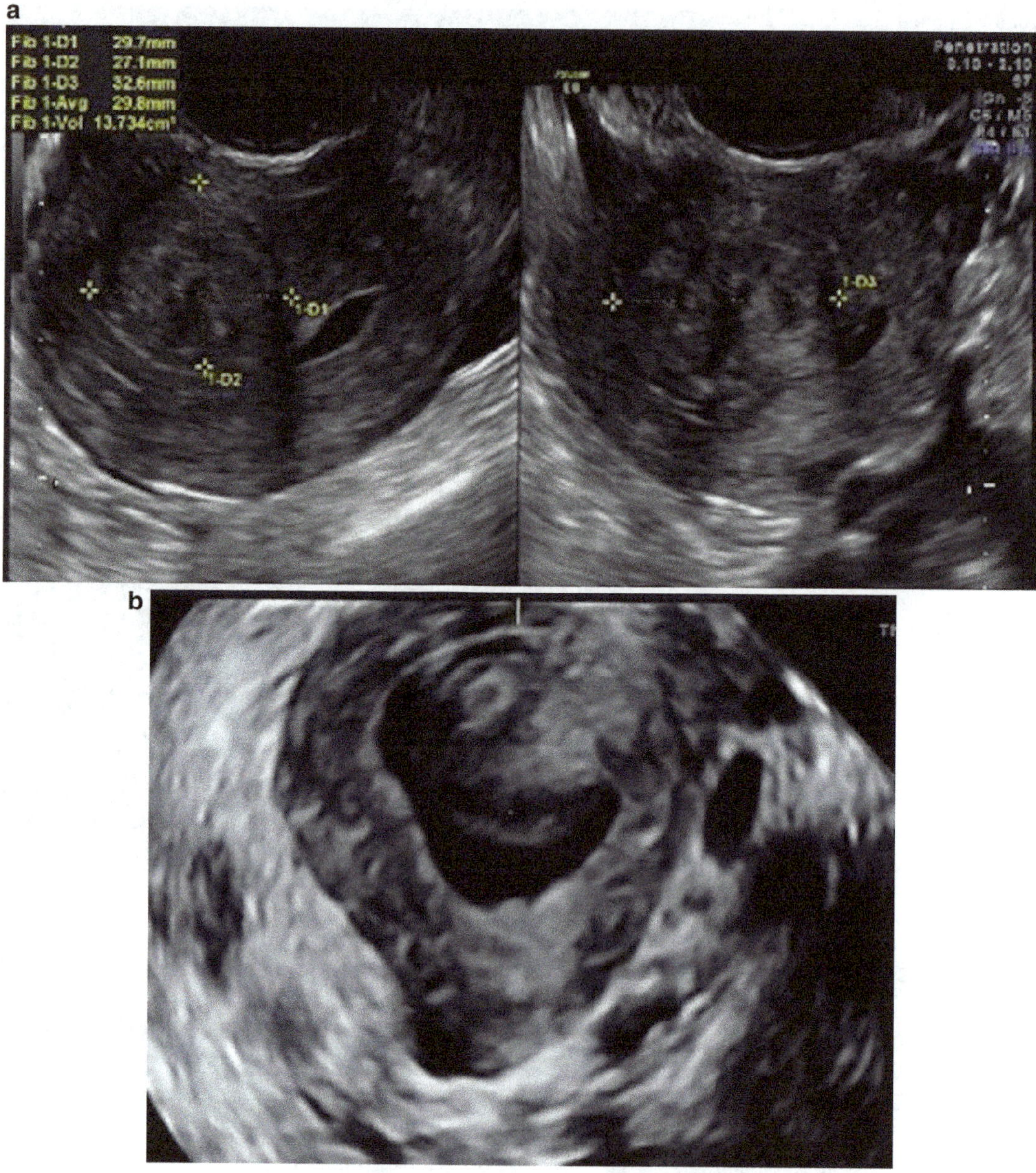

Fig. 6.4 Fibroid in a 34-year-old woman with dysmenorrhea and menorrhagia. (**a**) Gray scale images of 3 cm anterior myoma. (**b**) Saline sonohysterography reveals an intracavitary myoma. This fibroid was removed hysteroscopically with complete resolution of symptoms

peritoneal washings significantly increases the stage of disease. Both of the aforementioned studies concluded that SIS should not be performed in this population of women due to the risk of malignant cell dissemination. However, other studies have found the risk of cancer cell dissemination during this procedure to be smaller, with positive cancer cells after transtubal spill in only 2–12.5 % of patients [27, 28]. These studies concluded that SIS has a low probability of cancer cell dissemination. In addition, it is unclear whether positive peritoneal washings due to SIS have the same prognostic value as typical positive peritoneal cytology

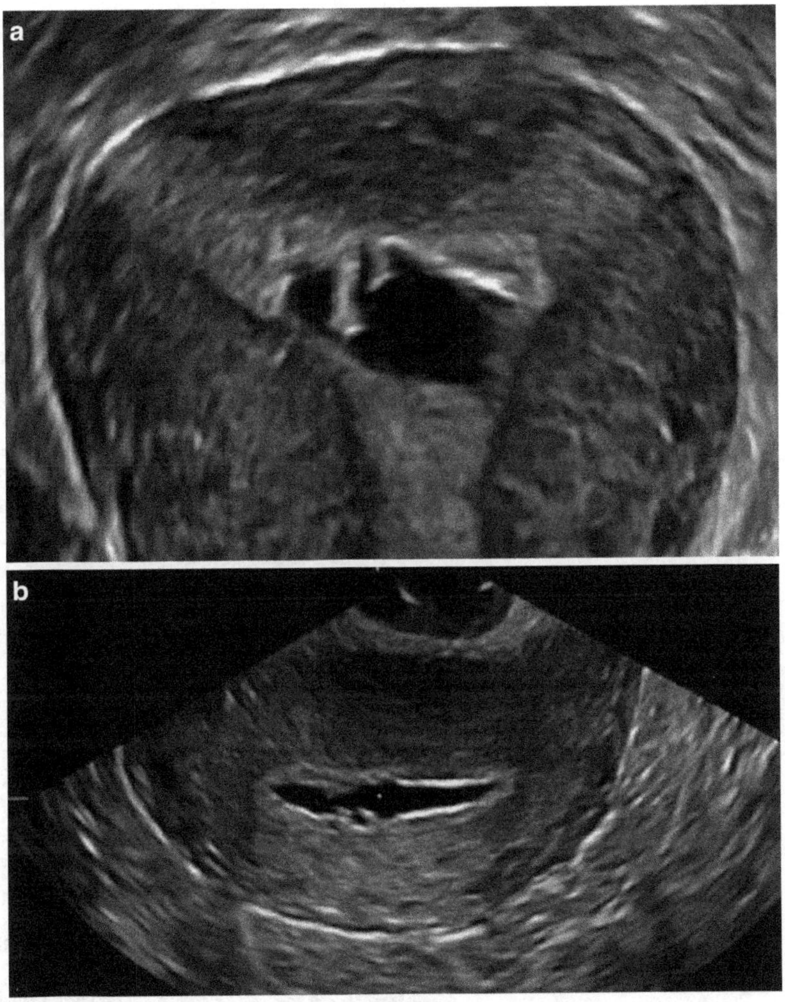

Fig. 6.5 Asherman's Syndrome in a patient with multiple intrauterine procedures. (**a**) Saline sonohysterography shows echogenic foci within the endometrium. (**b**) 3D SIS demonstrates intrauterine adhesions at the right cornual region of the uterus

encountered in endometrial cancer staging. We encourage the clinician to consider this area of controversy prior to performing SIS in populations of women at high risk for endometrial cancer, such as in women with postmenopausal bleeding. Figure 6.6 illustrates a thickened endometrium found during SIS in just such a patient with postmenopausal bleeding.

Equipment

One of the advantages of SIS is the minimal amount of equipment needed. Although many types of transcervical catheters have been proposed of various complexities, all can be effective in experienced hands [29]. The cost for specialized catheters can vary, with the most expensive approaching $100. However, even a pediatric Foley catheter, the least costly option, can be used to instill fluid into the endometrium and provide good quality images if needed. The major difference between catheters is the presence or absence of an intrauterine balloon; when inflated and positioned at or in the cervix, the balloon can prevent loss of distending fluid from the uterus. In some cases, such as the multiparous cervix, the balloon is especially useful; however, it should be noted that most studies also associate balloon use with increased discomfort during the procedure [29, 30]. Beyond the transcervical catheter, a 20–30 mL syringe with sterile saline

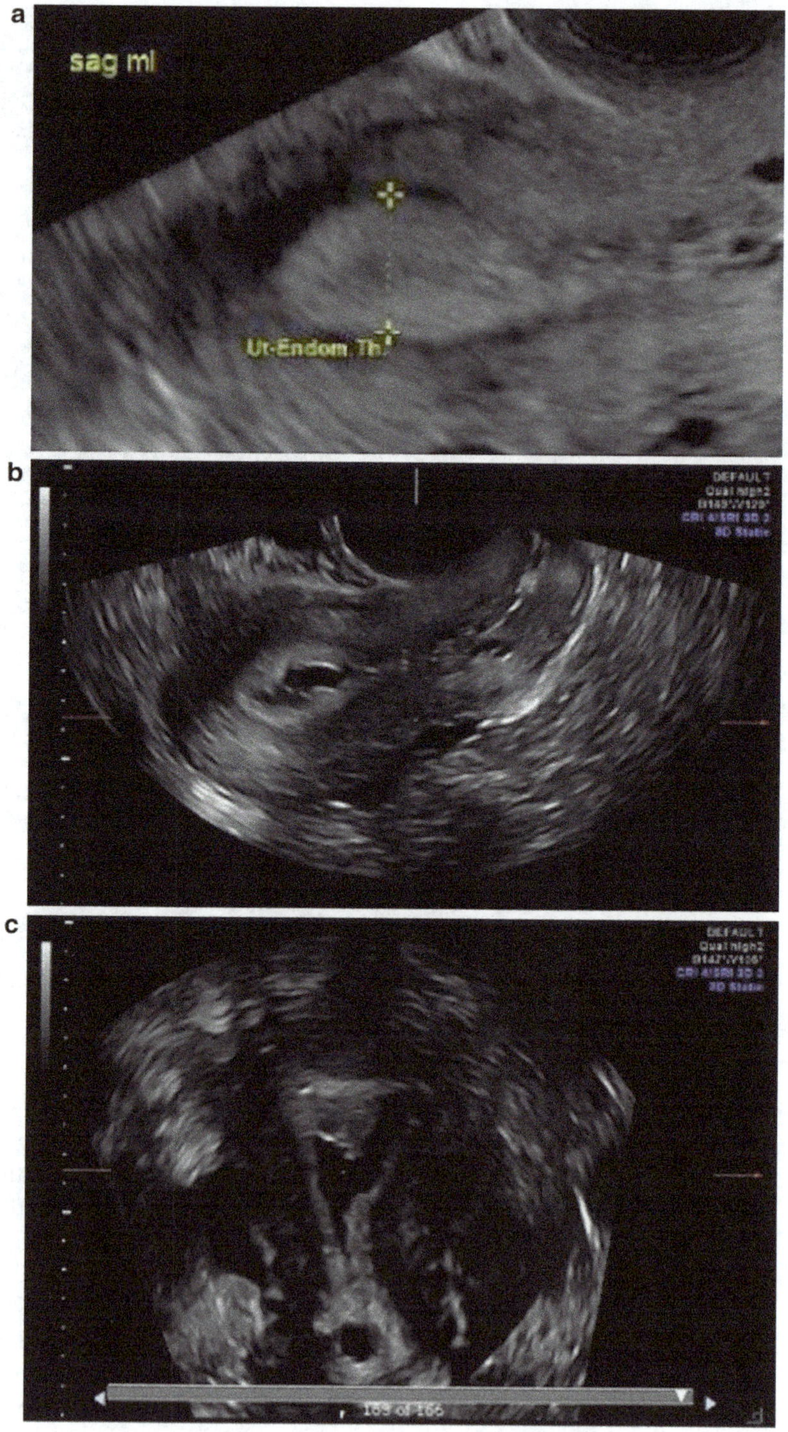

Fig. 6.6 Thickened endometrium in a patient with postmenopausal bleeding. (**a**, **b**) 2D images with and without saline demonstrate areas of irregular endometrial thickening. (**c**) 3D SIS shows with a focal area of thickening in the right fundus. The lesion was removed hysteroscopically and pathology confirmed a benign intrauterine polyp

or sterile water, a speculum and light source as well as a ring forceps or uterine forceps to assist in placement of the catheter are all necessary. Lastly, a high frequency transvaginal US probe and high resolution ultrasound machine are required to perform SIS. A cervical dilator probe and/or a single tooth tenaculum may be used in cases where passage of the catheter is difficult.

Three-dimensional (3D) sonohysterography is a useful tool to increase the sensitivity for intrauterine lesions [31] and assist in more fully evaluating Mullerian anomalies. 3D SIS does require special training other than having an ultrasound machine with 3D capabilities.

When making a distinction between anomalies (e.g., septate versus bicornuate uterus), the assessment of fundal contour with 3D imaging is invaluable and clearly superior to HSG images. Another helpful feature of modern ultrasonography is the cine loop or volume imaging, which allows rapid acquisition of images that can be manipulated or reviewed in different planes after the exam is complete. This property is beneficial when the cavity can only be distended for a minimum amount of time due to rapid fluid leakage from the cervix or in rare cases of patient discomfort.

Patient Preparation and Selection

Optimal timing of the procedure in reproductive aged women is during the first half of the menstrual cycle, after menstrual bleeding has stopped but before ovulation has occurred. For most women, this corresponds to cycle days 5–10. Performing the study during the follicular phase after cessation of normal menses helps ensure that a viable embryo is not flushed out with saline instillation. In women with irregular menstrual cycles, reliable contraception and/or a negative pregnancy test may be required before undergoing SIS. Additionally, timing the study after menses is complete ensures that bleeding and clots are not misconstrued as intrauterine pathology. In menopausal women, SIS can be scheduled at any time.

Patients should be advised that some cramping may occur during the procedure and pretreatment with nonsteroidal anti-inflammatories (NSAIDs) 30–60 min prior to SIS may help to lessen this discomfort. Patients should also be counseled that the cervix is cleaned with betadine or other appropriate antiseptic solution to decrease the small risk of pelvic infection associated with SIS [32]. In addition, routine transvaginal ultrasound should be performed prior to instillation of saline so that hydrosalpinx may be identified and antibiotic treatment considered. The complete series of steps required to perform SIS are listed in Table 6.1.

Helpful Tips

Although most SIS procedures are easily completed, the two most common technical issues relate to difficulties with transcervical catheter placement and acquisition of optimal images. A few simple strategies can help to overcome these obstacles while performing the SIS exam.

When placing the transcervical catheter, remember that the path from cervix to uterus is rarely straight; with patience and gentle repositioning, the catheter will often find its course. Careful placement of the speculum to orient the cervix to midposition can also straighten the cervix and uterus and facilitate easier passage of the catheter. Therefore, knowing whether the uterus is anteverted or retroverted before beginning the procedure can be helpful. For a mobile cervix, either a long cotton swab or a catheter guide can be used to stabilize the cervix while inserting the catheter. As a last resort, a single-toothed tenaculum (with or without cervical lidocaine injection) can be placed at the 12- or 6-o'clock position to provide traction against which the catheter can be gently introduced. For a stenotic cervix, pretreatment with misoprostol or gentle use of cervical dilators during the procedure can be beneficial. On the other hand, for a patulous cervix, use of a balloon type catheter is often required and the balloon

Table 6.1 Steps for SIS

Steps of procedure	Notes
1. Obtain consent and perform appropriate time out procedure as indicated	Risks of bleeding, discomfort, and infection should be discussed
2. Position patient in semi-upright dorsal lithotomy	Ensure buttocks are slightly beyond end of examination table
3. Perform Bimanual examination	Assess for pelvic tenderness, which may signal pelvic infection and need to postpone procedure
4. Survey with transvaginal (TV) ultrasound	Obtain and record measurements of the endometrium, uterus, and ovaries, and look for pelvic free fluid
5. Place speculum vaginally and clean external cervical os	Note any pain, cervical lesions, or purulent discharge which may signal pelvic infection and need to postpone procedure
6. Introduce 5 or 7 French catheter through cervix into uterus using aseptic technique and slowly inflate intrauterine balloon (if applicable) with 1–2 mL of saline; ring forceps or uterine forceps may be used to guide the catheter	Flush catheter prior to procedure to reduce air bubbles entering the uterus. If using a balloon, it should be deflated at the end of the procedure to fully view the lower uterine segment.
7. Remove speculum, reintroduce the TV probe, and manually instill sterile fluid into the uterine cavity slowly while acquiring real time images of the endometrial canal and cervix	Slow introduction of a minimal amount (usually <10 mL, but can range 5–30 mL) of sterile normal saline or water will reduce discomfort
8. Consider obtaining 3D images if possible	3D imaging coupled with SIS minimizes procedure time and can provide more complete information about intrauterine pathology
9. Remove the transvaginal probe and the transcervical catheter after deflating the balloon when appropriate	Review expectations after the procedure such as watery discharge, spotting, and cramping

may need to be held in place during the procedure to ensure a complete seal for better distention of the cavity.

Transvaginal imaging of enlarged uteri or uteri with multiple myomas may not yield satisfactory visualization. Instead, a lower-frequency transabdominal approach during SIS may produce better images of the endometrium. Another factor which frequently affects image quality is the presence of air in the uterine cavity; air is introduced unintentionally through the catheter at the start of the exam or when changing syringes. Air appears ultrasonographically as bright echoes inside the cavity and can either be mistaken for pathology or obscure abnormal findings. This problem can be alleviated by flushing the catheter prior to starting the procedure, careful syringe changes, and inflating the catheter balloon (if employed) with fluid rather than air. If using a balloon with a catheter, the balloon should be deflated at the conclusion of the procedure to ensure complete evaluation of the lower uterine segment. Rapid image acquisition with cine loop or volume imaging at this point can be helpful before the cavity loses distention.

A final impediment to proper visualization is the presence of blood or clot within the uterine cavity. Although SIS is ideally performed after cessation of menstrual flow, blood in the endometrial cavity may be unavoidable during SIS for women being evaluated for continual or unpredictable bleeding patterns. In these cases, the clinician should assess whether the lesion appears to be mobile, as would be expected of a blood clot. In these cases, it can even be completely dislodged with more forcible injection of fluid or with the catheter itself. Color Doppler imaging can also be used in these cases to determine whether the lesion has a vascular pedicle, a finding which would be typical of an intrauterine polyp rather than a blood clot.

AIUM Guidelines

Saline sonohysterography should be carried out according to the SIS guidelines set forth by the American Institute of Ultrasonography in Medicine (AIUM) [24]. For documentation of the study, both precatheterization images (in at least two planes) should be recorded to demonstrate both normal and abnormal findings. The thickest measurement of the endometrial stripe should be captured in the sagittal view whenever possible. Images from the SIS that represent normal or abnormal findings should also be saved and stored once the cavity is distended with fluid. If using a transcervical catheter with a balloon, the balloon should be deflated at the end of the study to allow images of the lower endometrial and endocervical canals to be obtained. Images using 3D sonohysterography or Doppler flow should also be recorded. For documentation purposes, normal and abnormal images should be permanently archived with appropriate labeling and an interpretation provided. Images of abnormalities should include measurements. Patient identification, facility, date, and side (right or left) should be clearly indicated with the name of the structure (ovary, uterus, fibroid) if possible. The final report with the interpreting physician's official findings should be entered into the patient's permanent medical record. The AIUM Practice Guideline recommendations for documenting an ultrasound examination should be followed [33].

Complications and Post-procedure Instructions

SIS is a safe procedure, with few, mild side effects and a very low incidence of serious complications. Most commonly, patients may experience cramping pain after the procedure that is best treated with NSAIDS. They may also expect to have some spotting and watery discharge [21]. An advantage of SIS is that patients may return home and resume their normal activities following the procedure.

The most common serious complication following SIS is pelvic infection. This occurs less than 1 % of the time, and appears more commonly in women with preexistent fallopian tube disease [21]. Warning signs include fever, persistent or worsening pain, or a change in the amount or type of vaginal discharge the day or two after returning home. Patients should be instructed to call their health care provider if they develop any of these symptoms following their procedure.

Conclusions

SIS is a procedure that that is simple, inexpensive, low-risk, and easy to perform in the office. It provides valuable information to the clinician on a wide range of gynecologic pathologies such as polyps, leiomyomata, adhesions, anomalies, and endometrial hyperplasia or cancer, all without the invasiveness of HSG or hysteroscopy. SIS clearly offers additional information beyond standard 2D transvaginal sonography. When coupled with newer modifications such as 3D sonography or tubal patency evaluation, it becomes an even more powerful tool. In sum, SIS is an essential imaging technique for gynecologists in their evaluations of the female reproductive system.

References

1. Parsons AK, Lense JJ. Sonohysterography for endometrial abnormalities: preliminary results. J Clin Ultrasound. 1993;21:87.
2. Neele SJ, Marchien van Baal W, van der MJ, et al. Ultrasound assessment of the endometrium in healthy, asymptomatic early post-menopausal women: saline infusion sonohysterography versus transvaginal ultrasound. Ultrasound Obstet Gynecol. 2000;16:254–9.
3. Goldstein S. Modern evaluation of the endometrium. Obstet Gynecol. 2010;116:168–76.
4. Grimbizis F, Tsolakidis D, Mikos T, et al. A prospective comparison of transvaginal ultrasound, saline infusion sonohysterography, and diagnostic hysteroscopy in the evaluation of endometrial pathology. Fertil Steril. 2010;94:2720–5.
5. Nannini R, Chelo E, Branconi F, et al. Dynamic echohysteroscopy: a new diagnostic technique in the

study of female infertility. Acta Eur Fertil. 1981;12:165–71.
6. Bingol B, Gunenc Z, Dekikbasi A, et al. Comparison of diagnostic accuracy of saline infusion sonohysterography, transvaginal sonography, and hysteroscopy. J Obstet Gynaecol. 2011;31:54–8.
7. Erdem M, Bilgin U, Bozkurt N, et al. Comparison of transvaginal ultrasonography and saline infusion sonohysterography in evaluating the endometrial cavity in pre- and postmenopausal women with abnormal uterine bleeding. Menopause. 2007;14:846–52.
8. Yildizhan B, Yildizhan R, Ozkesici B, et al. Transvaginal ultrasonography and saline infusion sonohysterography for the detection of intra-uterine lesions in pre- and post-menopausal women with abnormal uterine bleeding. J Int Med Res. 2008;36:1205–13.
9. Van den Bosch T, Verguts J, Daemen A, Gevaert O, et al. Pain experienced during transvaginal ultrasound, saline contrast sonohysterography, hysteroscopy, and office sampling: a comparative study. Ultrasound Obstet Gynecol. 2008;31:346–51.
10. Vilela JR, Cardoso MT, Franco Junior JG, et al. Sonohysterography accuracy versus transvaginal ultrasound in infertile women candidate to assisted reproduction techniques. Rev Bras Ginecol Obstet. 2012;34:122–7.
11. Maheux-Lacroix S, Boutin A, Moore L, Bergeron ME, Buiold E, Laberge PY, Lemyre M, Dodin S. Hysterosalpingosonography for diagnosing tubal occlusion in subfertile women: a systematic review protocol. Syst Rev. 2013;2:50.
12. Ludwin A, Ludwin I, Banas T, et al. Diagnostic accuracy of sonohysterography, hysterosalpingography and diagnostic hysteroscopy in diagnosis of arcuate, septate and bicornuate uterus. J Obstet Gynaecol Res. 2011;37:178–86.
13. Soares SR, Barbosa dos Reis MM, Camargos AF. Diagnostic accuracy of sonohysterography, transvaginal sonography, and hysterosalpingography in patients with uterine cavity diseases. Fertil Steril. 2000;73:406.
14. Lindheim SR, Morales AJ. Comparison of sonohysterography and hysteroscopy: lessons learned and avoiding pitfalls. J Am Assoc Gynecol Laparosc. 2002;9:223.
15. van Dongen H, de Kroon CD, van den Tillaart SA, et al. A randomised comparison of vaginoscopic office hysteroscopy and saline infusion sonography: a patient compliance study. BJOG. 2008;115:1232.
16. Wildrich T, Bradley LD, Mitchinson AR, et al. Comparison of saline infusion sonography with office hysteroscopy for the evaluation of the endometrium. Am J Obstet Gynecol. 1996;174:1327.
17. de Vries L, Dijkhuizen F, Mol B, et al. Comparison of transvaginal sonography, saline infusion sonography, and hysteroscopy in premenopausal women with abnormal uterine bleeding. J Clin Ultrasound. 2000;28:217–23.
18. de Kroon CD, Jansen FW, Louwe LA, et al. Technology assessment of saline contrast hysterosonography. Am J Obset Gynecol. 2003;188:945.
19. Dijkhuizen FP, Mol BW, Bongers MY, Breolmann HA, et al. Cost-effectiveness of transvaginal sonography and saline infused sonography in the evaluation of menorrhagia. Int J Gynaecol Obstet. 2003;83:45–52.
20. Choudry A, Shukr I, Khan S, et al. Acceptability and accuracy of saline infusion sonohysterography in women with postmenopausal bleeding. J Coll Physicians Surg Pak. 2010;20:571–5.
21. Dessole S, Farina M, Rubattu G, et al. Side effects and complications of sonohysterosalpingography. Fertil Steril. 2003;80:620.
22. Jacques E, Verma U, Whitted RW. Accuracy of saline infusion sonohysterography in diagnosis of uterine intracavitary pathology. Obstet Gynecol. 2001;97: S18.
23. American College of Obstetricians & Gynecologists. ACOG technology assessment in obstetrics and gynecology no. 5: sonohysterography. Obstet Gynecol. 2008;112:1467.
24. American Institute of Ultrasound in Medicine, American College of Radiology, American College of Obstetricians and Gynecologists, Society of Radiologist in Ultrasound. AIUM practice guidelines for the performance of sonohysterography. J Ultrasound Med. 2012;31:165.
25. Dessole S, Rubattu G, Farina M, et al. Risks and usefulness of sonohysterography in patients with endometrial carcinoma. Am J Obstet Gynecol. 2006;194:362.
26. Bese T, Demirkiran F, Guralp O, et al. Transtubal transport of carcinoma cells into the peritoneal cavity after saline infusion via transcervical route in patients with endometrial carcinoma. Int J Gynecol Cancer. 2009;19:682–5.
27. Berry E, Lindheim SR, Connor JP, et al. Sonohysterography and endometrial cancer: incidence and functional viability of disseminated malignant cells. Am J Obstet Gynecol. 2008;199:240.
28. Takac I. Saline infusion sonohysterography and the risk of malignant extrauterine spread in endometrial cancer. Ultrasound Med Biol. 2008;34:7–11.
29. Dessole S, Farina M, Capobianco G, Nardelli GB, Ambrosini G, Meloni GB. Determining the best catheter for sonohysterography. Fertil Steril. 2001;76 (3):605–9.

30. Snyder JT, Anasti J. A comparison of two saline infusion sonography catheters. Obstet Gynecol. 2000;95 Suppl 1:S31.
31. Sylvestre C, Child TJ, Tulandi T, Tan SL. A prospective study to evaluate the efficacy of two- and three-dimensional sonohysterography in women with intrauterine lesions. Fertil Steril. 2003;79(5):1222–5.
32. Bonnamy L, Marret H, Perrotin F, Body G, Berger C, Lansac J. Sonohysterography: a prospective survey results and complications in 81 patients. Eur J Obstet Gynecol Reprod Biol. 2002;102:42–7.
33. American Institute of Ultrasound in Medicine. AIUM practice guideline for documentation of an ultrasound examination. J Ultrasound Med. 2009;28(1):110–3.

7 Office Diagnostic Hysteroscopy

Jonathan D. Emery

Introduction

Hysteroscopy has been increasingly accepted as the "gold standard" for direct visualization of the uterine cavity in order to correctly diagnose and treat menstrual and reproductive abnormalities. Transfer of this technique from the operating room to the office has been taking place since the 1980s due to advances in technology in instrumentation and fiberoptics. The introduction of small-caliber hysteroscopes with an outer diameter of 5–6 mm or less has aligned the procedure even more. Further refinements include development of the "vaginoscopic" technique of Bettocchi in 1995 [1] and the "see and treat" approach which integrated diagnostic and operative modalities, using the operative channel of the hysteroscope.

The ability to use this technology in the office allows the gynecologist to make the correct diagnosis in the office without subjecting the patient to more invasive techniques or those that require anesthesia. Office hysteroscopy has been shown to be well tolerated with a minimum of pain [1, 2] and allows for more accurate diagnoses than a "blind" D&C [3] by using a guided biopsy. Thus, patients benefit from an expedited approach to diagnosis and treatment and a more rapid return to normal functioning. Thus, one might consider office hysteroscopy to be the "perfect" office diagnostic procedure on par with office cystoscopy. This chapter will focus on the development of diagnostic hysteroscopy in the office setting, evaluation of appropriate indications, instrumentation, and techniques.

Indications for Office Hysteroscopy

Evaluation of the uterine cavity with hysteroscopy has a multitude of indications (Table 7.1). The most common of these is abnormal uterine bleeding. Publication of the FIGO classification system of PALM-COEIN for classification of abnormal uterine bleeding in 2011 has helped to refine and standardize the nomenclature for disorders of menstrual bleeding [4]. Using this classification system, the "PALM" group represents structural entities that may be easily diagnosed by office hysteroscopy, at times in conjunction with other imaging modalities. This group includes *P*olyp, *A*denomyosis, *L*eiomyoma, and *M*alignancy/hyperplasia (Table 7.2). As up to 30 % of reproductive age women may have menstrual irregularities, office hysteroscopy can help to diagnose endometrial polyps, type 0 and 1 myomas (Figs. 7.1a, b and 7.2) as well as endometrial hyperplasia and cancer which may require guided biopsy.

Abnormalities of reproduction also serve as an indication of office hysteroscopic surgery.

J.D. Emery, M.D., F.A.C.O.G. (✉)
Department of Obstetrics & Gynecology,
Women's Health Institute, Cleveland Clinic,
2550 SOM Center Road, Suite 100,
Willoughby Hills, OH 44094, USA
e-mail: emeryj@ccf.org

J.D. Emery and M.F.R. Paraiso (eds.), *Office-Based Gynecologic Surgical Procedures*,
DOI 10.1007/978-1-4939-1414-2_7, © Springer Science+Business Media New York 2015

Table 7.1 Indications for office hysteroscopy

Evaluation of abnormal bleeding
• Premenopausal anovulatory women
• Premenopausal ovulatory women
• Postmenopausal bleeding
Evaluation of infertility
• Routine infertility work-up
• Abnormal HSG
• Pre-IVF evaluation
• Recurrent spontaneous abortion
Evaluation of abnormal TVUS or SIS when endometrium is:
• Not visualized
• Indeterminate
• Indistinct
• Not visualized in its entirety
Localization of foreign body
• Lost IUD
• Migration of cerclage
Postoperative evaluation
• Inspection of cavity following hysteroscopic myomectomy or polypectomy
• Inspection of cavity following abdominal myomectomy entrance into endometrial cavity
• Difficult postpartum D&C to evaluate for Asherman syndrome
• After removal of indwelling Foley catheter following adhesiolysis
• Inspection of cesarean scar
• Inspection following septum repair
• Recurrent bleeding after endometrial ablation
• Inspection of Essure device if migration of the device suspected or for irregular bleeding
Classification of submucosal fibroids
• Class I
• Class II
• Class III
Evaluation of the endometrium following UFE
• Evaluate complaints of amenorrhea
• Evaluate complaints of post-UFE cramping
• Evaluate complaints of chronic or episodic leukorrhea
• Evaluate the endometrium for submucosal fibroids when MRI is equivocal
Evaluation of the pregnant patient
• IUD localization in early pregnancy
• Retained products of conception
• Postpartum hemorrhage
• Ectopic pregnancy (tubal or interstitial)
• Failed termination of pregnancy
• Persistent bleeding after termination of pregnancy

(continued)

Table 7.1 (continued)

Endometrial cancer
• Staging
• Evaluation of cervical involvement
• Second look after nonsurgical treatment
Hysteroscopic tubal occlusion
• Determine if there is any obstruction to tubal ostia
• Determine if there are other intracavitary lesions that need removal

Legend: *D&C* dilatation and curettage, *IUD* intrauterine device, *HSG* hysterosalpingogram, *IVF* in vitro fertilization, *MRI* magnetic resonance imaging, *SIS* saline infusion sonography, *TVUS* transvaginal ultrasound, *UFE* uterine fibroid embolization

Adapted from: Bradley LD. Indications and Contraindications for Office Hysteroscopy. Chapter 3. In: Bradley LD, Falcone T (ed). Hysteroscopy: Office Evaluation and Management of the Uterine Cavity. Philadelphia, PA. Mosby;2009, used with permission

Table 7.2 PALM-COEIN basic classification system

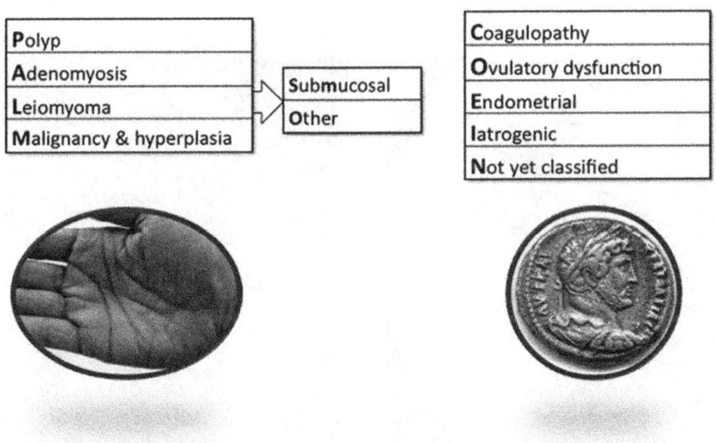

(Adapted from: Munro MG, Critchley HOD, Broder MS et al. FIGO classification system (PALM-COEIN) for causes of abnormal uterine bleeding in nongravid women of reproductive age. Int J Gynecol Obstet 2011; 113:3–13.)—used with permission

Both the evaluation of infertility or subfertility can be assisted by endometrial evaluation with hysteroscopy which may show intrauterine synechae or adhesions or a uterine septum. Evaluation of abnormal hysterosalpingography (HSG) is another indication as well as final appraisal of the intrauterine environment prior to beginning of in vitro fertilization (IVF). Also, tubal blockage may be identified and treated with office techniques. Post reproductive complications such as retained placenta postpartum or incomplete pregnancy termination can be diagnosed using office hysteroscopy. This is especially important in patients who may have a negative urine or serum hcg (human chorionic gonadotropin) level on laboratory testing but where office hysteroscopy reveals retained gestational tissue which is causing abnormal bleeding or impaired subsequent fertility.

Other indications for office hysteroscopy include inspection of the uterine cavity after operative hysteroscopy for large polyps or submucosal leiomyoma or evaluation of abnormal bleeding after global endometrial ablation. Difficult or complicated surgery for pregnancy loss with dilatation and curettage (D&C) can lead to

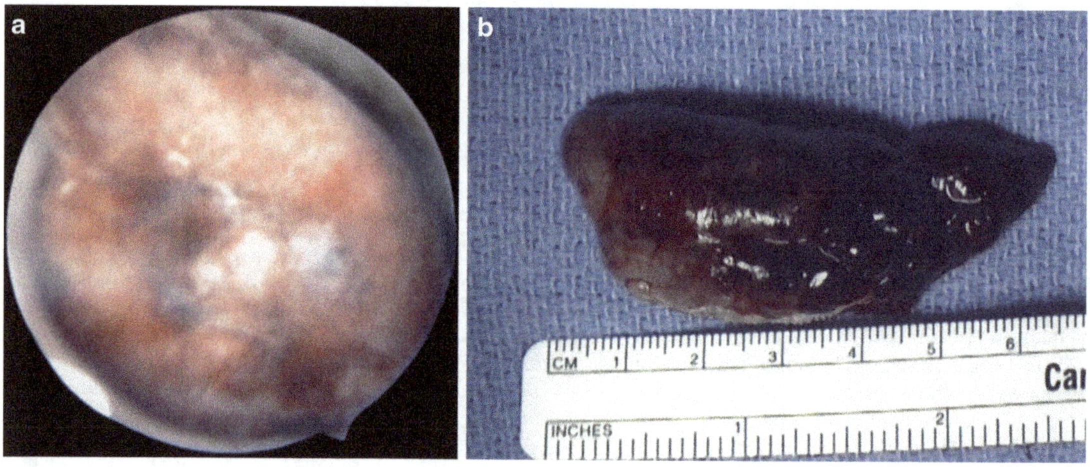

Fig. 7.1 (a) Endometrial polyp filling the endometrial cavity. (b) Gross specimen of endometrial polyp from (a)

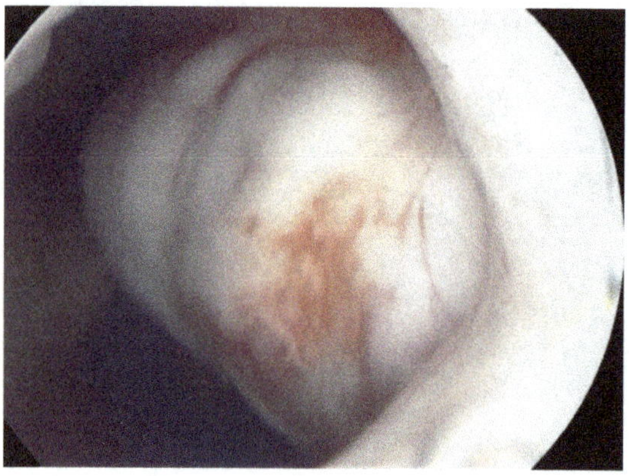

Fig. 7.2 Submucosal leiomyoma

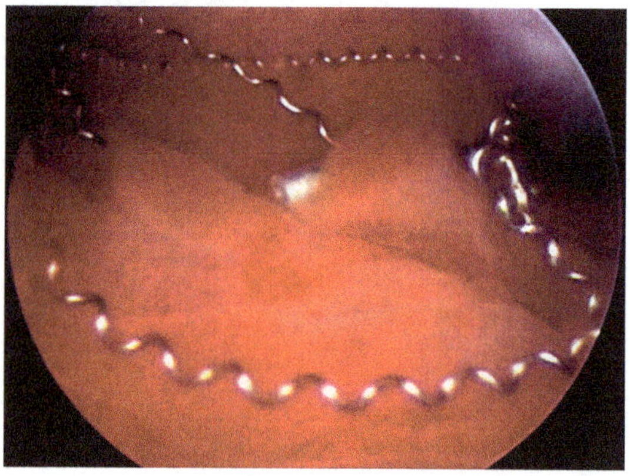

Fig. 7.3 Example of unwound Essure™ microcoils displaced throughout the endometrium in a patient with heavy menses after hysteroscopic sterilization

adhesions or after D&C for postpartum bleeding in order to assess removal of all gestational tissue. Lastly, after tubal sterilization, endometrial appraisal may be helpful to assess placement or disturbance from the microcoil inserts (Fig. 7.3).

Uterine fibroid embolization (UFE) is increasingly becoming a procedure to decrease menstrual bleeding from symptomatic uterine leiomyomata. After the procedure, the leiomyomata and surrounding uterine muscular and secretory tissue can become hypoperfused, leading to atrophy and pale, nonviable endometrium: adhesions, fibrosis, and calcifications may also develop. All of these factors can lead to development of an onerous vaginal discharge, at times described as clear, yellow, brown, or rusty. Office hysteroscopy is the ideal tool to evaluate these complaints. The performance of this can help in diagnosis and to decide what, if any, therapy is needed. Commonly, expectant management is all that is needed but patients can respond well to operative hysteroscopic resection of the necrotic tissue [5]. Also, after UFE, one study showed that up to 22 % of patients will require subsequent surgery months or years after UFE, with many of the surgeries hysteroscopic in nature [6].

Table 7.3 Incidence of hysteroscopically confirmed endometrial polyps in women receiving tamoxifen

Author	Year	No. patients on tamoxifen	No. patients with polyp (%)
DeMuylder et al.	1991	23	13 (57)
Lahti et al.	1994	49	17 (35)
Mouritas et al.	1999	22	7 (32)
Leidman	2000	35	18 (51)

Adapted from: Emery JD, Falcone T. Effects of Drugs on the Uterus, chapter 8. In Baggish MS, Valle RF, Guedj H eds. Hysteroscopy: Visual Perspectives of Uterine Anatomy, Physiology and Pathology, 3rd ed. 2007. Lippincott Williams & Wilkins. Philadelphia, PA, used with permission

Planning for hysteroscopic resection of submucosal leiomyomata based on transvaginal ultrasound or saline infusion sonography (SIS) would benefit from office hysteroscopy prior to the operative resection: hidden pathology in the form of multiple fibroids, polyps, or adhesions can be identified and the surgical approach may be modified if needed. For instance, a multiple stage resection may be needed for large or multiple submucosal myomas if the risk of hyperosmotic fluid absorption puts the patient at risk. As noted hysteroscopist Dr. Linda Bradley recommends, "Avoid surprises in the operating room" [7].

Evaluation of postmenopausal bleeding can be easily accomplished in the office, especially when the patient may have comorbid medical conditions making operative evaluation in the OR or ASC more problematic. Bleeding can occur within the first few years after the menopause transition or may not occur until 20–25 or more years past menopause. While not all postmenopausal bleeding indicates malignancy or even endometrial hyperplasia, suspicion of this type of pathology should be increased in the face of risk factors including obesity, diabetes mellitus, hypertension, and unopposed estrogen replacement therapy. Patients with these factors or those with transvaginal ultrasound showing double layer endometrial thickness of greater than 5 mm should undergo office endometrial biopsy. However, office pipelle biopsy has shown to miss focal lesions in the endometrium, with a sensitivity ranging from 83 to 98 % [8, 9]. Thus, office hysteroscopy is strongly recommended in patients who have continued postmenopausal bleeding after a negative endometrial biopsy. Focal and specific hysteroscopic directed biopsies can be performed at the time of office hysteroscopy, providing an accurate diagnosis.

Women taking tamoxifen for adjunct therapy for breast cancer also can benefit from office hysteroscopy. Tamoxifen, a nonsteroidal triphenylethylene derivative, has been shown to increase survival in patients with estrogen receptor-positive tumors. In the breast, tamoxifen works as an estrogen antagonist but in the endometrium, it has a weak estrogen agonistic effect and is thus a mixed agonist/antagonist. Women taking tamoxifen need monitoring during and after therapy for the development of atypical endometrial hyperplasia and malignancy. Routine screening with ultrasound and/or endometrial biopsy is not recommended as false positive rates are increased [10]. In patients who are currently or have ever received tamoxifen develop frank vaginal bleeding, spotting/staining or even brown or unusual vaginal discharge should undergo direct visualization of the endometrium with hysteroscopy as visualization is more accurate in diagnosing frank pathology. In these women, a variety of endometrial patterns can be seen on hysteroscopy, including pale atrophy or alternatively, a hypervascularized pattern in addition to a cystic appearance reported to be from activation of subendothelial adenomyotic glands and cysts [11, 12]. Also, the incidence of endometrial polyps is significantly increased in women receiving tamoxifen: reported incidences of 32–57 % have been reported [13] (Table 7.3).

Also, evaluation of an abnormal transvaginal ultrasound result may benefit from office hysteroscopic assessment in addition to or in place of endometrial sampling. Given increasingly specific ultrasound reports, not only may double layer endometrial thickness be reported, but other endometrial findings such as endometrial or subendometrial cysts, calcifications, or endometrial fluid may be described as well as less well-defined terms such as "space-occupying lesion." These descriptions may indicate polyps, submucosal leimyomata, malignancy or atypical hyperplasia or adenomyosis. Fluid in the endometrium has been described by many and can be associated with cervical stenosis as well as endometrial pathology. Vuento and colleagues reported that in a group of over 1,000 asymptomatic postmenopausal women, 12 % had fluid in the endometrium with 5 % of these patients having endometrial pathology, including cancer [14]. Techniques are available to assist in the office with overcoming cervical stenosis if present and then office hysteroscopy can be done along with directed biopsies and/or endometrial biopsy as indicated.

Lastly, patients will present with an intrauterine device (IUD) where the stings have been withdrawn into the endometrial cavity or are missing. Also, older models such as the Lippes loop or those from manufacturers outside the United States may not have strings attached, thus requiring either blind uterine manipulation or hysteroscopy to remove them. Alternatively, an IUD with visible strings that is difficult to remove due to cervical stenosis or possible uterine embedment will be easily assessed with office hysteroscopy. In the United States, IUD use is increasing for both contraception as well as for gynecologic treatment with the levonorgestrel releasing IUD (LNG-IUD). As such, complications with IUD can be more easily diagnosed in office with hysteroscopy. Also, if one has a sheath with an operating channel in office, utilizing the operating channel with hysteroscopic grasping forceps can be utilized to remove the IUD in one setting in the office, providing another example of a "see and treat" philosophy of office hysteroscopic surgery. The strings can be moved to the ectocervix while leaving the IUD in utero or the IUD can be removed if it has expired, is causing complications or if the patient desires pregnancy. Office hysteroscopy can also determine if the IUD is embedded into the myometrium (Fig. 7.4). At times, the initial evaluation in office can determine if removal of the embedded IUD can be accomplished in office with an operative approach or if a more involved surgery with hysteroscopy (and or laparoscopy if needed) is required to remove the impacted IUD. Other types of foreign bodies that may be retrieved with the in-office technique of hysteroscopy include lost laminarium or portions of laminaria, surgical gauze, Essure™ microcoil and fetal bone after incomplete pregnancy termination.

Contraindications to Office Hysteroscopy

There are several major contraindications to office diagnostic hysteroscopic surgery. Current pelvic inflammatory disease (PID) is the leading absolute contraindication. If PID is suspected (fever, uterine tenderness, and/or adnexal masses), the procedure should be postponed and evaluation to confirm the diagnosis and establish treatment should be initiated. Past episodes of PID may predispose to hydrosalpinx or other obstructions of the endometrium or salpinges, thus consideration of pre and postoperative antibiotics should be considered.

Recent cervical infection, if treated, is not a contraindication though if compliance with treatment is suspected, the office procedure should be delayed until negative cervical cultures are verified. Current or active herpesvirus infection is another absolute contraindication to the performance of hysteroscopy. Vigilance when obtaining a patient history is required to be certain an asymptomatic herpes infection is not present and if lesions are seen when prepping the patient, delaying the hysteroscopy is important. The presence of cervical cancer has been proposed as an absolute contraindication as concern about dissemination of malignant cells. Pregnancy is a relative contraindication to performance of hysteroscopy in the office. While a hysteroscopic procedure may be needed in early pregnancy to remove an IUD, it is suggested to perform this in the operating room under low

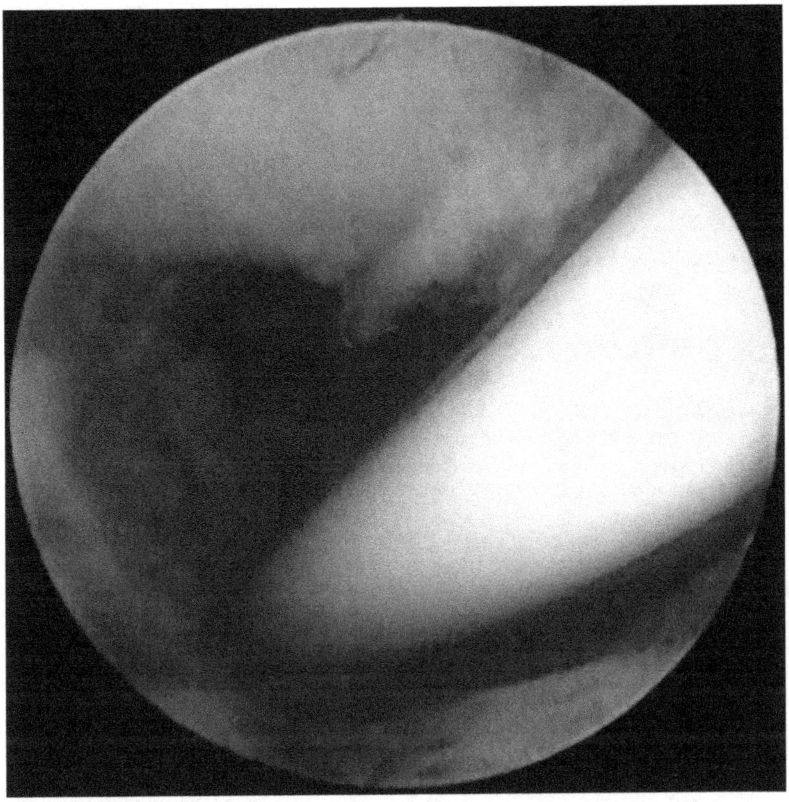

Fig. 7.4 Embedded levonorgestrel IUD

pressure using only saline for distention (carbon dioxide poses risk of gas embolism). In the presence of heavy and profuse vaginal bleeding, office hysteroscopy may be difficult with smaller caliber hysteroscope (so-called "mini-hysteroscopes") due to problems maintaining adequate irrigation and uterine insufflation. An uncooperative patient is another relative contraindication as patient compliance with ability to remain relatively still during the procedure and tolerate the possibility of mild discomfort is needed: discussion of the benefits of office hysteroscopy must be weighed with a patient's ability to cooperate.

Instrumentation for Office Hysteroscopy

As mentioned, office hysteroscopy has evolved with improvements in technology and the development of small diameter hysteroscopes and improved fiberoptics and video monitoring. Instrumentation for office hysteroscopy has two options: rigid and flexible. There are documented benefits of each type of equipment in addition to the experience and training of the physician performing the office procedure.

Rigid hysteroscopy has been used the longest with reports generated from the late 1970s and early 1980s reporting on office hysteroscopy in-office. Advances since then have yielded current rigid hysteroscopes for use in office have a diameter ranging from 1.2 to 4 mm with continuous flow features as well as improved visualization and coupled with the diagnostic sheath, these scopes have a final diameter that does not exceed 5 mm (Fig. 7.5). Nagele et al. demonstrated success in outpatient diagnostic hysteroscopy in 2,500 patients of over 96 % using a 4-mm telescope with a 5-mm diagnostic sheath [2]. With these smaller diameter telescopes, there are different angled lenses that can help facilitate visualization of the endometrial cavity: 30, 12, and 0-degree objective lens angulations are available, with 12 and

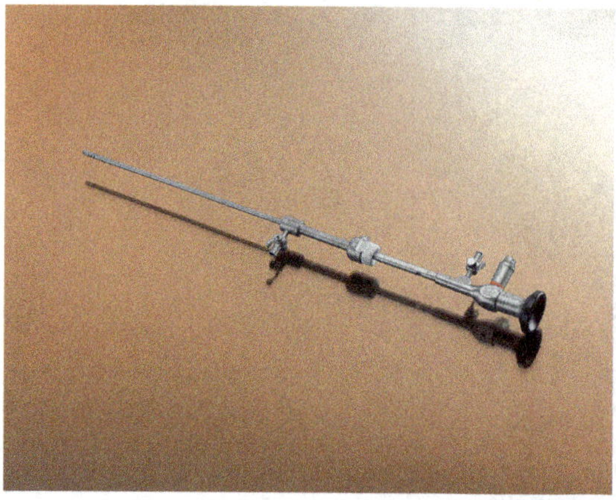

Fig. 7.5 Karl Storz rigid hysteroscope (copyright 2014 photo courtesy of KARL STORZ Endoscopy-America, Inc.)

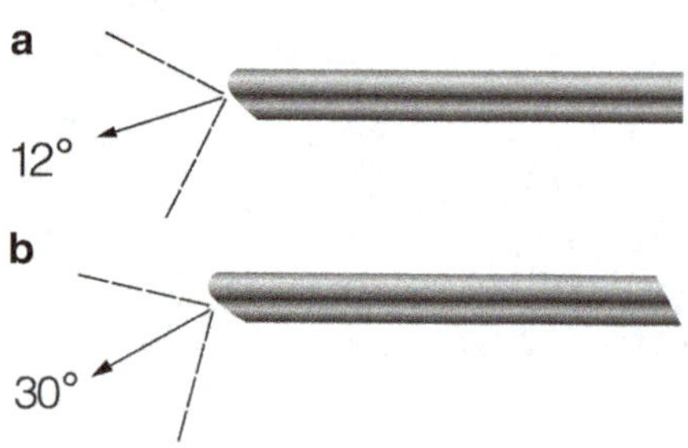

Fig. 7.6 Example of hysteroscope with a 12° deflected view (**a**) and a 30° deflected view (**b**) (copyright 2014 photo courtesy of KARL STORZ Endoscopy-America, Inc.)

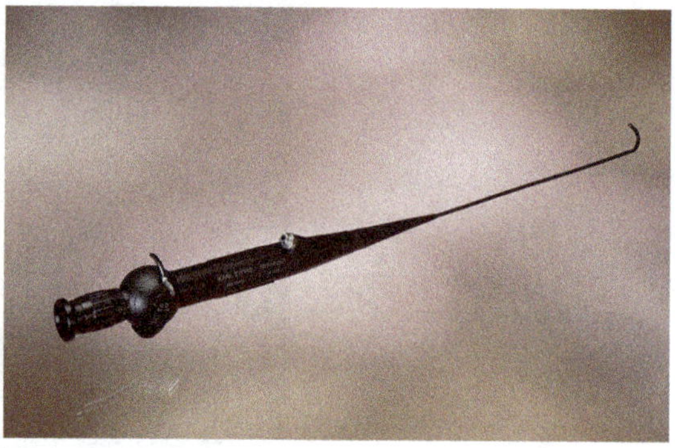

Fig. 7.7 Karl Storz flexible hysteroscope (copyright 2014 photo courtesy of KARL STORZ Endoscopy-America, Inc.)

Table 7.4 Comparison of rigid versus flexible hysteroscopy

Rigid hysteroscopy
• Improved visualization and image with saline distending media.
• Use of operating channel for ability to "see and treat" pathology if present
• Easier to maintain; less expensive to purchase
Flexible hysteroscopy
• Easier and less painful to perform in a very anteverted or retroverted uterus
• Easier to maneuver around intracavity lesions or through a tortuous endocervix
• Extended working length of scope: easier in obese patients
• Use of carbon dioxide or saline for distention

30-degree being used more commonly in the office setting (Fig. 7.6a, b).

Flexible hysteroscopy utilizes zero degree lens with a bendable tip that allows a bidirectional mode allowing for up to a 120-degree field of vision along a long working sheath that includes a channel for distending media (Fig. 7.7). There are adaptors available which will create an ancillary port, which when used as an operative channel, can be used to obtain directed biopsies or to retrieve IUD strings or remove small polyps. Bradley demonstrated in over 400 women that office flexible hysteroscopy is well tolerated and cost effective for evaluation of menstrual disorders [15].

Table 7.4 lists some basic advantages of each type of hysteroscope. When setting up an office hysteroscopy program, the physician must keep in mind issues concerning their own training and skill set in each technique as well as issues regarding maintenance and sterilization of the equipment. Also, recent introduction of single use office hysteroscopes have been introduced which may be applicable to certain practices based on cost, reimbursement, and office-based efficiency factors.

Patient Preparation

Once a patient has been identified as needing office hysteroscopy for diagnostic and/or possible therapeutic purposes, certain criteria should be met and procedures in place in the office in order to make the process smooth and acceptable to the patient as well as to allow for accurate diagnostic efficiency for the physician. Patient selection is critical: patients who do not tolerate speculum exam well or who have debilitating anxiety may not be good candidates for an office procedure. For more details, see Chap. 1. Prior to the hysteroscopy, educating the patient on expectations both during and after the procedure is tantamount: warning her of possible points of the procedure where mild pain, discomfort, or cramps may be encountered should be discussed. Letting the patient know about the procedure with educational materials (printed or online) will also decrease potential questions about the office surgery as well.

Informed consent should also take place prior to the procedure, either the day of, or preferably at an appointment before, the actual procedure. This process is reviewed more thoroughly in Chap. 3: however, discussion of the risks, benefits, and complications of the hysteroscopy should be reviewed and appropriate documentation should be made as well. Side effects of the procedure and post-procedure should also be reviewed—this can help to decrease post procedural telephone calls to the office. Also, the patient should be made aware that the procedure will stop at any time if she becomes too uncomfortable or anxious—reassuring her of permission to stop the procedure at any time gives the patient a sense of autonomy.

Optimally, the patient will be seen in the office at a time before the actual procedure. This will be helpful for several reasons. First, informed consent can take place as discussed above. Secondly, choosing an appropriate date for hysteroscopy can be accomplished. This is especially true for women in their reproductive years in order to perform the hysteroscopy during the proliferative phase of the cycle in order to better identify true pathology. Proliferative endometrium can be best encountered 7–10 days after the last menstrual period in patients who have documented ovulation. Also, need for urine or even serum pregnancy testing can also be ascertained at this time. If there is confusion about whether the patient may be pregnant, defer the procedure until lab testing can clearly show that the patient is not pregnant. Patients who are postmenopausal may be scheduled at any time.

If there is concern about the possibility of cervical stenosis—such as a patient who is nulliparous or postmenopausal—consideration for the use of misoprostol is recommended. Misoprostol, a prostaglandin E1 analogue, has been shown to be useful in preparing the cervix prior to hysteroscopic surgery. Studies have shown that pre-procedural use of this medication can decrease cervical resistance during hysteroscopy and decrease cervical dilatation [16, 17]. Misoprostol 200–400 μg can be given orally or vaginally 9–24 h before office hysteroscopy to help prepare the cervix and facilitate endocervical entry, especially at the internal os. This will improve the experience for both patient and physician. Warn patients of mild side effects such as vaginal spotting or bleeding and lower abdominal cramps. Diarrhea or other gastrointestinal side effects are rare. Also, if patients are concerned about pain or discomfort, advising them to take a nonsteroidal (such as ibuprofen 400–600 mg or naproxen sodium 500 mg) up to 60 min prior to the office surgery can help to decrease pain associated with the office procedure.

Equipment and Office Setup

In order to establish a hysteroscopy program, an office will need to obtain some basic equipment required to safely and successfully perform the procedure in the office setting.

The initial decision should be whether to use a rigid hysteroscope or a flexible hysteroscope. The merits of each are discussed above in the "Instrumentation" section.

Surgeon preference, cost to rent or purchase as well as costs of maintenance will also need to be considered.

Also, deciding upon which distention medium to use is important. In rigid office hysteroscopy, normal saline is most commonly used. Carbon dioxide may also be used but should be used for only diagnostic hysteroscopy as blood and endometrial debris can collect and cause problems with visualization when using carbon dioxide. Some hysteroscopists prefer carbon dioxide for improved visualization and ease of use. Risks of CO_2 include diaphragmatic irritation with subsequent shoulder pain cited [18]. Also, risk of air embolism, while small at 0.51 %, is a concern to keep in mind with using either medium [19]. There are two randomized controlled trials [20, 21] which showed that normal saline has less pain, shorter procedure times, and greater patient satisfaction when compared with CO_2.

Equipment for the distending medium chosen would include the medium itself (1 L intravenous bag of saline or CO_2 cannister) as well as tubing and appropriate measuring device. AAGL has issued guidelines for management and utilization of distention media [22]. These discuss the use of pumps for fluid and measuring systems but also note that with simple diagnostic procedures, "there is little value to using these systems for diagnostic hysteroscopy or even for simple procedures" but use of simple gravity to create an intrauterine pressure that is at a level below the patient's mean arterial pressure. It should be noted, however, that having a "perineal drape" that can collect the extruded fluid is recommended in case one suspects increased fluid absorption during the procedure. This way the physician and office staff will be able to assess fluid intake versus output for office procedures that take more time than anticipated.

Regardless of the type of scope to be used or the choice of distending media, the necessary accessories needed to maintain visualization of the uterus and cervix are needed. These include a light source with appropriate fiberoptic cables and a camera and monitor to take still images at a minimum (Fig. 7.8). Many offices will also utilize a digital printer and/or a video digital recorder to document and preserve the procedure and important images of pathology identified. Many offices will have this equipment all present on one mobile cart which contains other needed supplies such as specula, cleansing solution, tenaculum, and dilator probes. Having all equipment in one location will help the nursing and other office staff to have the necessary materials on hand in case problems or complications arise during the hysteroscopy procedure.

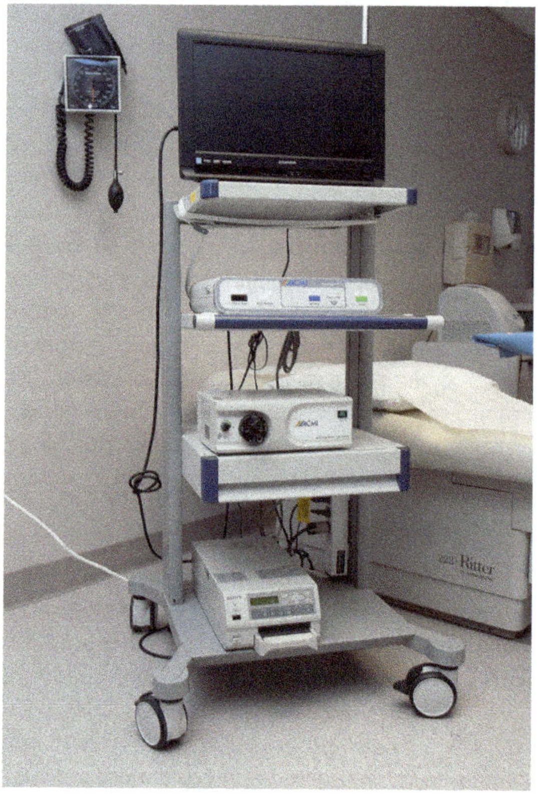

Fig. 7.8 Office hysteroscopy tower with video monitor, lightsource, video adaptor, and printer on mobile tower cart

Hysteroscopic Procedure

Rigid or Flexible Hysteroscopy: Standard Technique

After appropriate pre-procedure evaluation, informed consent and procedural "time out," the in-office procedure may proceed. Assessment of complete operational aspects of the hysteroscope and needed equipment should be undertaken before proceeding to assure no equipment malfunctions or absence of needed equipment is identified mid-procedure. Also, "white balancing" and focusing the scope should be undertaken to confirm appropriate visualization is achieved. Lastly, flush or purge the tubing with the distention medium (saline or CO_2) prior to beginning the procedure to reduce the risk of air embolism.

The patient is placed in the dorsal lithotomy position, with adequate drapes or chux pads in place to absorb extruded saline or other fluid if liquid distention medium is used. A speculum (preferably one sided) is placed and the cervix is visualized. Cleansing the cervix, while not required, is appropriate with approved antiseptic solution. If using a paracervical anesthetic block, it may be administered at this time. Some have advocated using only a "small dot of anesthetic (0.5 mL).... Placed at the anterior cervical lip where the tenaculum is placed" [23]. Placement of a single tooth tenaculum at the 12 o'clock position of the cervix is then done. If cervical stenosis is present or if the patient is nulliparous or postmenopausal, consideration of a minimal cervical dilation may be considered at this time.

Then after assuring the anesthetic has had adequate time to take effect, the hysteroscope may be introduced. Fluid or CO_2 distention through the hysteroscope should be initiated just as the scope is being placed into the external cervical os. Once inside the external os, follow the endocervix by direct visualization while slowly advancing the hysteroscope. If adequate distention is not present, slowly closing the outflow channel may help to improve visualization. By following the endocervical canal, the internal cervical os will then be reached. Once past the internal os, entry into the uterine cavity will require a brief pause to completely distend the cavity. At this time, a complete survey of the uterine cavity should be performed including anterior and posterior walls, uterine fundus and both corneal regions with notation of bilateral tubal ostia (Fig. 7.9). Video photos can be taken at this time to provide documentation of both a normal cavity or to identify and denote any pathology seen.

In some patients, the anatomic position of the uterus (anteverted or retroverted) may require the surgeon to manipulate the hysteroscope in order to accomplish an adequate uterine evaluation. This may require gentle removal of the speculum (warning the patient of this occurrence during the procedure will help to decrease the patient's possible startle reflex) to allow more anterior, posterior, or lateral movement of the hysteroscope. If the patient is on an electrically driven table, adjusting the table position or height during the procedure may also allow for improved visualization and patient comfort. Also, if using a 30° or 70° lens, rotation of the hysteroscope can allow for adequate visualization while decreasing undue movement of the scope. The surgeon should also be aware that with a 12° or 30° hysteroscope, the image seen on the monitor is not directly in front of the scope and so adjusting movements during the procedure may be needed. With flexible hysteroscopes, however, the angle of view is zero degrees, so one should keep the cervix and uterine cavity in the center of the field of view.

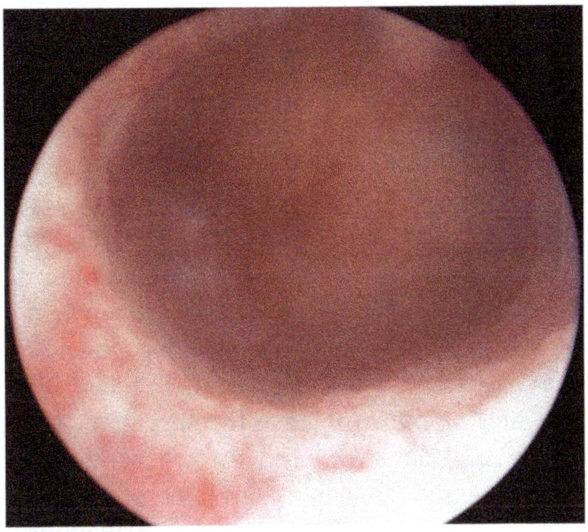

Fig. 7.9 Panoramic view of endometrium from lower uterine segment

If endometrial pathology is identified, targeted biopsies may be undertaken if the hysteroscope has attached biopsy channel. This allows for what has been described as "see and treat" approach: Bettocchi et al. have noted, "in this situation, there is no longer a distinction between diagnostic and operative procedure, because a single procedure is performed in which the operative part is perfectly integrated in the diagnostic work-up" [24]. Further description of office operative hysteroscopic techniques are described in Chap. 9. Otherwise, complete the procedure by slowly withdrawing the hysteroscope and viewing the uterine cavity and the endocervix. Stop the distending medium flow as the scope is exiting the external os. Remove any excess fluid in the vagina, remove the tenaculum (and check for excessive bleeding at the tenaculum site), and then remove the speculum. If an endometrial biopsy is needed for general endometrial sampling (such as suspicion of endometritis or other general endometrial pathology), performance of the biopsy may be undertaken immediately after completing the hysteroscopy and before removal of the vaginal instruments.

After the procedure, assure that the patient is comfortable. Before discharging her from the office, it is beneficial to review the findings including review of photos taken during the procedure. Many women will be able to observe the procedure in "real time" by viewing the monitor during the procedure. This both allows for a visual "distraction" from any minor discomfort she may be experiencing as well as allowing her to be invested in the findings of the procedure. Review of post-procedure instructions about activity, diet, and recovery from any required analgesics or sedatives is recommended at this time as well. Usually, most patients may resume normal activity the day of or just after the procedure. Recommendations about resumption of intercourse vary according to surgeon preference but this may be allowed within the first few days post-procedure provided the patient is comfortable.

Vaginoscopic Technique for Office Hysteroscopy

The Vaginoscopic (or "no touch") technique of hysteroscopy was developed by Bettocchi and Selvaggi in 1995 and describes a method of office hysteroscopy that does not require a vaginal speculum or cervical tenaculum [1]. This technique has been studied against the traditional office hysteroscopy and has been shown to be effective: reported procedural times are faster [25] and procedural pain scores are reduced [26] when compared to traditional office hysteroscopy. This technique avoids the need to both introduce the vaginal speculum to visualize the cervix and place the single tooth tenaculum to grasp the cervix. Bettocchi has noted that this approach "requires a good knowledge of anatomy and of the instrumentation, as well as dexterity on the part of the operator" [27]. While this technique has been described using rigid hysteroscopy, flexible hysteroscopy may be used with this approach as well.

As with the traditional approach, assure initial steps of patient evaluation, consent, time out, and equipment setup are in place. With the patient in the dorsal lithotomy position, no speculum is placed. Instead, the hysteroscope is placed into the lower vagina followed by initiation of distention with saline (or CO_2) within the vagina. Since the vaginal axis is generally directed posteriorly, the saline will accumulate in the posterior vaginal fornix and allow for subsequent vaginal distention. Then the hysteroscope may be advanced toward the cervix and the external cervical ostium is visualized and the scope is guided into the endocervix *without* the use of a tenaculum. Distention of the endocervical canal will then allow the hysteroscope to be directed through the internal os into the uterine cavity. Survey of the uterine cavity and the remainder of the procedure is the same as described above in the traditional approach.

Complications of Office Diagnostic Hysteroscopy

Office hysteroscopy is a safe procedure but it is not without complications. There have been many studies that have reviewed complications associated with hysteroscopic surgery, but many of these have been studies of procedures done in a hospital or ASC and have included operative hysteroscopies: these have been shown to have increased risks due to potential complications with larger sizes of hysteroscopes needed to perform the surgeries as well as those associated with increased quantities of distention media and use of surgical energy during hysteroscopic surgery [28]. Office diagnostic hysteroscopy, however, is a safe procedure with few minor complications: Naegele et al. estimated an overall morbidity from outpatient diagnostic hysteroscopy at 2.3 % [2]. These complications include pain during and after, vasovagal episodes, uterine perforation and distention media complications (both saline and CO_2).

While diagnostic office hysteroscopy is generally very well tolerated, occurrence of pain during and after the procedure has been documented and studied. There is a wide variation on quoted rates of pain from 0.1 % with "severe pain" [2] to 16.5 % [18] with rigid traditional hysteroscopy. A recent meta-analysis showed that the vaginoscopic or "no-touch" technique of office hysteroscopy has a significant reduction in pain compared to the traditional hysteroscopy using a speculum and/or cervical tenaculum [26] and Bettocchi et al. reported that the vagnoscopic technique used on over 11,000 patients, only 0.9 % described pain [24]. When using flexible hysteroscopy, results have been similar with Bradley reporting 3.6 % incidence of "intolerable" pain in an observational trial of office-based flexible diagnostic hysteroscopic procedures [15]. One aspect of use of carbon dioxide for distention in either rigid or flexible diagnostic hysteroscopy is the incidence of shoulder pain associated with this medium. Post procedural pain is typically managed with nonsteroidal medications and rarely are narcotic medications needed.

Vasovagal episode is likely the most common complication of office-based diagnostic hysteroscopy. It occurs in approximately 0.5–2.3 % [18, 29] with increased risk associated with use of a rigid hysteroscope (1.9 %) and with CO_2 as the distention medium (2.3 %). Use of smaller caliber hysteroscopes (3.5 mm or less) as well as use of local anesthesia can reduce the risk [30, 31]. Treatment of vasovagal episodes is supportive; use of ammonia or other noxious inhalants is rarely needed and only if syncope occurs.

Uterine perforation is also a recognized but rare complication of office-based hysteroscopy. There are few studies looking specifically at office-based procedures but most studies of diagnostic hysteroscopy done in the operating room finds a risk of uterine perforation at 0.13–1.2 % [32]. With all likelihood, the risk of uterine perforation may be lower in office-based procedures. Also, similar to perforation is the risk of cervical trauma related to cannulation of the external, or more commonly, the internal cervical os from office hysteroscopy. While the true incidence of this is uncertain, it is a potential complication either from the hysteroscope or from a cervical dilator or "os finder" which may cause inadvertent bleeding upon cervical entry. Also, creation of a false passage may occur during initial dilatation of the cervix or at the time of hysteroscopic entry, especially in a cervix affected by stenosis, scarring, nulliparity or significant postmenopausal state.

Both cervical trauma and false passage creation may be lessened by "priming" or pretreating the cervix in the hours to days before the office procedure. Use of misoprostol has been shown to improve cervical dilatation and decrease resistance upon cervical entry [17, 18]; dosing was previously discussed in the "Patient Preparation" section. Also, use of laminaria placed the day prior to surgery will also help to provide mechanical dilation of the cervix but should be avoided in patients with an iodine or shellfish allergy. If perforation is encountered during a diagnostic hysteroscopy, identification of and observation of the perforation should be undertaken to evaluate bleeding. If no operative instruments or electrical energy was used, cessation of the procedure and patient observation, either in office or in hospital, should be considered. If there is a suspicion of active bleeding or injury to a vital pelvic organ, immediate transfer to a hospital with necessary hematologic and imaging modalities used to evaluate the patient. Laparoscopy or laparotomy should be considered if the patient becomes unstable. Lastly, external trauma to the stroma of the vaginal portion of the cervix may be encountered with use of a single tooth tenaculum, especially during difficult cervical entry or with a severely an anteverted or retroverted uterus. Treatment with silver nitrate or placement of a suture may be required to stop bleeding if encountered.

Bleeding during in-office surgery may be encountered either due to cervical trauma, uterine perforation or from disruption of the endometrium during the procedure. Rarely does the procedure need to be stopped but if such bleeding occurs, identification and treatment of the source of bleeding should be undertaken before discharging the patient from the office. There is a small chance of infection from office-based diagnostic hysteroscopy. The exact incidence is unknown, again due to few solely office-based studies but it is also unlikely in absence of patient risk factors due to the relatively short time it takes to perform office diagnostic hysteroscopy, the small amount of distending media used and absence of concomitant operative or energy related procedures. Loffer notes that infection is seldom a concern when strictly considering diagnostic hysteroscopy as many studies do not report such complications but notes an estimate of 0.2 % [33]. While ACOG does not recommend prophylactic antibiotics, in patients with a history of PID or significant hydrosalpinx, consideration of pre- and post-procedure antibiotics can reduce the risk of development of post hysteroscopy tubo-ovarian abscess [34] though these cases were associated with operative and not diagnostic, hysteroscopic surgery.

Complications associated with distention media in office diagnostic hysteroscopy are few and infrequent (estimated to be between 0.2 and 1.1 %0 [32, 33] but require diligence and effective office-based protocols to first prevent and secondly, recognize and treat if they occur. In-office diagnostic hysteroscopy will utilize physiologic solutions (such as physiologic saline or lactated ringers) or carbon dioxide gas almost exclusively. The cost and ease of use make these good options for office-based diagnostic procedures. Use of carbon dioxide is safe and embolization of CO_2 in small amounts is not dangerous [33]. Increased instillation pressure (greater than 60 mmHg) and flow rates will increase the risk of intravasation of the gas which may lead to severe or fatal carbon dioxide embolism. This is treated by immediate cessation of the procedure, ventilation support, placing the patient on her left side with immediate transfer to a hospital for further management. When using saline, air embolism can occur and the risk may be decreased by purging all air from the hysteroscopic tubing before beginning the procedure. Also, avoiding steep Trendelenberg position (where the uterus may be elevated over the heart) will decrease this risk: rarely is this position needed in office-based diagnostic procedures. Lastly, while physiologic solutions used in the office setting are safe, rare cases of increased fluid intravasation may lead to fluid overload with resultant pulmonary edema and congestive heart failure [35]. This complication, while less likely during short office-based cases, can be avoided by monitoring fluid deficits during surgery and stopping the procedure if the deficit reaches 1,500 mL of physiologic fluid. Post procedural monitoring of vital signs in office is strongly encouraged if such an event occurs and prompt evaluation of any pulmonary symptoms such as shortness of breath occurs.

Tips and Tricks for Office Diagnostic Hysteroscopy

1. *Practice Specific Technique*: Prior to transitioning to the office, perform diagnostic hysteroscopy in an OR or ASC with only minimal anesthesia and or just a paracervical block to get acclimated to your technique. Also, use of a hysteroscopic simulator can help to provide practice for the technique prior to undertaking office surgery.
2. *Patient Selection*: Selecting patients who easily tolerate pelvic examination or previous endometrial biopsy or colposcopy are likely good candidates for office hysteroscopy. Also, patients with significant anxiety may be better served in an operating theater though mild anxiety may be overcome with oral medication 1 h prior to the procedure (see Chap. 4: Anesthesia and Analgesia). Also, the first two to three patients who undergo office surgery should be those who are well known by the surgeon and staff.

3. *Timing of the procedure*: Office hysteroscopy may be performed at any time but typically in the first 1–2 weeks after cessation of menses will allow for best visualization.
4. *Show her the hysteroscope*: Certainly the scope is long but stress how small the *tip* is: smaller than a pencil but just larger than the tip of a pen. This will help to allay potential anxiety.
5. *"Vocal Local"*: During the procedure, having the nurse or assistant talk to or converse with the patient while the procedure is ongoing. This will distract the patient from portions of the procedure so as to decrease her anxiety and possibly her discomfort. Also, allow her to view the monitor as seeing the procedure may also improve a patient's experience.
6. *After the Procedure*: Go over any pathology, if found. Assess any pain, discomfort, and anxiety and treat accordingly. Go over post-procedure instructions and be certain the office staff knows to take any post-procedure phone calls seriously: post-operative phone calls from the patient means she is concerned and you and your staff should be as well.
7. *Elicit Feedback*: Both from the patients and from your staff. Find out what helps the patients and build on that. Track outcomes and complications and assess how to improve.

Conclusion

Diagnostic hysteroscopy is an ideal tool to use to diagnose a myriad of menstrual concerns, infertility questions, and uterine conditions. Performing this as an office-based procedure is safe and effective and can provide needed diagnostic information, with the possibility of concomitant operative procedures as needed. Establishing this procedure in the gynecology office can also be the gateway to advanced hysteroscopic procedures such as in-office sterilization. Both traditional and vaginoscopic techniques are associated with minimal pain and few complications.

References

1. Bettocchi S, Selvaggi L. A vaginoscopic approach to reduce the pain of office hysteroscopy. J Am Assoc Gynecol Laparosc. 1997;4:255–8.
2. Nagele F, O'Connor H, Davies A, et al. 2500 outpatient diagnostic hysteroscopies. Obstet Gynecol. 1996;88:87–92.
3. Epstein E, Ramirez A, Skook L, et al. Dilation and curettage fails to detect most focal lesions in the uterine cavity in women with postmenopausal bleeding. Acta Obstet Gynecol Scand. 2001;80:1131–6.
4. Munro MG, Critchley HOD, Broder MS, et al. FIGO classification system (PALM-COEIN) for causes of abnormal uterine bleeding in nongravid women of reproductive age. Int J Gynecol Obstet. 2011;113:3–13.
5. Bradley LD. Indications and contraindications for office hysteroscopy. Chapter 3. In: Bradley LD, Falcone T, editors. Hysteroscopy: office evaluation and management of the uterine cavity. Philadelphia, PA: Mosby; 2009.
6. Park AJ, Bohrer JC, Bradley LD, et al. Incidence and risk factors for surgical intervention after uterine artery embolization. Am J Obstet Gynecol. 2008;199:671.e1–6.
7. Bradley LD. Hysteroscopic sterilization, Chapter 8. In: Bradley LD, Falcone T, editors. Hysteroscopy: office evaluation and management of the uterine cavity. Philadelphia, PA: Mosby; 2009.
8. Guido RS, Kanbour-Shakir A, Rulin MC, et al. Pipelle endometrial sampling. Sensitivity in the detection of endometrial cancer. J Reprod Med. 1995;40:553–5.
9. Stovall TG, Photopulos GJ, Poston WM, et al. Pipelle endometrial sampling in patients with known endometrial cancer. Obstet Gynecol. 1991;77:954–6.
10. Love CD, Muir BB, Scrimgeour JB, et al. Investigation of endometrial abnormalities in asymptomatic women treated with tamoxifen and an evaluation of the role of endometrial screening. J Clin Oncol. 1999;17:2050–4.
11. Perez-Medina T, Salazar FJ, San-Frutos E, et al. Hysteroscopic dynamic assessment of endometrium in patients treated with long-term tamoxifen. J Minim Invasive Gynecol. 2011;18:349–54.
12. Mouritas MJ, Van der Zee AGJ, Willemse PHB, et al. Discrepancy between ultrasonography and hysteroscopy and histology of endometrium in postmenopausal breast cancer patients using tamoxifen. Gynecol Oncol. 1999;73:21–6.
13. Emery JD, Falcone T. Effects of drugs on the uterus, Chapter 8. In: Baggish MS, Valle RF, Guedj H, editors. Hysteroscopy: visual perspectives of uterine anatomy, physiology and pathology. 3rd ed. Philadelphia, PA: Lippincott Williams & Wilkins; 2007.

14. Vuento MH, Pirhonen JP, Makinen JI, et al. Endometrial fluid accumulation in asymptomatic postmenopausal women. Ultrasound Obstet Gynecol. 1996;8:37–41.
15. Bradley LD, Widrich T. State-of-the-art flexible hysteroscopy for office gynecologic evaluation. J Am Assoc Gynecol Laparosc. 1995;2:263–7.
16. El-Mazny A, Abou-Salem N. A double-blind randomized controlled trial of vaginal misoprostol for cervical priming before outpatient hysteroscopy. Fertil Steril. 2011;96:962–5.
17. Ngai WS, Chan YM, Liu KL, et al. Oral misoprostol for cervical priming in non-pregnant women. Hum Reprod. 1997;12:2373–5.
18. DeIaco P, Marabini A, Stefannetti M, et al. Acceptability and pain of outpatient hysteroscopy. J Am Assoc Gynecol Laparosc. 2000;7:71–5.
19. Bradner P, Neis KJ, Ehmer C. The etiology, frequency, and prevention of gas embolism during CO2 hysteroscopy. J Am Assoc Gynecol Laparosc. 1999;6:421–8.
20. Brusco GF, Arena S, Angelini A. Use of carbon dioxide versus normal saline for diagnostic hysteroscopy. Fertil Steril. 2003;79:993–7.
21. Pellicano M, Guida M, Lavitola G, et al. Carbon dioxide versus normal saline as a uterine distension medium for diagnostic vaginoscopic hysteroscopy in infertile patients: a prospective randomized multicenter study. Fertil Steril. 2003;79:418–21.
22. AAGL Advancing Minimally Invasive Gynecology Worldwide. Munro MG, Storz K, Abbott JA, et al. AAGL practice report: practice guidelines for management of hysteroscopic distending media. J Minim Invasive Gynecol. 2013;20:137–48.
23. Valle RF. Office hysteroscopy. Chapter 17. In: Baggish MS, Valle RF, Guedj H, editors. Hysteroscopy: visual perspectives of uterine anatomy, physiology and pathology. 3rd ed. Philadelphia, PA: Lippincott Williams & Wilkins; 2007.
24. Bettocchi S, Nappi L, Ceci O, et al. Office hysteroscopy. Obstet Gynecol Clin N Am. 2004;31:641–54.
25. Sharma M, Taylor A, di Spiezio Sardo A, et al. Outpatient hysteroscopy: traditional *versus* the 'no-touch' technique. BJOG. 2005;112:963–7.
26. Cooper NA, Smith P, Khan KS, et al. Vaginoscopic approach to outpatient hysteroscopy: a systematic review of the effect on pain. BJOG. 2010;117:532–9.
27. Bettochhi S, Di Spiezio SA, Ceci O. Instrumentation in office hysteroscopy: rigid hysteroscopy. Chapter 1. In: Bradley LD, Falcone T, editors. Hysteroscopy: office evaluation and management of the uterine cavity. Philadelphia, PA: Mosby Inc.; 2009.
28. Propst AM, Liberman RF, Harlow BL, et al. Complications of hysteroscopic surgery: predicting patients at risk. Obstet Gynecol. 2000;96:517–20.
29. Agostini A, Bretelle F, Ronda I, et al. Risk of vasovagal syndrome during outpatient hysteroscopy. J Am Assoc Gynecol Laparosc. 2004;11:245–7.
30. Cicinelli E, Didonna T, Ambrosi G, et al. Topical anaesthesia for diagnostic hysteroscopy and endometrial biopsy in postmenopausal women: a randomised placebo-controlled double blind study. BJOG. 1997;104:316–9.
31. Cicinelli E, Schonauer LM, Barba B, et al. Tolerability and cardiovascular complications of outpatient diagnostic minihysteroscopy compared with conventional hysteroscopy. J Am Assoc Gynecol Laparosc. 2003;10:399–402.
32. Jansen FW, Vredevoogd CB, Ulzen K, et al. Complications for hysteroscopic surgery: a prospective, multicenter study. Obstet Gynecol. 2000;96:266–70.
33. Loffer FD. Complications of hysteroscopy—their cause, prevention, and correction. J Am Assoc Gynecol Laparosc. 1995;3:11–26.
34. McClausland VM, Fields GA, McClausland AM, et al. Tubo-ovarian abscesses after operative hysteroscopy. J Reprod Med. 1993;38:198–200.
35. Emery J, Falcone T. Complications of hysteroscopic surgery, Chapter 20. In: Bradley LD, Falcone T, editors. Hysteroscopy: office evaluation and management of the uterine cavity. Philadelphia, PA: Mosby, Inc.; 2009.

Hysteroscopic Tubal Sterilization

8

Jonathan D. Emery

Introduction

Successful development of female sterilization using reliable hysteroscopic techniques has allowed for tubal sterilization to be moved from the operating room to the office setting. Since 2002 in the United States [1, 2], hysteroscopic sterilization methods have been Food and Drug Association (FDA) approved and continued development of this technique has permitted performance in the office. Advantages of hysteroscopic sterilization include minimal to no anesthesia, ability to perform the procedure in women with significant comorbid medical conditions as well as in women with multiple prior abdominal or pelvic surgeries. Introduction of hysteroscopic sterilization to the office setting has been shown to have minimal pain, a shorter recovery time with expedited return to normal activities as well as increased patient satisfaction [3, 4]. Arjona et al. reported that women undergoing the procedure believe that the most positive aspect of having in-office hysteroscopic sterilization was "the absence of the operating room" with almost 20 % of patients verifying it as a "quick and comfortable procedure" [5].

In the United States during the years 2006–2008, female surgical sterilization of any type was the second most common form of contraception utilized, closely following oral contraceptive pill: 17.3 % of women using the pill followed by 16.7 % choosing sterilization [6]. While the majority of female sterilization procedures in the United States are performed after delivery in the peripartum period, interval sterilization can now be performed in the office with the hysteroscopic technique rather than subjecting patients to the surgical risks of laparoscopy. Effectiveness of female sterilization as quoted by the CREST data is very high (cumulative 10-year probability of pregnancy post tubal ligation was 18.5 per 1,000 procedures) [7] and it appears, based on recent data, that effectiveness of hysteroscopic sterilization is similar or even better than tubal ligation. Both the Essure Pivotal Trial and the Phase II trial [1, 2] reported zero pregnancies in 643 women who did not report pregnancy in the follow-up period. Others, however, have reported pregnancies following transcervical sterilization with one author estimating effectiveness at 99.74 % for preventing pregnancy [8, 9].

Historical Perspective

In the United States, hysteroscopic sterilization has been an approved technique by the United States Food and Drug Association (FDA) since 2002. That year, the Essure™ Permanent Birth Control System (Conceptus, Mountain View, CA) was approved for use in the United States.

J.D. Emery, M.D., F.A.C.O.G. (✉)
Department of Obstetrics & Gynecology,
Women's Health Institute, Cleveland Clinic,
2550 SOM Center Road, Suite 100, Willoughby Hills,
OH 44094, USA
e-mail: emeryj@ccf.org

J.D. Emery and M.F.R. Paraiso (eds.), *Office-Based Gynecologic Surgical Procedures*,
DOI 10.1007/978-1-4939-1414-2_8, © Springer Science+Business Media New York 2015

Subsequently, in 2009, the Adiana® Permanent Contraception system (Hologic™, Inc., Malborough, MA) was approved for use in the United States for hysteroscopic sterilization as well but was discontinued for use by the manufacturer in 2012. Thus, hysteroscopic sterilization in the office today consists of use of the Essure™ system.

Prior to 2002, attempts at transcervical or hysteroscopic sterilization had been attempted by a variety of methods including chemical (quinacrine hydrochloride), electrosurgical, and multiple mechanical (silicone, polyethylene, nylon, and polytetrafluoroethylene) techniques [10]. These previous methods were felt to have increased failure rates due to tubal migration or expulsion or incomplete tubal occlusion. Cooper had emphasized the need for an implant or device to be anchored in the uterine portion of the fallopian tube as it is less compliant and serves as an ideal location to anchor an implant [10]. Both the Essure™ and Adiana® systems accomplished this requirement by placing mechanical inserts in the uterotubal junction: the Adiana system utilizes insertion of polymer matrix after inducing thermal injury to uterotubal junction while the Essure™ system places a metal–polymer insert at this critical anatomic location.

The Essure™ microinsert is a metal–polymer combination consisting of an inner coil of polyethylene terephthalate (PET) fibers admixed with stainless steel and an outer coil of nickel–titanium (nitinol) (Fig. 8.1). Once placed, this microinsert elicits a local tissue inflammatory response which causes tissue in-growth, fibrosis, and subsequent tubal occlusion over a 6–12 week period [11]. As the Adiana system is no longer available in the United States since May 2012, the remainder of this chapter will focus on data and techniques of the Essure™ system.

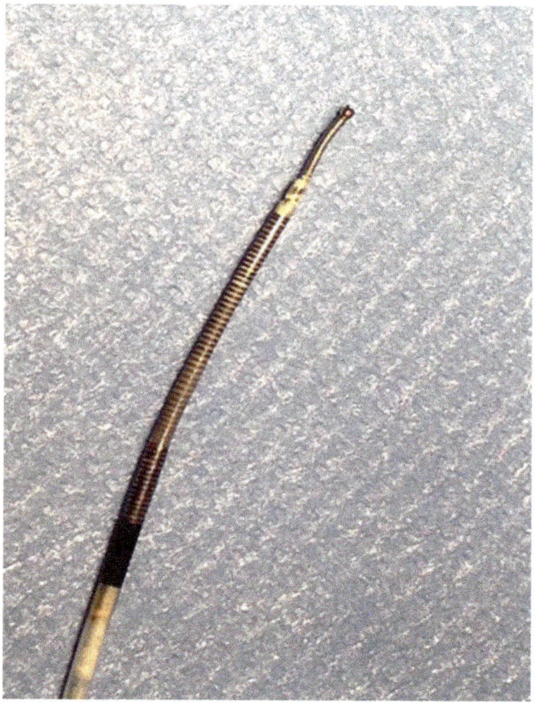

Fig. 8.1 Tip of Essure™ delivery catheter with loaded nitinol microcoil insert

In-Office Application

Since FDA approval of a device for transcervical sterilization in 2002, the number of tubal sterilizations accomplished by the hysteroscopic approach has increased significantly, mostly at the expense of laparoscopic sterilization. It has been reported at one institution that laparoscopic sterilization decreased significantly over a 5-year period with the introduction of hysteroscopic sterilization, such that after 5 years, the hysteroscopic approach was more common than laparoscopic tubal ligation, 51–49 % [12]. While this shift has not yet occurred nationally at this time, physician adoption of and patient acceptance of hysteroscopic sterilization is increasing.

This increase in utilization of the Essure procedure has been accelerated by transfer of the technique from the operating room (OR) or ambulatory surgery center (ASC) to the office setting. In-office gynecologic surgical procedures are increasing in number, led by the adoption of this technique. In order for any surgical procedure to be transferred from the OR/ASC to the office, both physician and patient factors must be considered and be shown to equal to or supersede statistics of the same procedure when performed in OR or ASC. This has been the case with hysteroscopic sterilization.

Factors that affect physician adoption of this technique in the office include the procedure's ease of use. For hysteroscopic sterilization, this would encompass ease of placement of the microcoils, overall procedure time, minimizing procedural complications, and cost of the procedure in-office. More important, however, are the factors affecting the patient's experience of having the procedure done in the office versus in the operative setting. For hysteroscopic sterilization these include, but are not limited to, minimizing pain and discomfort, decreasing inconvenience, faster return to normal activities and overall satisfaction with the procedure.

Prior to considering performance of the procedure in-office, however, the physician must be adequately trained on and familiar with the procedure as performed in the operating room or ASC. Proper operative experience with hysteroscopic sterilization will ensure a smooth transition to the office once the surgeon has gained appropriate knowledge and skill with the procedure in order to anticipate and manage perioperative, intraoperative, and post-procedural problems and complications. While a surgeon may have "privileges" to perform the procedure in the OR/ASC setting, this does not equate to clinical competence. The granting of privileges is based on satisfactory training, experience and demonstration of contemporary clinical competence [13]. Achieving clinical competence has been studied and it has been suggested that in order to gain competence with a procedure, the surgeon should have performed a minimum of 20–25 procedures. Thus, performance of an adequate number of operative hysteroscopic sterilization procedures in the OR/ASC should be mandated prior to the transition of the skill to the office setting. Also, the surgeon should be certain to practice good clinical judgment as to which patients will be most successfully treated with in-office sterilization versus those who should undergo hysteroscopic (or even laparoscopic) sterilization in the setting of the ASC or operating room with adequate anesthesia and postoperative monitoring. For instance, patients who have difficulty with standard speculum or pelvic exams, patients with significant anxiety disorders and patients with "low pain tolerance" should be considered for surgical sterilization with anesthesia.

Data supporting transfer of this technique to the office setting has been well documented in recent years. From the physician perspective, ease of use has been established primarily through prospective clinical trials. Review of in-office procedures shows the placement rate of the coils in both tubal ostia ranges from 89 [14] to 98.6 % [3]. These placement rates compare favorably with the Phase III trial which showed a placement rate of 92 % [1]. One study noted that the placement failure rate was higher in the first 25 % of cases performed in-office during the study period [3], suggesting that as operator experience increases, placement rates may improve, correlating with a "learning curve" effect. This effect is also seen when considering time to perform the procedure. Studies have shown a range of time of procedure from 6.8 to 12.4 min [3, 15] with Levie noting a learning curve effect after the first 13 cases. Overall, when the procedure is done in-office, the complication rate is very low, ranging from 0 to 5 % for procedural complications [5, 14–16] with several studies noting a very small rate of vasovagal related incidents, being reported at 1–5 %. One study looked at the surgeon's perception of difficulty with the procedure and 85 % noted the procedure to be of low to medium difficulty [3]. Placement rates and procedural difficulties were noted in several studies to be correlated with uterine and endometrial anatomic changes as well as tubal spasm. Lastly, once the procedure is completed, tubal occlusion rates as shown on hysterosalpingography (HSG) range from 98 to 100 % in published studies of the in-office procedure [14, 15].

The patient experience with any minimally invasive procedure should be equal to or superior to the more standard techniques and application of in-office hysteroscopic sterilization has been shown to be well accepted by patients. Several studies have reviewed patient's perception of pain; while the scales used to assess pain have differed, all have shown pain to be at the level of or less than the pain experienced during that woman's menstrual cycle. Levie et al. showed a rate of 70 % for perception of pain less than a menstrual cycle and Mino et al. reported that 84 % of women experienced "little or no discomfort" during the procedure [3, 17]. While studies varied in assessments of pain, several reviewed patients use of pain medication associated with the in-office procedure with one study showing that only 9 % of patients took any pain medication following the procedure [3] and another study showed only 17 % of patients were given pain medication after the procedure [14]. Both of these findings are superior to the Phase III trial where 25 % of patients received post-procedural pain medication [1]. Several studies assessed patients "return to normal activities" which was 84 % on the day of the procedure [3] to 100 % within 24 h of the procedure [14]. Finally, overall patient satisfaction was evaluated in the post-procedure period by varying methods, with 94–100 % of patients expressing high satisfaction with the Essure procedure [3, 5, 14, 16, 18]. Again, these findings show high correlation with the Phase III trial which reported that 98 % of women in that study were satisfied or very satisfied, when questioned on follow-up studies [1]. Interestingly, Sinha et al. reported that on post-procedure questionnaire, the most common reason for choosing Essure method of sterilization in their in-office trial was "the desire to avoid general anaesthetic" in 72 % of patients followed by avoidance of surgical incisions (59 %) and lack of hospital stay (50 %) [16].

Lastly, the cost advantage of in-office female sterilization has been demonstrated in studies [19, 20]. Cost advantages for the in-office procedure versus laparoscopic sterilization in the operating room or ASC are incurred due primarily due to the absence of the operating room and associated anesthesia charges—both pharmacologic and personnel-related. The primary in-office expense needs for the procedure include costs associated with the disposable microinserts as well as for the office hysteroscopic equipment and maintenance. Levie and Chudnoff [19] performed a detailed cost analysis which included evaluation of the office hysteroscope and associated equipment including the tower stand, video monitor, light source and cable, video printer, and camera. Their analysis assumed that the equipment was used for sterilizations only at a rate of 100 sterilization procedures/year and included added costs for maintenance. Their estimate was for $325 per-procedure hysteroscope cost. Obviously, costs could be lowered by performing more procedures and by utilizing the equipment for other office-based hysteroscopic procedures, both diagnostic and therapeutic (see Chaps. 7 and 9).

Patient related costs can be lowered by the office procedure which may reduce patient and insurance expenses. Also, physician related costs can be lowered due to ease of scheduling (including no need for travel time to hospital or ASC).

Patient Preparation

Prior to having the patient arrive on the day of the procedure, several factors should be addressed with her before hysteroscopic sterilization should proceed. These include pre-procedural counseling about both sterilization and the hysteroscopic procedure itself, endometrial preparation and post-procedural concerns.

Initial screening in the office must include screening for appropriateness of the patient to have the procedure performed: a list on contraindications for the procedure is listed in Table 8.1. When discussing sterilization with the patient, assessing the patient's readiness for the procedure is important. If there are concerns about future fertility, suggesting long-acting reversible contraception (LARC) would be recommended. The American College of Obstetricians and Gynecologists (ACOG) recommends all patients undergoing sterilization be counseled on "risk of regret" [21]. This is due to a documented incidence of regret after sterilization of up to 20 % [22]. This is more common among women under age 30 and in those with less than two children, amongst others; women over age 40 have been shown to have the least regret.

Table 8.1 Contraindications to hysteroscopic sterilization

• Pregnancy or suspected pregnancy
• Use within 6 (six) weeks of delivery or pregnancy termination or miscarriage
• Desire for future fertility and/or uncertainty about whether to be sterilized
• Previous tubal ligation or other tubal surgery, such as treatment for ectopic pregnancy
• Current active or recent upper or lower pelvic infection, including herpes simplex infection
• Patients in whom only one microcoil can be placed due to
– Contralateral proximal tubal occlusion or spasm
– Unicornuate uterus or bicornuate uterus with inaccessible rudimentary horn
– Lateral tubal ostium anatomic location
– Severe intrauterine adhesions preventing access to tubal ostia
• Known allergy to contrast dye
• Inability to return for 3-month HSG

(Adapted from Conceptus Incorporated. Essure: instructions for use. Mountain View (CA): Conceptus Inc.; 2012. Available at: http://www.essuremd/Portals/essuremd/PDFs/TopDownloads/Essure%20IFU.pdf. Retrieved October 10, 2013)

Also, counseling on the risk of future pregnancy after in-office sterilization should be discussed. This counseling is predicated on the fact that the patient undergoes the 3-month confirmation HSG showing bilateral tubal occlusion. In the CREST study of tubal ligation performed by all methods, risk of pregnancy following tubal ligation was 1.85 % (cumulative 10 year rate for all types of tubal sterilization) [7]. Published failure rates with hysteroscopic sterilization have been similar. In patients followed from the Phase II and III trials, the manufacturer of the Essure system claims a 0 % pregnancy rate on participants in their study [1, 2]. Recent case reports and other studies have shown that pregnancies do occur after the procedure, even in those who have completed appropriate confirmation with HSG [23, 24] though these studies suggest misinterpretation of HSG may play a role. The crude pregnancy rate has been reported to be between 0.1 and 0.2 % with Essure [25, 26] with Munro et al. suggesting an age-adjusted effectiveness of the procedure of 99.74 % at 5 years [8]. The patient should be notified of this rate prior to the procedure. Reports of ectopic pregnancies following Essure sterilization have been reported in the manufacturer and user facility device experience (MAUDE) database [27], so counseling about possible ectopic pregnancy if sterilization failure occurs is important.

Informed consent for the procedure is also recommended to be accomplished prior to the day of the procedure but may be accomplished just before the procedure itself if adequate counseling was performed beforehand. A full description of and details incumbent of Informed Consent are detailed in Chap. 3. The five main points to discuss before any procedure include: (1) Risks of the actual procedure, (2) Benefits of the procedure, (3) Alternatives to the procedure, (4) Complications of the procedure and (5) Personnel involved during the procedure. Items especially pertinent to hysteroscopic in-office include possibility of the inability to place the microcoils either due to inadequate visualization or tubal spasm, pain with endometrial insufflation and with tubal microcoil placement and possibility of inadequate occlusion on HSG. Benefits, while seemingly self-explanatory with a sterilization procedure also include ability to assess the endometrium for any undiagnosed pathology. Alternatives include other forms of sterilization including laparoscopic tubal sterilization and male partner sterilization, if acceptable. Also, the alternative of performing the procedure in the OR or ASC should also be discussed and offered to the patient if she has concerns about undergoing the procedure in the office, whether real or perceived. Surgical complications to hysteroscopic sterilization are listed below and should be explained.

Lastly, office personnel who will be assisting during the procedure and recovery in the office should be reviewed and introduced prior to the procedure as well.

Optimally, informed consent should be reviewed at a time prior to the actual procedure. This is also a good time to be certain the patient has adequate endometrial preparation for the procedure as well as review the need for contraception before having the confirmatory HSG. This is of utmost importance as one of the two most important aspects of in-office sterilization is the ability to see and access the tubal ostia (the other being minimizing patient discomfort). Therefore, scheduling the patient during the early proliferative phase of her menstrual cycle is important or having the patient undergo medical treatment to ensure endometrial thinning may also be considered. Hormonal management with combination oral contraceptive pills, progestin-only contraceptives (pill, injection or subdermal) or progesterone containing intrauterine systems are all considered appropriate prior to female sterilization. All will allow for development of endometrial thinning due to atrophy: a pale, thin endometrial cavity will allow for maximal visualization of the tubal ostia and increase successful microcoil placement (Fig. 8.2). Also, instituting these therapies prior to the procedure visit allows these therapies to be utilized for contraception in the 3-month period until the confirmatory HSG can be performed.

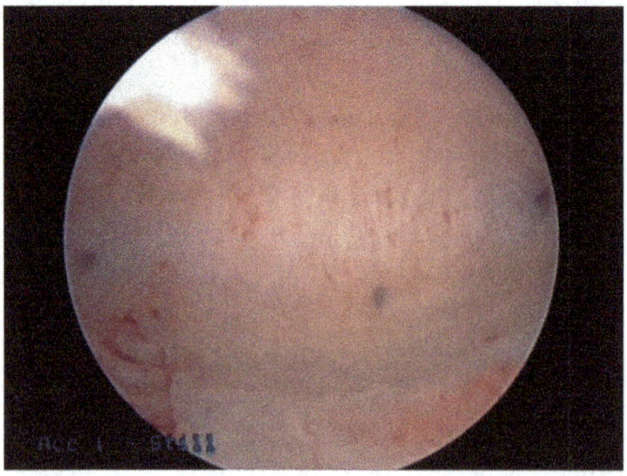

Fig. 8.2 Endometrial atrophy with uniform pale endometrium at uterine fundus showing both tubal ostia

Pretreatment with medications before arriving at the office is important to consider. Having the patient take a pre-procedure dose of ibuprofen 600–800 mg (or other equivalent nonsteroidal anti-inflammatory drug (NSAID)) orally approximately 1 h before the procedure is encouraged. For patients with anxiety concerns, consideration of oral benzodiazepine may also be prescribed; in this case, signing any informed consent documents should have taken place prior to this time. Misoprostol is an effective medication to consider for assistance in cervical ripening prior to any hysteroscopic surgery, in-office or otherwise. Misoprostol is a prostaglandin E1 analogue which has been shown in studies to be effective at promoting cervical preparation before procedures with a decreased need for cervical dilatation and decreased operative times as well [28, 29]. Note that misoprostol used in this fashion is an "off-label" indication from FDA guidelines and consideration should be given to informing patients of this off-label use if misoprostol is prescribed.

Procedural issues that should be discussed prior to the in-office technique include those inherent to the procedure itself. Encountering unexpected endometrial pathology when entering the endometrium may be a cause of obstruction of one or both of the tubal ostia. This may not allow for placement of the microcoils or make the cannulation of the ostium technically difficult. Some have recommended a preoperative saline infusion sonogram or office hysteroscopy be considered prior to sterilization in patients with heavy, prolonged or irregular menses in order to diagnose and remove pathology so as to "avoid surprises at the time of the sterilization technique" [30]. Also, studies have demonstrated a high microcoil placement rate using the in-office technique [5, 15, 31] but there is a possibility of inability to place the microcoils due to pathology, unusual anatomy, tubal spasm, or patient discomfort. If patients are unable to have one or both microcoils placed, alternatives for contraception or alternative sterilization procedures should be discussed.

Post-procedural issues to review with the patient include that of pain relief, needs for back-up contraception and scheduling of the confirmation HSG. Many studies have shown the procedure to be well tolerated in-office with a minimum of pain relief as discussed previously. However, due to endometrial insufflation and tubal spasm, patients may experience pain at the time of and after the procedure. Most commonly, only oral NSAIDs may be needed after surgery but other medications may be considered relative to patient preference, allergies, or response to discomfort (see Chap. 4). The need for contraception is mentioned above and the contraceptive of choice should be ascertained from the patient. Lastly, scheduling the 3-month confirmatory HSG is strongly recommended before the patient leaves the office once the hysteroscopic microcoil application is completed. This works to establish a time for follow-up and to confirm tubal occlusion. Studies have shown that noncompliance with the HSG can lead to unintended pregnancies and that in certain patient populations, the follow-up rate for this can be as low as 13 % [32]. Therefore, assuring that the patient is able to return for the HSG is important because if she is unable to return to confirm occlusion, consideration of an alternative form of sterilization such as laparoscopic tubal ligation may be a more appropriate, though more invasive, procedure where sterilization is immediate. Also, as shown in the contraindications, it should be discussed at this time if the patient has a true allergy to contrast dye or iodine as she will not be able to undergo the HSG and should be offered alternative sterilization (laparoscopic) or long-acting contraception.

Lastly, performing the procedure in-office in patients who are utilizing an intrauterine device (IUD) for contraception can be easily performed. Placement of the microcoils can be performed with the IUD in place as demonstrated by several authors [33–35] but in some patients, the IUD may have to be removed in order to facilitate bilateral microcoil placement [34]. The IUD remains in place for 3 months and then can be removed either before or after HSG confirmation of bilateral tubal occlusion. It should be noted, however, that the manufacturer's Instructions for Use [11] excludes IUD use for contraception for the 3-month interval before confirmatory HSG though studies listed above have shown this to be a safe and reliable option.

Equipment and Personnel

Performance of hysteroscopic sterilization in the office requires some basic equipment needed for the performance of the procedure. Any small rigid hysteroscope, generally with an outer diameter of less than 6 mm can be utilized for the procedure, provided it has a continuous flow system (in-flow and out-flow channels) and a 5-Fr operating/biopsy channel (Fig. 8.3). Multiple brands of hysteroscopes are available in the market today, which meet these specifications, including newer "mini" hysteroscopes. Also, the hysteroscope should have a 12° or 30° lens so as to allow for easier lateral visualization of the tubal ostia. One author has recommended that included with the operative hysteroscope, having hysteroscopic graspers available is advised so that if unexpected pathology such as a polyp or a fragment of detached endometrium is encountered, it can be grasped and removed so that tubal cannulation may proceed. Also, graspers may be used to grasp a microcoil that is abnormally deployed and is free in the endometrial cavity. Lastly, "testing" the operating channel with the graspers prior to starting the actual procedure can be beneficial to ascertain that the channel is free from obstruction: this is important as damage to the tip of the microcoil during delivery through the operating channel can bend or damage the microcoil, thus making it unusable to place in the tubal ostia.

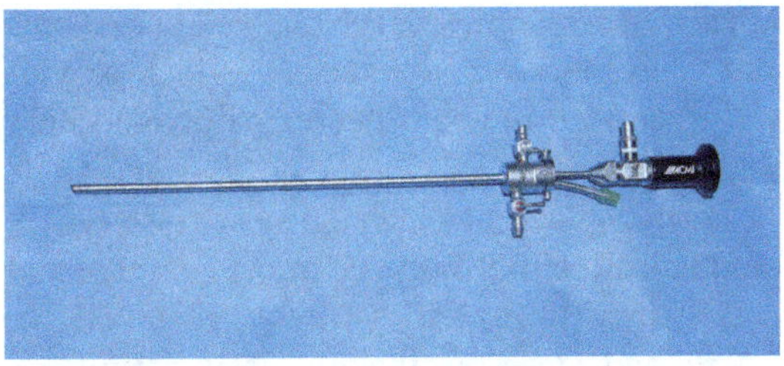

Fig. 8.3 Hysteroscope with 5 Fr operating channel

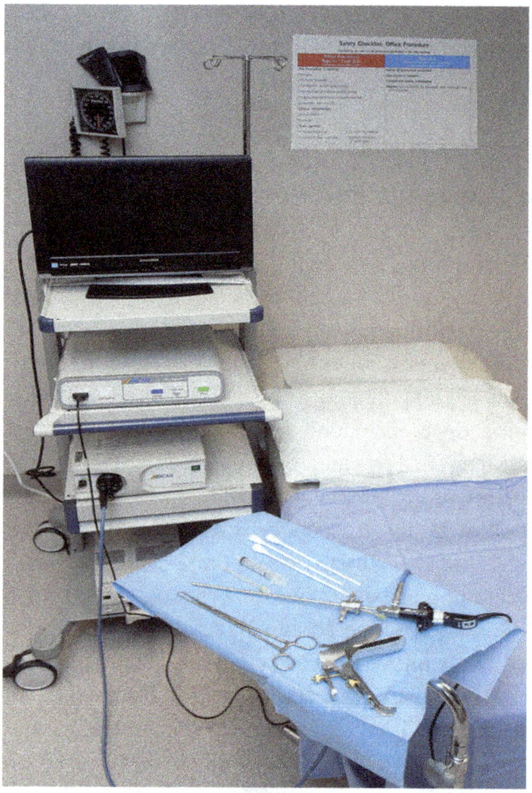

Fig. 8.4 Office setup for hysteroscopic sterilization with hysteroscope, ancillary equipment, and video and light tower

Associated equipment needed includes the light source or light generator and fiberoptic cable for illumination as well as a video camera and monitor in order to provide real time visualization; most come with photographic capabilities and as such, either a printer or computerized image storage system is recommended in order to document images of the microcoils deployed in the tubal ostia at the close of the procedure. Finally, the equipment is typically all placed on a cart or in sequence in a "tower" which is typically stationed in one office exam or procedure room (Fig. 8.4).

Lastly, a fluid management system is needed. Normal saline (0.9 %) is the most common and easiest fluid to use, with its low cost, relative safety, and clean-up, though lactated Ringer's solution may also be considered. Typically, 1 L or less is needed for the procedure as well as the appropriate tubing; warmed solution is recommended as it helps to minimize tubal spasm. Continuous flow systems are recommended to be used as they allow for attainment and maintenance of interuterine pressures of between 25 and 45 mmHg. A fluid management system to record media in-flow and out-flow is recommended as well. In absence of this system, a single flow sheath on the hysteroscope may be used, with the saline solution placed 1.5 m above the patient to provide adequate flow and endouterine pressure; also, others have used a medium-sized blood pressure cuff around a 1 L bag of saline with pressure applied to the bag in order to maintain flow. Both of these methods, however, do not allow for accurate measurement of flow of the media and may result in higher intrauterine pressures that increase intrauterine saline absorption during the procedure. AAGL recommends has issued recommendations for monitoring and management of distending media used in hysteroscopy; in terms of isotonic fluids used for hysteroscopic sterilization, "Excessive absorption of isotonic fluids such as normal saline can cause severe complications". Although isotonic fluids do not cause cerebral edema, there is still a mandate for continuous and accurate measurement of input and output for the calculation of fluid absorption [36].

Once the office has the appropriate equipment needed for performance of hysteroscopic procedures, the sterilization device is needed. As of 2013, there is currently one device available in the market. The third generation Essure™ system (ESS305) comes in a package of two [2] individually wrapped microinsert devices each with one microcoil insert within the disposable delivery catheter attached to an ergonomic hand piece and one disposable introducer. It is also recommended that the gynecologist be familiar with and read through the manufacturer's instructions included with the devices.

Lastly, necessary equipment and medication for local anesthetic are needed if a paracervical block or other local anesthetics are utilized. Some gynecologists will also add other oral or intravenous medications to their office protocols to assist in patient comfort or to decrease anxiety. Knowledge of the pharmacologic properties of these medications as well as awareness and compliance with national, state, and local government agencies regarding in-office medication is required. Details concerning this are found in Chap. 4.

Performing this female sterilization technique in the office requires a minimum of two people: the gynecologic surgeon and an assistant. The role of the assistant is to provide the sterilization catheters to the surgeon and help guide the tip into the operating channel when instructed. The assistant should wear sterile gloves and utilize sterile techniques as to mimic an operating room in the office procedure room. Some surgeons have found that a three-person team works more efficiently with a second assistant providing supplies and adjustment of the hysteroscopic equipment and attending to the patient as needed. Many times the second assistant can provide "vocal-local" anesthetic to the patient to decrease anxiety and at times distract her from the procedure as well.

Lastly, as with any in-office procedure, ensuring appropriate documentation of the procedure as well as the reference lot numbers of the microinserts is recommended. Having a standardized office procedure checklist is also recommended to reduce medical errors as well as to ensure patient safety. Consideration of annual quality review of this procedure as well as "mock drills" of complications with office staff is tantamount to patient safety. ACOG recommends application of activities and tools from the inpatient setting be applied to office-based procedures, such as team and office meetings, time-outs, checklists, mock drills, and measurement and reporting systems [37].

Procedure

Performance of the hysteroscopic procedure in the office setting should be done as similarly to how the procedure is performed in the operating room or ASC. Of course, transition from the operating room to the office requires that the gynecologist has been instructed about and performed a minimum number of cases in surgery before attempting to move the procedure to the office. As with any new procedure there is a learning curve, so that anticipation of potential problems should be undertaken to allow for ease of procedure in-office for both surgeon and patient. One suggestion is to perform the surgery in the OR or ASC with the patient receiving only "monitored anesthesia care" for several cases and utilizing the procedure as one would in the office. That way, the surgeon may gain the confidence needed to perform the procedure in the office setting.

The equipment needed to perform the procedure is listed in Table 8.2 and the steps of the procedure are listed in Table 8.3 but are reviewed here as well.

Once the patient is positioned accordingly in the office procedure room, standard procedural steps to place the speculum (an open sided speculum is recommended) and to visualize the cervix are undertaken. The cervix and vagina are cleansed with standard solution. A paracervical block may be placed at this time as outlined in Chap. 4. Once the block is placed, the surgeon should allow at least 5 min for the local anesthetic to set in. Then, a 5.5 mm or small rigid hysteroscope is introduced (with a 5-Fr or greater operating channel in place) using a physiologic saline solution through the cervix to allow adequate visualization of the endometrium. Avoiding cervical dilation or "sounding the uterus" if possible, as an undilated cervix will allow for greater uterine cavity distention. Measuring the uterine cavity may be undertaken prior to beginning hysteroscopy though it is the author's opinion that this is not necessary and may in fact damage or obscure one of the tubal ostia. Once inside the endometrial cavity, perform a panoramic and complete survey of the endometrial cavity, noting both tubal ostia and any pathology present. Also, at this time, be certain adequate endometrial insufflation pressure is present in order to allow for easier placement of the microcoils.

Table 8.2 Equipment needed for hysteroscopic sterilization

• Operative hysteroscope (12° or 30° lens) with 5 Fr operating channel with:
– Light source and light cord
– Camera and video monitor
• Hysteroscopic fluid (normal saline or lactated ringers) with appropriate tubing
• Appropriate draping to collection excess distending media
• Fluid monitoring system or measurement device to calculate fluid deficit
• Essure™ system (including two catheters with attached hand pieces and introducers) or other FDA-approved hysteroscopic sterilization system
• Speculum (one-sided speculum preferred)
• Cleansing solution for cervix
• Sterile gloves
Optional:
• Single toothed tenaculum
• Uterine sound or dilator
• Hysteroscopic grasper
• Equipment needed for paracervical or intracervical local anesthetic block (Chap. 4)

Table 8.3 Procedural steps for performing hysteroscopic sterilization with microcoil device

1. Obtain or confirm informed consent
2. Complete appropriate "Sign-In" or "Time-Out" protocols
3. Correctly position patient in lithotomy position
4. Place speculum and cleanse cervix
5. Place paracervical or intracervical block as appropriate (may skip previous two steps if performing the "Vaginscopic technique")
6. Perform hysteroscopy with insufflation and visualization of uterine cavity
7. Identify BOTH tubal ostia
8. Once ascertaining that BOTH ostia are visualized, have assistant open first catheter
9. Place introducer into operating channel
10. Insert first delivery catheter through working channel while visualizing tubal ostium
11. Be certain to slowly advance microcoil catheter once the tip is in view inside the uterine cavity: adjust the hysteroscope as needed while advancing the catheter into the tubal ostium
12. Advance the Essure™ catheter to the black positioning marker ("black line") and stabilize the hand piece
13. Rotate thumbwheel on the hand piece backwards to a hard stop: note that the black line moves toward the surgeon during this step
14. Verify correct position of the microcoil at this time the gold "notch" just outside the tubal ostium with the green catheter in view: adjust the hand piece slowly to reposition the catheter as needed
15. Depress the button on hand piece
16. Rotate the thumbwheel a second time to withdraw the internal guidewire and to fully deploy the microcoil and remove the hand piece from the working channel after the coils are expanded
17. Document the number of "trailing coils" in the uterine cavity and take video photos if needed: also record the lot number of the catheter in operative note
18. Repeat process for the remaining tube after adjusting the position of the hysteroscope to fully visualize the second tubal ostium
19. Record and document trailing coils and lot number for second tube
20. Remove hysteroscope and vaginal instruments/speculum after completion of procedure
21. Document operative note including any complications of the procedure or with equipment and if any patient related complications occurred

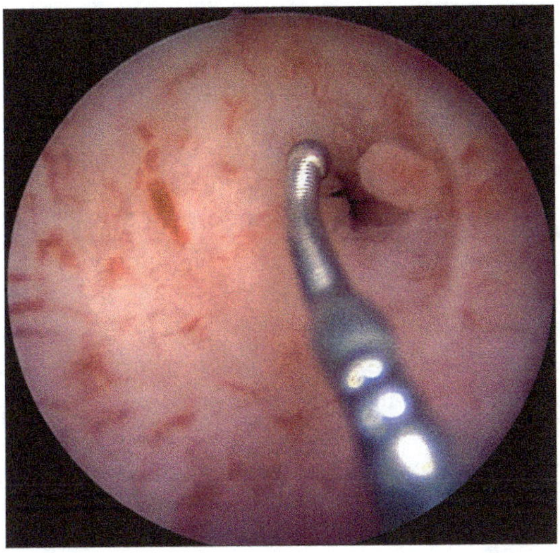

Fig. 8.5 Tip of delivery catheter about to enter tubal ostium

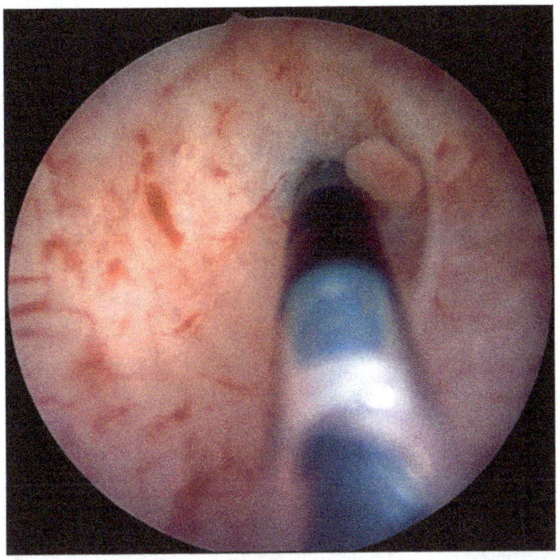

Fig. 8.6 "Black Line" on delivery catheter at correct position just outside tubal ostium

Once certain the tubal ostia are seen and easily accessible and that the patient will be able to tolerate the complete procedure, have the assistant open the first catheter. If however, the surgeon cannot ascertain that the procedure will be successful at this time, then the decision must be made at this point if the procedure can be completed with *both* tubal ostia treated. If so, then place the introducer into the working channel. Have your assistant then hand the tip of the catheter so it can easily be placed through the introducer and into the working channel. Slowly advance the catheter through the hysteroscope being aware of and visualizing the tubal ostium to be cannulated first; it is best to place the catheter in the "more difficult" ostium first. Slowly advance the catheter out of the visual end of the hysteroscope until the tip of the catheter is seen. Once the tip is in view, adjust the hysteroscope to where the catheter can easily be advanced into the ostium (Fig. 8.5). Once inside the ostium, advance the catheter to the level of the black positioning marker reaches the ostium (Fig. 8.6). The patient may experience some mild discomfort at this time—be ready to assess her discomfort and reassure her (the assistant can also provide some "vocal-local" as well). At this time, the operator should also be grasping the catheter handle adjacent to the hand grasping the hysteroscope. Once at the black marker, rotate the thumbwheel on the handle back towards the operator to a hard stop. The surgeon should keep the catheter handle steady by stabilizing it against the hysteroscope or camera so as to prevent moving the insert as the outer sheath of the catheter is removed in this step. At this time, visualization of the gold band just outside the tubal ostium should be present as well as the slightly more proximal green release catheter: these two landmarks on the delivery system will help to ensure proper positioning (Fig. 8.7).

After confirming that the positioning of the delivery system has the microcoil in the correct position of the uterotubal junction, only then should the button on the delivery handle be pressed. Then the thumbwheel on the hand piece should be rolled back a second time until it stops—this will withdraw the inner guidewire and deploy the microinsert which will expand once released. Remove the hand piece and withdraw the guidewire through the working channel. Note how many "trailing coils" are present:

optimum placement will reveal 3 (three) to 8 (eight) expanded outer coils of the Essure microinsert trailing into the endometrial cavity [11] (Fig. 8.8).

Complete the procedure a second time with the remaining tubal ostium. Video photos of both ostia with properly placed microinserts is recommended to document placement and all for appropriate documentation and assertion of placement. Also, it is recommended to keep a procedural log in the office with documentation of procedure, device serial numbers and complications (see Chap. 2). Once the procedure is completed, remove the hysteroscope and all vaginal instruments. Assess the patient's level of discomfort and if prolonged recovery time is needed: most women will be able to be discharged from the office with a minimum of recovery time needed. Be certain to provide and review appropriate discharge and follow-up instructions including a follow-up date in 3 months to return for the confirmatory HSG to assure bilateral tubal occlusion. Lastly, record an operative or procedure report in the patient's medical record with notation of number of trailing coils from each tubal ostium.

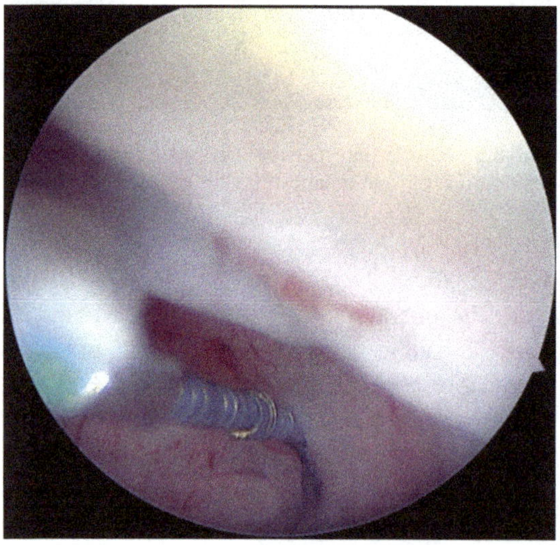

Fig. 8.7 Essure™ delivery catheter with correct positioning of the catheter at the "gold band"; note *green* release catheter to *left*

Tips and Tricks

Several points are made by the manufacturer in the *Instructions for use* [11] that accompany the device, which will aid in proper use of the procedure as well as expedite the ease of application of the microinserts. Some of these include:

- Performance of the procedure in the early proliferative phase of the menstrual cycle.
- Administer a NSAID 1–2 h prior to the procedure (the patient may take the medication at home) which has been shown to significantly increase the likelihood of success of placement.

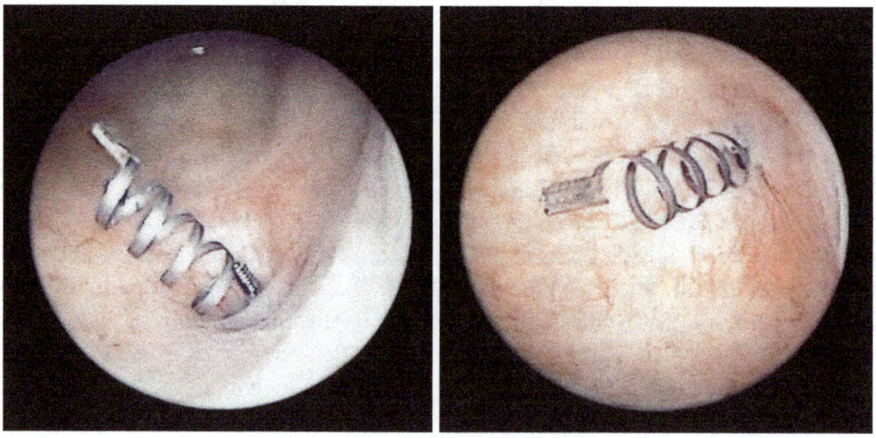

Fig. 8.8 Correct placement of microcoils at the tubal ostium with "trailing" coils

- The amount of time required to complete the hysteroscopic portion of the procedure should not be greater than 20 min.
- The saline solution used for distention should be pre-warmed to 37 °C or less to help minimize tubal spasm.
- The procedure should be discontinued if the fluid deficit exceeds 1,500 cm^3.
- If the microinsert is inadvertently deployed in the uterine cavity and not in the tube, the microinsert should be removed from the uterus and another attempt made at microinsert placement in the tube.

Aside from the manufacturer's recommendations, there are other practical suggestions to help provide a successful procedure for the physician as well as an excellent experience for the patient which is the desired outcome:

- Have a nurse or assistant in the room provide "vocal-local" assistance to the patient to allay fears and anxieties.
- Invite the patient to watch the procedure on the video monitor which may also distract her from the actual procedure itself.
- Consider removing the speculum (remember a one-sided speculum) to help facilitate hysteroscope placement at an appropriate position or angle to allow the microinsert to exit the working channel and glide easily into the tubal ostium.
- Keep the distending medium flowing at a steady rate through the procedure: this includes the 1–2 min during which your assistant is opening and placing the catheter into the surgeon's hands. This will allow continued visualization of the tubal ostium and expedite placement of the microinsert.
- If tubal spasm occurs, decrease the fluid pressure to allow for opening of the tube and consider giving intramuscular ketorolac or glucagon to relieve spasm.
- After the procedure is completed, recommend abstinence from intercourse of douching for a matter of days (physician preference) in order to decrease risk of possible intrauterine infection.
- Be certain to remind the patient to use contraception for the 3 months following the procedure and to schedule the confirmation HSG prior to leaving the office.

Complications

Both short-term and long-term complications may occur after in-office hysteroscopic sterilization and are similar in scope and dimension to those found in surgery or in ASC with a few exceptions. In the office, the possibility of a vasovagal reaction from either the paracervical block or the procedure itself may be encountered; Arjona found this occurred in approximately 1 % of over 1,600 in-office procedures [5] while Povedano et al. reported a rate of 1.9 % in over 4,300 procedures [4]. This is easily treated with lying supine, rest, oral fluids and time. Most if not all cases will resolve, though, on occasion, providing an intramuscular injection or oral dose of an anti-nausea medication may rarely be needed. Poor distention during the procedure was noted in one study [31] which may happen more often in obese patients as higher intrauterine pressures may be needed to maintain uterine insufflation. Another important short-term complication includes inability to place the microinserts. This complication has been reported in both OR-based and office-based procedures and varies between 1.4 and 11 % [3, 14]. Infection and bleeding are possible post procedurally and should be managed according to personal preference and office protocols. Abdominal pain on the day of and several days after the procedure may be reported by patients and should be managed accordingly; Povedano reports approximately 15 % of patients will experience moderate to severe pain [4]. Chapter 4 addresses medications for this purpose. It should be noted, however, that office staff should be counseled to take seriously patient calls to the office in the hours and days after the procedure in order to effectively diagnose and treat these complications.

Longer term complications are similar to those reported in published studies and may include device expulsion, tubal perforation, and abdominal pain [4]. Connor noted persistence of pelvic pain post hysteroscopic sterilization which may be related to malpositioned device, cornual perforation, concomitant global endometrial ablation or to unknown causes [26]. Pelvic pain and dysmenorrhea have been reported as long-term complications (up to 12 months) in patients who received the polymer matrices for tubal sterilization [38]. Mild changes in menstrual flow have been noted as well, with Cooper [1] noting 2.2 % increase in menstrual flow and 1.5 % reduction in flow.

Confirmation of Tubal Occlusion

The success of hysteroscopic tubal sterilization depends upon assuring complete tubal occlusion with the confirmatory hysterosalpingogram (HSG), performed post microinsert placement. The purpose of the HSG is to both document correct microinsert placement and assure bilateral tubal occlusion. In the United States, Essure™ package labeling requires an HSG up to 3 months after the procedure. After performing the procedure in the office, assuring patient compliance with both the need for other contraceptive use for the next 3 months AND scheduling the patient for the HSG test is of paramount importance. While need for interval contraception should optimally have taken place at the pre-procedure office visit, confirming this with the patient on the day of office tubal sterilization is needed. Compliance with both parameters is an issue and studies have addressed concerns of compliance with the HSG both in terms of scheduling and patient acceptance of the procedure [32, 39]. Physicians should be knowledgeable about imaging requirements of the post sterilization HSG which are detailed in the Essure™ package insert and are beyond the scope of this chapter.

There are, however, reminders about this procedure which merit discussion. First, the HSG should be done as a low pressure test. This is recommended as increased pressure during HSG can cause tubal spasm and produce a false positive occlusion. Minimal uterine pressure is recommended with just enough applied to provide contrast fill of the endometrium. Secondly, ideal microinsert location to be confirmed by imaging is such that the inner coil of the microinsert crosses the uterotubal junction (Fig. 8.9). Failure to fully address abnormally placed inserts places the patient at risk for sterilization failure and subsequent pregnancy as mentioned by studies [8, 23, 24]. Management of unsatisfactory microinsert placement can be found in the Essure™ Instructions for Use [11].

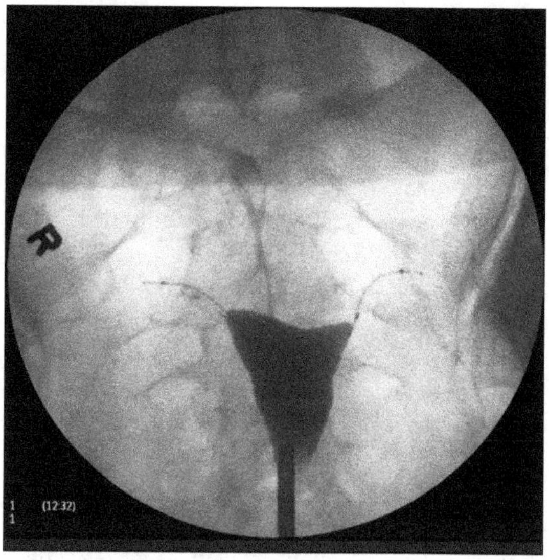

Fig. 8.9 Hysterosalpingogram showing bilateral tubal occlusion and correct microcoil placement at the uterotubal junction

Establishing a protocol for scheduling and reminding patients of the HSG test is strongly encouraged and tracking compliance with this necessary test should be established.

Summary

Hysteroscopic transcervical sterilization can be safely performed in the office setting once the physician has shown clinical competence of the procedure in the OR/ASC setting. There are advantages to the patient including convenience and less time away from daily activities, less pain and post-procedural convalescence, avoidance of incisions and reassurance of a post-procedural confirmation test (HSG). Establishing an in-office hysteroscopic sterilization program is easily obtained and requires little extra expense if a standard diagnostic hysteroscopy program is in place. Ensuring an optimal patient experience in-office requires planning and team adherence to office protocols. Knowledge, patient selection, and prior experience are important as well as several office-based guidelines to assist in successful office performance. Ensuring patient adherence to need for post-procedure pain relief, contraception and follow-up is imperative for both the physician and the patient.

References

1. Cooper JM, Carnigan CS, Cher D, et al. Microinsert nonincisional hysteroscopic sterilization. Obstet Gynecol. 2003;102:59–67.
2. Kerin JF, Cooper JM, Price T, et al. Hysteroscopic sterilization using a micro-insert device: results of a multicentre Phase II study. Hum Reprod. 2003;18:1223–30.
3. Mino M, Arjona JE, Cordon J, et al. Success rate and patient satisfaction with the Essure™ sterilisation in an outpatient setting: a prospective study of 857 women. BJOG. 2007;114:763–6.
4. Povedano B, Arjona JE, Velasco E, et al. Complications of hysteroscopic Essure® sterilisation: report on 4306 procedures performed in a single centre. BJOG. 2012;119:795–9.
5. Arjona JE, Mino M, Cordon J, et al. Satisfaction and tolerance with office hysteroscopic tubal sterilization. Fertil Steril. 2008;90:1182–6.
6. Mosher WD, Jones J. Use of contraception in the United States: 1982-2008. National Center for Health Statistics. Vital Health Stat. 2010;23(29):1–44.
7. Peterson HB, Xia Z, Hughes JM, et al. The risk of pregnancy after tubal sterilization: findings from the U.S. collaborative review of sterilization. Am J Obstet Gynecol. 1996;174:1161–70.
8. Munro MG, Nichols JE, Levy B, et al. Hysteroscopic sterilization: ten-year retrospective analysis of worldwide pregnancy reports. J Minim Invasive Gynecol. 2014;21(2):245–51. doi:10.1016/j.jmig.2013.09.016. pii: S1553-4650(13)012880.
9. Ory EM, Hines RS, Cleland WH, et al. Pregnancy after microinsert sterilization with tubal occlusion confirmed by hysterosalpingogram. Obstet Gynecol. 2008;111:508–10.
10. Cooper JM. Hysteroscopic sterilization. Clin Obstet Gynecol. 1992;35:282–98.
11. Conceptus Incorporated. Essure: instructions for use. Mountain View (CA): Conceptus Inc. 2012. http://www.essuremd/Portals/essuremd/PDFs/TopDownloads/Essure%20IFU.pdf. Accessed 10 Oct 2013.
12. Shavell VI, Abdallah ME, Shade GH, et al. Trends in sterilization since the introduction of Essure hysteroscopic sterilization. J Minim Invasive Gynecol. 2009;16:22–7.
13. American College of Obstetricians and Gynecologists: quality and safety in women's health care. 2nd ed. Part 3. Assessing clinical competence; 2010. p. 43–9.
14. Litta P, Cosmi E, Sacco G, et al. Hysteroscopic permanent tubal sterilization using a nitinol-dacron intratubal device without anaesthesia in the outpatient setting: procedure feasibility and effectiveness. Hum Reprod. 2005;12:3419–22.
15. Levie MD, Chudnoff SG. Prospective analysis of office-based hysteroscopic sterilization. J Minim Invasive Gynecol. 2006;13:98–101.
16. Sinha D, Kalathy V, Gupta JK, et al. The feasibility, success and patient satisfaction associated with outpatient hysteroscopic sterilization. BJOG. 2007;114:676–83.
17. Levie M, Weiss G, Kaiser B, et al. Analysis of pain and satisfaction with office-based hysteroscopic sterilization. Fertil Steril. 2010;94:1189–94.
18. Ubeda A, Labastida R, Dexeus S, et al. Essure®: A new device for hysteroscopic tubal sterilization in an outpatient setting. Fertil Steril. 2004;82:196–9.
19. Levie MD, Chudnoff SG. Office hysteroscopic sterilization compared with laparoscopic sterilization: a critical cost analysis. J Minim Invasive Gynecol. 2005;12:318–22.
20. Kraemer DF, Yen PY, Nichols M. An economic comparison of female sterilization of hysteroscopic tubal occlusion with laparoscopic bilateral tubal ligation. Contraception. 2009;80:254–60.
21. American College of Obstetricians and Gynecologists. Benefits and risks of sterilization. Practice bulletin 133. Obstet Gynecol. 2013;121:392–403.
22. Hillis SD, Marchbanks PA, Tylor LR, et al. Poststerilization regret: findings from the United States collaborative review of sterilization. Obstet Gynecol. 1999;93:889–95.
23. Veersema S, Vleugels MP, Moolenaar LM, et al. Unintended pregnancies after Essure sterilization in the Netherlands. Fertil Steril. 2010;93:35–8.
24. Cleary TP, Tepper NK, Cwiak C, et al. Pregnancies after hysteroscopic sterilization: a systematic review. Contraception. 2012;87:539–48.
25. Jost S, Huchon C, Legendre G, et al. Essure® permanent birth control effectiveness: a seven-year survey. Eur J Obstet Gynecol Reprod Biol. 2013;168:134–7.

26. Connor VF. Essure: a review six years later. J Minim Invasive Gynecol. 2009;16:282–90.
27. Al-Safi ZA, Shavell VI, Hobson DT, et al. Analysis of adverse events with Essure hysteroscopic sterilization reported to the manufacturer and user facility device experience database. J Minim Invasive Gynecol. 2013;20:825–9.
28. Preutthipan S, Herabutya Y. Vaginal misoprostol for cervical priming before operative hysteroscopy: a randomized controlled trial. Obstet Gynecol. 2001;97:640–1.
29. Thomas JA, Leyland N, Durand N, et al. The use of oral misoprostol as a cervical ripening agent in operative hysteroscopy: a double-blind, placebo controlled trial. Am J Obstet Gynecol. 2002;186:876–9.
30. Bradley LD. Hysteroscopic sterilization, Chapter 17. In: Bradley LD, Falcone T, editors. Hysteroscopy: office evaluation and management of the uterine cavity. Philadelphia, PA: Mosby, Inc.; 2009. p. 187–200.
31. Nichols M, Carter JF, Fylstra DL, et al. A comparative study of hysteroscopic sterilization performed in-office versus a hospital operating room. J Minim Invasive Gynecol. 2006;13:447–50.
32. Shavell VI, Abdallah ME, Diamond MP, et al. Post-Essure hysterosalpingography compliance in a clinic population. J Minim Invasive Gynecol. 2008; 15:431–4.
33. Augostini A, Crochet P, Petrakian M, et al. Hysteroscopic tubal sterilization (Essure) in women with an intrauterine device. J Minim Invasive Gynecol. 2008;15:277–9.
34. Mascaro M, Marino M, Vicens-Vidal M. Feasibility of Essure placement in intrauterine device users. J Minim Invasive Gynecol. 2008;15:485–90.
35. Tatalovich JM, Anderson TL. Hysteroscopic sterilization in patients with a Mirena intrauterine device: transition from extended interval to permanent contraception. J Minim Invasive Gynecol. 2010;17:228–31.
36. AAGL. AAGL practice report: practice guidelines for the management of hysteroscopic distention media. J Minim Invasive Gynecol. 2013;20:137–48.
37. Erickson TB, Kirkpatrick DH, DeFrancesco MS, et al. Executive summary of the American College of Obstetricians and Gynecologists Presidential Task Force on patient safety in the office setting: reinvigorating safety in office-based gynecologic surgery. Obstet Gynecol. 2010;115:147–51.
38. Vancaillie TG, Anderson TL, Johns DA. A 12-month prospective evaluation of transcervical sterilization using implantable polymer matrices. Obstet Gynecol. 2008;16:1270–7.
39. Tagoe UJ, Della Badia C, Chaudhari A. Post-operative compliance with a 3-month hysterosalpingogram alter Essure hysteroscopic tubal occlusion. J Minim Invasive Gynecol. 2006;13(5S):S107.

Office Operative Hysteroscopy: Polyp and Submucosal Fibroid Removal

9

Mona E. Orady and Rakshanda Aslanova

Introduction

Today's advancements in hysteroscopic tools allow physicians to minimize patient morbidity and health care costs while still improving clinical outcomes. Increasing comfort with office hysteroscopy and availability to patients has improved diagnostic methodologies utilized to assess abnormal bleeding. Office hysteroscopy was found to be more accurate in the evaluation of endometrial pathology, including polyps, submucous myomas, structural abnormalities, hyperplasia, and endometrial cancer in symptomatic women compared to transvaginal sonography (TVS) and saline infusion sonography (SIS) [1, 2]. This has allowed previously blindly performed manipulations to be transformed into more accurate evaluation methods which include direct visualization of the uterine cavity. Moreover, it gives the opportunity for targeted biopsy providing more precise histologic results [3–5].

Now that comfort with utilizing this technology for diagnosis is increasing, the need for extending the utilization of this approach to the thereapeutic realm becomes natural. The goal would be to apply diagnostic and surgical procedures simultaneously in the outpatient setting. This opportunity to "see and treat" became more feasible after operative hysteroscopes with a final diameter of <6 mm as well as mechanical tools and bipolar electrosurgical systems were developed. Application of mechanical tools like scissors and graspers permit the removal of small cervical polyps, endometrial polyps, and treatment of filmy intrauterine adhesions, whereas the advent of bipolar electrosurgical technology gave office hysteroscopy potential for the treatment of large polyps, small (<1 cm) submucosal myomas, uterine adhesionolysis, and guided endometrial biopsies.

The advent of bipolar resection tools and mechanical hysteroscopic morcellation equipment allows normal saline distention media instead of nonionic distention media (glycine, sorbitol, or mannitol) and thus decreases complications related to fluid balance or energy spread. This thus enhanced the safety of the office hysteroscopic procedures increasing the potential transition of some surgical manipulations from the operating room to a gynecologic office setting. This decreases the need for anesthesiologist, anesthesia, surgical assistants, or specialized nursing thus improving cost and time efficiency of these procedures compared to the operating room setting [6–9]. This chapter will discuss the application of office hysteroscopy to the removal of polyps and small fibroids. Patient selection, preparation, anesthesia, techniques, and tools available will be reviewed.

M.E. Orady, M.D., F.A.C.O.G. (✉)
Department of Obstetrics and Gynecology & Women's Health Institute, Cleveland Clinic, 9500 Euclid Ave., Suite A81, Cleveland, OH 44195, USA
e-mail: oradym@ccf.org

R. Aslanova, M.D.
Department of Obstetrics and Gynecology, Faculty of Medicine, Trakya University, Cleveland, Edirne 22030, Turkey
e-mail: rahshanda@yahoo.com

J.D. Emery and M.F.R. Paraiso (eds.), *Office-Based Gynecologic Surgical Procedures*,
DOI 10.1007/978-1-4939-1414-2_9, © Springer Science+Business Media New York 2015

Preoperative Evaluation

History

Abnormal uterine bleeding affects 10–30 % of reproductive-aged women and up to 50 % of perimenopausal women [10, 11] Evaluation of patients with abnormal uterine bleeding in childbearing-age includes ruling out pregnancy-associated bleeding causes, exogenous hormone use, bleeding due to intrauterine device (IUD), cervicitis or coagulation disorders. Anatomic causes such as endometrial polyps or fibroids frequently appear in women of reproductive age. Endometrial polyps are characterized with a shorter term history of intermenstrual and irregular bleeding and menorrhagia (Fig. 9.1). Endocervical polyps usually cause intermenstrual spotting and postcoital bleeding. Fibroids tend to present as a longstanding, but progressively worsening menorrhagia. Submucosal fibroids especially cause menorrhagia disproportionate with the size of the uterus (Fig. 9.2). A primary complaint of progressively worsening dysmenorrhea coupled with menorrhagia beginning after childbearing is more suggestive of adenomyosis. Endometrial pathology such as endometrial hyperplasia and endometrial cancer causes more irregular and heavy bleeding. Postmenopausal bleeding, in the absence of hormone therapy, should be carefully evaluated because 5–10 % of these cases can be caused by endometrial cancer. Infertility complaints may also be caused by intrauterine pathology including endometrial polyps, fibroids, intrauterine sinechiae, or congenital anomalies of uterus. Thus, hysteroscopic procedures may also be employed in the evaluation and treatment of these patients. Characteristic symptoms of intrauterine adhesions include amenorrhea, irregular menstrual bleeding, and recurrent pregnancy loss. Uterine congenital anomalies are associated with increased rate of spontaneous abortion or could be incidental finding during infertility investigation.

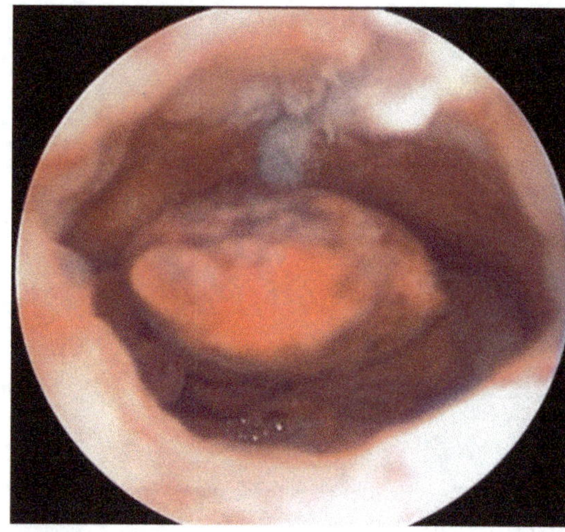

Fig. 9.1 Endometrial polyp occupying >50 of endometrial cavity

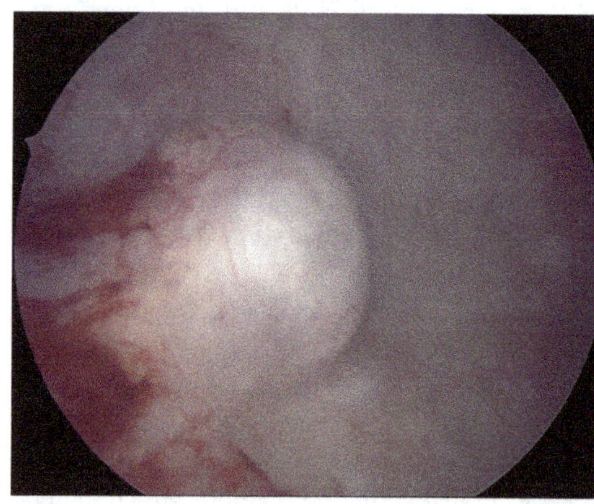

Fig. 9.2 Submucosal Type I leiomyoma seen in right cornual region of postmenopausal women

Physical Examination

Careful gynecologic examination should be included in the evaluation of all patients with the above complaints, and is useful for pre-procedure assessment and planning. Visualization of vagina and cervix are both necessary and must be easily obtainable if an office hysteroscopic procedure is to be considered. Cervix must be of normal shape and configuration without distorting features or severe stenosis. Vaginal discharge could be a symptom of pelvic inflammatory disease, which is an absolute contraindication for office hysteroscopy and must be evaluated and treated prior to procedure scheduling. The presence of cervical polyps can be an indication of endometrial polyps. Enlarged or irregular uterus may indicate the presence of uterine fibroids. Cervical pathologies such as cervical cancer must also be excluded. Bimanual pelvic examination allows assessment of the size and position of the uterus and any severe deviation or tethering which may have resulted secondary to prior cesarean sections, severe endometriosis or pelvic adhesive disease, adnexal pathology or fibroids. Severe enlargement of the uterus or deviation of the path of the cervical canal may indicate difficulty obtaining access and visualization of the endometrial cavity. Thus patients with these findings may be better suited to hysteroscopic procedures in the operating room. Patients should only be considered candidates for office hysteroscopic procedures if the cervix is easily visualized and accessible without severe distortion, deviation, enlargement, or stenosis. Endometrial cavity should also be felt to be of relatively normal positioning, shape and configuration such that the hysteroscope may be introduced into it with relative ease. If the examination indicates otherwise, then it is better to take the patient into the operating room under a deeper level of anesthesia which can allow a greater amount of manipulation of the cervix or uterus in order to accomplish the procedure.

Imaging

Assessment of endometrial and uterine pathology can benefit from well-established diagnostic tools, such as Transvaginal ultrasound (TVS) and Saline infusion sonography (SIS). Transvaginal ultrasound, in particular, is an inexpensive and noninvasive initial evaluation procedure for uterine diseases. It has sensitivity of 56 % and specificity of 72 % for the detection of any endometrial pathology. Saline infusion sonohysterography was introduced as an improved method for the diagnosis of endometrial diseases. In the evaluation of any endometrial pathology SIS has a sensitivty of 81% and a specificity of 100% [12]. For the evaluation of intracavitary masses, like submucous myomas and endometrial polyps Bonnamy et al. found sensitivities of 57 % and 95 % and specificities of 69 % and 77 % for TVS and SIS respectively [13]. The diagnosis of endometrial diseases such as hyperplasia or endometrial cancer cannot be distinguished by TVS or SIS, but can be suspected by increasing of endometrial thickness. Krampl et al. showed TVS and SIS had sensitivities of 33 % and 33 % with specificities of 88 % and 92 % respectively in the diagnosis of uterine structural abnormalities [14]. Soares et al. found TVS and SIS had sensitivities of 75 % and 50 %, specificities of 82 % and 96 % respectively [15]. Therefore, SIS is overall more benefitial for differentiating between focal lesions and diffuse endometrial thickening and is more accurate in the diagnosis of intracavitary masses (See Chap. 6 for more details on SIS).

Utilizing imaging for evaluating patients preoperatively to determine the extent of their pathology and determination of candidacy for an office procedure is extremely important. Pelvic ultrasound can show just a thickened endometrial stripe or may actually delineate a polyp or fibroid. If suspicious enough to warrant diagnostic hysteroscopy, decision to proceed with excision of polyp or fibroid can be made at the time of the hysteroscopy itself. If a small (<1 cm) submucosal fibroid or polyp is seen on ultrasound one can use SIS if readily available at the time of ultrasonography to further characterize the size and location of the polyp and the size of the pedicle of the submucosal fibroid for preoperative assessment. In general, polyps or fibroids on the anterior or posterior walls of the uterus are more accessible and thus more amenable to an office procedure versus pathology near the cornua or protruding off the fundus. Saline infusion ultrasonography is thus highly recommended for detailed assessment of endometrial pathology preoperatively in order to determine whether a case is simple enough to perform in the office, or is more complex, indicating that the operating room setting would be better suited to the case.

Patient Selection

Patients that have small polyps or single polyps or very small (<1 cm) submucosal fibroids with >80 % protrusion into the cavity are good candidates for attempt at an office procedure. Preoperative evaluation of the size and location of the pathology is very important. In addition patients must not have severely distorted cervical or uterine anatomy, a large fibroid uterus, stenotic cervix, or complex pathology in order to be candidates for office hysteroscopic operative procedures. Patients must also be motivated, have an understanding of the procedure, and able to be cooperative and patient during the procedure. Thus patients with a language barrier, high anxiety levels, or inability to understand or cooperate with the procedure should not be considered candidates for office-based surgery. Also, office hysteroscopy cannot be performed on patients with current uterine bleeding because of hindrance to adequate visualization of the cavity and pathology. In these cases, only high flow irrigation could provide satisfactory view of uterine cavity, which it is generally not possible in this setting because of small diameter of office hysteroscopes. Also, when dilatation and curettage is required, this may also be too painful to perform in the office setting. Thus, exclusion of cervical stenosis, severe cervical canal deviation, and recent uterine perforation must be undertaken prior to the procedure in order to decrease the risk of perforation. Uncooperative patients, cardiorespiratory disorders, cervical cancer, pelvic infections, and known intrauterine pregnancy are other contraindications for office hysteroscopy (Table 9.1).

Table 9.1 Contraindications to office operative hysteroscopic procedures

Contraindications for office hysteroscopy
• Uncooperative patients
• Cardiorespiratory disorders
• Severely distorted cervical or uterine anatomy
• Stenotic cervix
• Cervical cancer
• Large fibroid uterus
• Current, active or heavy uterine bleeding
• Recent uterine perforation
• Pelvic infection
• Intrauterine pregnancy

Informed Consent

Once a patient is deemed a candidate for an office hysteroscopy procedure, a detailed discussion of the pathology and treatment options must be discussed with the patient. As in any surgical procedure, the reason for the procedure, risks, benefits, and alternatives to the procedure must be discussed and informed consent should be obtained; Chap. 3 provides a complete discussion of Informed Consent. Potential complications should be discussed. As the patient will be awake for the procedure, the expectations of the patient with regards to length of the procedure and any expected discomfort should be discussed. Motivation and cooperation of the patient and a desire to avoid anesthesia and the operating room setting must be present, as not all patients will wish to undergo an office procedure if given the option to go to the operating room. The patient must also know that the procedure may not be completed in the office setting and may be aborted at any point, and thus must understand that although the goal is to avoid going to the operating room, that this may still be a possibility if more extensive pathology is found.

The patient must also understand that mild cramping or bleeding after the procedure is not unusual after the office hysteroscopy, but that fever, severe abdominal pain, and heavy vaginal bleeding or discharge would be warning signs of complications or infection, and that the patient should immediately call the office or proceed to the emergency room if these develop. Although usually a safe procedure, complications including possible injury to the cervix or the uterus, infection, heavy bleeding, or side effects of medications used can occur and should be discussed with the patient.

Operative Procedure

Preop Preparation

History, physical examination, imaging, and discussion with the patient help determine what preoperative preparation, anesthesia requirements, and equipment may be required for the procedure. Adequate assessment and planning is truly what ensures the success of the procedure. Knowing what findings to expect and challenges that may be encountered allows the surgeon to anticipate and avoid difficulty or complications. For this reason, if an office procedure is desired, the extra step of performing a saline infusion sonogram in order to assess size and location of pathology can be worthwhile in most cases. Small polyps can generally be handled without energy or morcellation, whereas fibroids or larger polyps may need bipolar resection or morcellation and thus the equipment for these techniques must be readily available.

In order to reduce intraoperative pain and spasm of the uterus, preoperative treatment of the patient with nonsteroidal anti-inflammatory agents such as ibuprofen or naproxen may be utilized to suppress prostaglandin production and thus prevent cramping and spasm of the uterus. Thus, having pre-procedural treatment with nonsteroidal anti-inflammatory drugs (NSAIDs) may improve the success of an office procedure as a common reason for aborting the procedure is Inadequate pain control. Dilation of cervix is also a painful component of the procedure and also has potential complications such as uterine perforation and cervical laceration. Difficulty with dilatation and stenotic cervix is more common in postmenopausal or nulliparous women and those receiving GnRH agonists. Numerous studies have been performed to examine the effect of preoperative administration of misoprostol to the pain and cervical dilation. They concluded that the use of misoprostol before hysteroscopy eases cervical dilation beyond 5 mm, decreases complication rates and is effective in pain reduction [16, 17]. Misoprostol also causes myometrial contractions which may reduce bleeding and facilitate resection of fibroids. Although there is no unified dosing recommendation, application regimen, or route of misoprostol use, generally administration of 400 mg misoprostol vaginally 6 h before hysteroscopy is recommended as a minimum application [18, 19]. Please see Chap. 1 for a more detailed discussion of preoperative misoprostol and other concerns for patient preparation before an office-based surgery.

Anesthesia

Anesthetic options are dependent on the patient and procedure and the agents that are available. Oral or intramuscular medications that are frequently utilized include nonsteroidal anti-inflammatory agents, narcotics, and benzodiazepine anxiolytic agents. For most patients undergoing a short procedure (<10 min) a combination of oral ibuprofen or naproxen or intramuscular ketorolac combined with a paracervical block utilizing local anesthetic agents is adequate. For longer procedures or more anxious patients the addition of an oral benzodiazepine such as alprazolam or lorazepam with or without oral narcotics such as oxycodone or hydrocodone may be useful. Some offices have the capability of intravenous sedative techniques which may include intravenous midazolam and/or fentanyl which may be used for more extensive procedures such as in patients with multiple polyps or who require resection of fibroids with energy, during which patients must be more relaxed. These sedative techniques however require special training and certification in monitored anesthesia care. In all patients the utility of a good paracervical block is essential as most of the pain control and pre-emptive prevention of postoperative pain results from blocking the nerve plexus innervating the uterus which enter at the level of the cardinal ligaments. Becoming proficient and comfortable with this technique is thus important. Please refer to Chap. 4 for procedural points on paracervical block and more details regarding anesthesia during office hysteroscopy.

Instrumentation

Using rigid, semirigid, and flexible hysteroscopes with a small diameter gives physicians the opportunity to perform hysteroscopy without cervical dilatation. Since cervical dilatation is often the most painful part of hysteroscopy commonly causing procedure failure, this new instrumentation is allowing the increased use of office hysteroscopy for procedures beyond just diagnosis [20]. One of the first small diameter-rigid office hysteroscopes was the Office Continuous Flow Operative Hysteroscope, size 5 (Karl Storz, Tuttlingen, Germany). It consists of a 2.9 mm diameter rod-lens system with 30° vision angle and 5 mm sheath diameter. The newest version of this hysteroscope is Office Continuous Flow Operative Hysteroscope, size 4 (Karl Storz, Tuttlingen, Germany) which has thinner scope and outer diameter, 2 and 4 mm, respectively (Fig. 9.3). Both models include an oval shaped 5F operative channel through which small instruments such as graspers, biopsy forceps, or scissors can be placed (Fig. 9.4). The semirigid hysteroscope, Versascope (Gynecare, Ethicon Inc., Sommerville, NJ, USA) is characterized by 3.2 mm sheath diameter, 1.8 mm diameter, 28 cm length, 0° view scope and a single disposable outer sheath. An expandable working channel allows easy conversion from a diagnostic to a therapeutic procedure with 7F semirigid mechanical instruments or 5F bipolar electrodes. The flexible minihysteroscope is a more recent innovation. The new minihysteroscopes demonstrate similar benefits including less discomfort for patient [21]. The usefulness of flexible minihysteroscopes is restricted by higher costs for equipment; more difficult cleaning, disinfection, and sterilization; and reduced image size on the monitor screen compared with full-size standard hysteroscopy [21]. They do not yet accommodate operative instruments and thus are most useful as an initial step in evaluation of the cavity and extent of the pathology prior to proceeding with an operative procedure.

Initial operative instruments included graspers, scissors, and biopsy forceps which can fit through a small operative channel in the office hysteroscope (Fig. 9.4). These were first used in office procedures for dealing with extremely small pathological changes such as small polyps, syncytia or directed biopsy of endometrial tissue. Development of bipolar systems of resection also benefitted office hysteroscopy. One of the newest bipolar electrosurgical systems is the Versapoint, characterized by a 1.6-mm-diameter (5-F), 36-cm-long, flexible electrode (Gynecare Inc., Somerville, NJ, USA) (Fig. 9.5). The configurations of the electrode are spring, twizzle, and ball electrodes, which are intended for vaporizing, cutting, and coagulating of the tissue, respectively. The most important advantage is its allowance of the utilization of physiological saline as a distention medium, thus reducing the risk of fluid overload and hyponatremia when compared with the use of monopolar systems with hypotonic solutions like glycine, sorbitol, or mannitol. Minimization

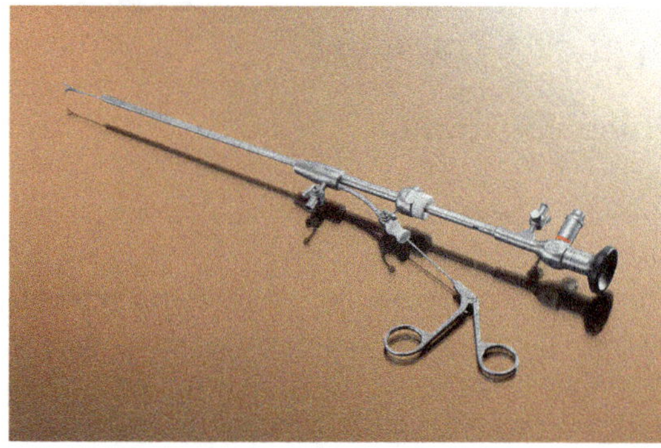

Fig. 9.3 Office continuous flow operative hysteroscope, size 4, with operating channel and hysteroscopic instrumentation (Copyright 2014 Photo Courtesy of KARL STORZ Endoscopy-America, Inc)

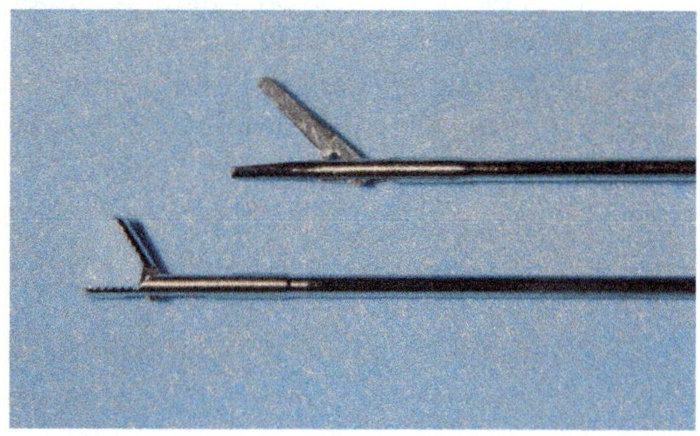

Fig. 9.4 Hysteroscopic scissors (*top*) and graspers (*bottom*) for use through operating channel of hysteroscope

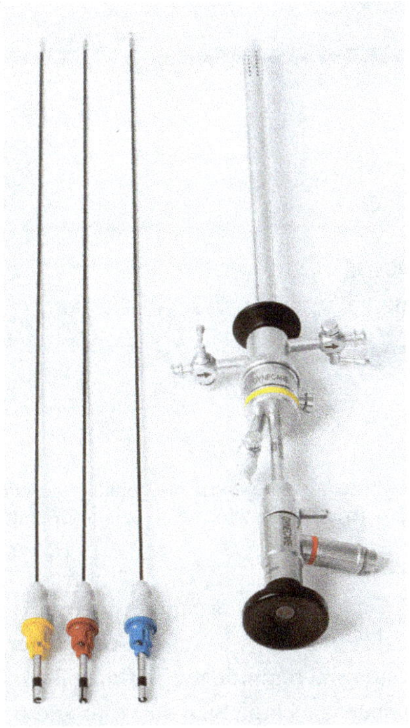

Fig. 9.5 Versapoint (TM) hysteroscopic system with operating channel and 5Fr bipolar electrodes. Copyright 2014 Ethicon US LLC, Somerville, NJ, USA, Used with permission

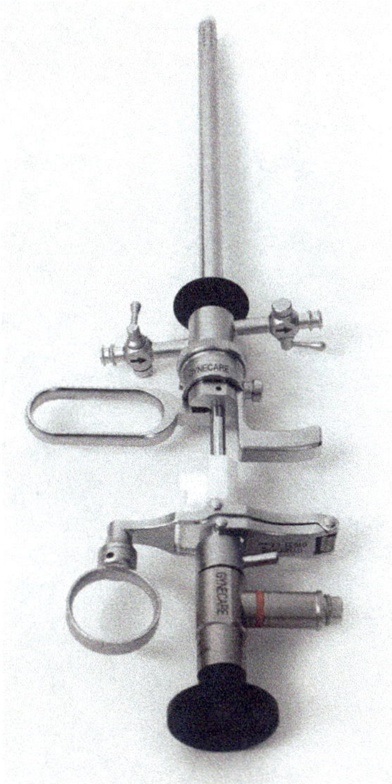

Fig. 9.6 Gynecare Versapoint™ resectoscope. Copyright 2014 Ethicon US LLC, Somerville, NJ, USA, Used with permission

of energy spread also makes procedures less painful and decreases the risk of skin burns at the bovine pad site [7].

The development of a bipolar resection system allowed for the utilization of safer bipolar energy with saline distention media for resection purposes. The use of the Gynecare Versapoint™ Bipolar Electrosurgery System has increased since its and it is the first bipolar system in the US market. It is used in combination with the Gynecare Versapoint™ Resectoscope which has a small 4 mm bore size and is available with either a 30° wide angle or a 12° lens (Fig. 9.6). By utilizing this system at the time of diagnostic hysteroscopy, it allows a single intervention to both diagnose and treat intrauterine pathology at the same time, thus reducing the cost. It can be utilized to remove submucosal myomas, polyps, intrauterine adhesions, or septa. Other bipolar resection systems are also now in development and becoming available on the market.

Even more recently, the advent of mechanical hysteroscopic morcellators can eliminate the need for use of any type of energy, thus increasing the safety of the procedure. However, length of time of the procedure must be balanced with the benefit of the elimination of energy use. Despite a generally slower rate of resection, most morcellators however remove specimen fragments via suction thus eliminating the need for removal of fragments which may often be difficult in a patient who is awake. Two hysteroscopic morcellators are currently on the market in the United States. The Truclear™ hysteroscopic morcellator (Smith & Nephew, Andover, MA) (Fig. 9.7a) was approved by the US Food and drug administration in 2005 followed by approval of the MyoSure® Tissue Removal System (Hologic, Bedford, MA) in 2009. Both rely on a suction-based mechanical energy for tissue removal, rather than bipolar energy resection.

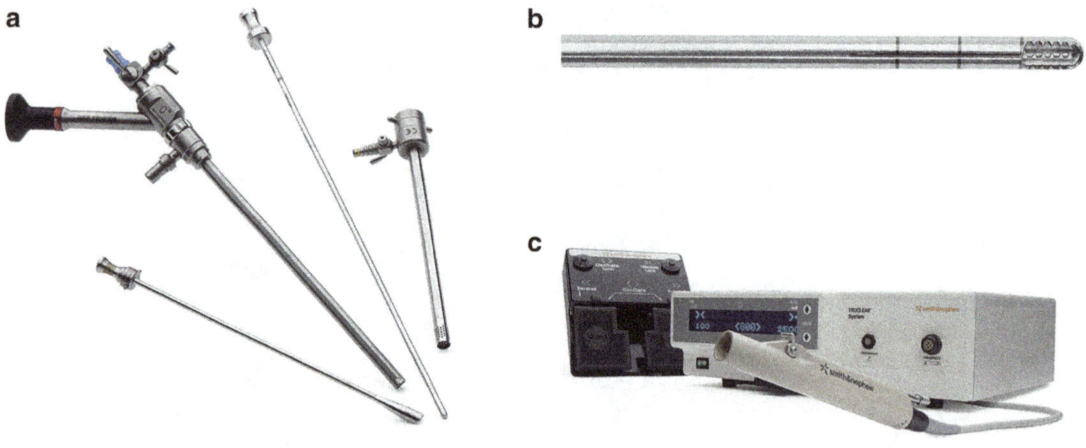

Fig. 9.7 (**a–c**) Truclear Hysteroscopic Morcellator: Smith & Nephew, Inc. Hysteroscopic morcellator showing basic equipment components (**a**), morcellator applicator with cutting window (**b**) and handpiece with (**c**) motor control unit (Copyright 2014 Smith&Nephew, Inc)

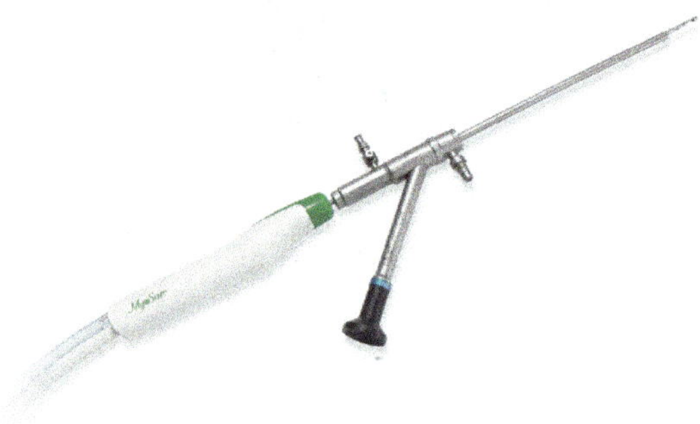

Fig. 9.8 MyoSure® tissue removal system (Hologic, Bedford, MA), courtesy of HOLOGIC, Inc. and affiliates

Truclear™ uses a single-use rigid metal inner tube with cutting edges that rotate and/or reciprocate within an outer tube with a side-facing cutting window at its distal end (Fig. 9.7b). The handpiece is reusable and is attached to a motor control unit (Fig. 9.7c). Suction is applied and tissue is pulled into the cutting window as the inner tube rotates at 1,100 rpm. The resected tissue is then aspirated through the device into a collecting pouch for later histopathologic analysis. For use in the office setting, rather than the original 9-mm outer diameter, rigid, continuous-flow, 0° hysteroscope, the newer 5.6 mm-diameter hysteroscope is used with the Truclear incisor plus blade 2.9. The MyoSure® system (Fig. 9.8) also relies on a suction-based, mechanical energy, rotating tubular cutter system to remove intrauterine tissue. It has a 2.5-mm inner blade that rotates and reciprocates within a 3-mm outer tube at speeds as high as 6,000 rpm and presents an outer bevel on the rotating blade edge. The blade and handpiece are combined into a single-use device that is then attached to suction and a motor control unit. An offset lens 6.25 mm, 0° continuous flow hysteroscope is used to introduce the unit into the endometrial cavity. With both devices, learning the correct resection technique, although not difficult, is of prime importance since the speed of morcellation is directly dependent on maintaining tissue contact between the cutting window and pathology, as well as the density of the pathology.

For polyps and Type I and Type II submucous myomas, hysteroscopic morcellation is a feasible alternative to traditional energy-based resection. Some studies have suggested that it can be both faster and easier to learn than traditional resectoscopy. Emanuel et al. showed a significant reduction in operating room time when removing polyps and Type I and Type II submucous myomas with a hysteroscopic morcellation device [22]. Ban Dongen and associates also randomized 60 patients with an endometrial polyp or a Type 0 or Type 1 myoma or Type I myoma to either hysteroscopic morcellation or loop-electrode resection by residents in training.

The morcellation group demonstrated a 38 % reduction in operating room (OR) time (17 vs. 10.6 min; $P = 0.008$), a 32 % reduction in distention media used (5,050 vs. 3,413 mL; $P = 0.041$), and a marked reduction in the number of insertions and reinsertions of the hysteroscope to remove chips when the morcellator was used (number of insertions = 1 [range, 1–2]) compared with the resectoscope (number of insertions = 7 [range, 3–50]) [23]. As far as average time for procedure, Miller et al. reported average polyp morcellation times of 37 s and average myoma morcellation times of 6.4 min for Type 0, I, and II myomas with a mean diameter of 31.7 mm [24]. Given this relatively fast morcellation time, for smaller pathology and a limited number of lesions, it becomes conceivable to perform some of these procedures in the office with oral sedation and a paracervical block, thus reducing cost. The diameter of either the MyoSure hysteroscope (6.25 mm) or the smaller Truclear hysteroscope (5.0 mm) allows either system to be utilized for office-based treatments of polyps and Type 0 or I submucosal fibroids.

Polyp Resection

Endometrial polyps could be associated with abnormal bleeding or be asymptomatic. They typically present with a short-term history of menorrhagia, intermenstrual spotting, or postmenopausal bleeding. The incidence of endometrial hyperplasia or cancer in seemingly benign endometrial polyps is 1.7 % and is associated with an 8.3-fold increased risk of preneoplastic and neoplastic lesions in patients over 60 years with postmenopausal bleeding [25].

If suspected on radiologic examination, like ultrasound, SIS or HSG, endometrial polyps are an indication for hysteroscopy. If they are (<5 mm) with a small stalk, they may be removed with mechanical tools such as hysteroscopic scissors or graspers especially if easily accessible on the anterior or posterior uterine walls or in the endocervical canal, allowing safe removal in the office [26]. If they are larger or located closer to the fundus or cornua, a hysteroscopic morcellator may provide easier access to shave them down. The bipolar electrosurgical system (VersaPoint, Gynecare Inc., Somerville, NJ, USA) permit excision of large polyps using physiologic saline as the dissension medium instead of hypotonic solutions used with monopolar energy increasing the safety of electrosurgical resection [27]. Electrosurgical resection, using the Twizzle electrode for cutting and the Spring electrode for diffuse tissue vaporization made possible the removal of endometrial polyps ranging in size from 5 to 50 mm [28, 29] Transection of sessile endometrial polyps is more difficult than pedunculated polyps. In these cases bending of the twizzle electrode 25–30° can facilitate cutting of the polyp's base in a similar fashion to the hook electrode resection technique [7]. Alternatively, large sessile endometrial polyps with thick stalks can be removed by mechanical hysteroscopic morcellators, using the TRUCLEAR™ hysteroscopic morcellator (Smith & Nephew, Andover, MA) or MyoSure® Tissue Removal System (Hologic, Bedford, MA) in 2009, as it is easier to gradually shave them down to the base with these instruments. Removal in the office should be restricted to the smaller polyps. If polyps are large, have a broad base, or are numerous, consider taking the patient to the outpatient operating room setting for more control and ability to perform a longer or more complex procedure.

Fibroid Resection

It is estimated that 25–50 % of women between ages 30 and 50 have fibroids. Fibroids can occur in many locations and are typically categorized as subserosal, intramural, or submucosal. Although, these fibroids are not typically associated with an increased risk of uterine cancer, they are a very common cause of abnormal uterine bleeding, and may possibly contribute to infertility. Submucosal fibroids in particular, even when small, often present with a history of gradually worsening menorrhagia, often leading to chronic iron deficiency anemia. Thus, patients typically present with bleeding gradually worsening over time, rather than acute bleeding, and a history of fibroids. Submucosal fibroids are further subcategorized into types dependent on the extent that the fibroid protrudes into the endometrial cavity. A categorization of submucosal fibroids is summarized in Table 9.2. They are classified as Type 0, Type I, or Type II, according to the degree of myometrial penetration. Only type 0 and type 1 submucosal fibroids tend to be amenable to resection. In type II submucosal fibroids, more than 50 % of a tumor penetrates the myometrium, increasing the risk of excessive intraoperative fluid absorption as well as bleeding. These types of tumors also increase operative time and the likelihood that additional procedures will be needed because of incomplete resection [30, 31]. Some of these resection procedures can be extensive, take a prolonged time, or may need to be performed over multiple procedures in order to limit the chances of fluid overload or excessive bleeding. Thus, selection of the appropriate patient for an office-based procedure based on prior imaging and other diagnostic procedures is even more important. Due to the time that it may take to resect fibroids, only smaller fibroids (<1 cm) and preferably those on a small stalk (Type 0) may be amenable to resection in the office with a hysteroscopic morcellator that provides suction to remove the fibroid fragments. All others should be taken to the operating room for resection purposes.

Table 9.2 Classification of uterine leiomyomata relative to position of tumor within the uterus

Classification of submucous myomas	
Type 0	Entirely within endometrial cavity No myometrial extension (pedunculated)
Type 1	<50 % myometrial extension (sessile) >90° angle of myoma surface to uterine wall
Type 2	>50 % myometrial extension (sessile) <90° angle of myoma surface to uterine wall

Table 9.3 Indications for office operative hysteroscopic surgery

• Abnormal uterine bleeding (premenopausal or postmenopausal)
• Endometrial polyps (<50 mm)
• Submucosal fibroids (Type 0, 1)
• Uterine septum
• Intrauterine synechia
• Foreign object removal or retrieval

Other Office-Based Hysteroscopic Procedures

In addition to removal of endometrial polyps and submucosal leiomyoma in the office, a complete list of indications for office-based operative hysteroscopy is reviewed in Table 9.3. Menstrual irregularities, dysmenorrhea, pelvic pain, amenorrhea, infertility, and pregnancy disorders like miscarriage, placenta accreta and intrauterine growth restriction are typical for patients with intrauterine adhesions [32]. Safe and effective division of intrauterine adhesions can be performed by office hysteroscopy, improving fertility and normal menstrual periods. However, intrauterine adhesions can reform in rates of 10 % and 60 % in patients with initially moderate and severe adhesions respectively, even following surgical treatment [33]. In outpatient settings, intrauterine adhesions can be removed using scissors or ball and twizzle electrodes [34, 35]. The studies evaluating methods to prevent recurrent adhesions following adhesiolysis, found that the insertion of an IUD or ballon catheter following lysis of adhesions is effective to prevent their reformation. Effectiveness of estrogens or combination of estrogens and progestins were also reported [36, 37]. Recent research has also advocated antiadhesive property of hyaluronic acid application to reduce adhesion development after surgery [38]. Similar to patient selection for polyp or fibroid resection, only patient with mild to moderate adhesions should be chosen for the office hysteroscopic approach. Dissection should be limited to sharp dissection with scissors, or if adhesions are slightly more dense, the operative hysteroscopic morcellator, or versapoint bipolar loop may be utilized to lyse adhesions. If at the time of the office procedure a more extensive procedure is felt to be necessary then the procedure should be aborted and transferred to the operating room at another time.

Uterine septa are the most common among mullerian fusion anomalies. About 20–25 % of patients with a uterine septum have infertility. Moreover, first or second trimester miscarriages, preterm delivery, and abnormal presentation are other concomitants of septate uterus. This is another uterine pathology that may be treated with office hysteroscopy [39–43]. Similar to treatment of submucosal fibroids, correction of a uterine septum has gone through an evolution from traumatic abdominal metroplasty to office hysteroscopic septum resection. Pretreatment of the patients with gonadotrophin-releasing hormone agonists for 3 months preoperatively, then performing the procedure during the early proliferative phase will help to avoid thickness of endometrium. Only small partial septae that are deemed to be thin are suited for the office. Thicker septa, or in patients where partial bicornuate uterus is suspected should be performed in the operating room with or without the assistance of laparoscopy to prevent resecting to much of the septum or causing perforation of the uterus [44, 45]. Three diagnostic criteria, established by Bettocchi in 2007, can be used in order to perform safe and effective office hysteroscopic metroplasty while differentiating septate from bicornuate uterus [44]. These criteria include the color, vascularization, and sensitive innervation of the tissue. Pinkish colored, rich vasculature, and sensitive tissue indicates myometrium rather than septa. While cutting through a septum, the appearance of two of these three criteria is a sign to stop. Application of these diagnostic criteria led to 93.1 % of septoplasties performed by a mechanical tool (5F sharp scissors) to be complete septum excisions with corrected uterine anatomy [44]. Recent studies have concluded that hysteroscopic metroplasty performed by resectoscope, microscissors or fiberoptic lasers improve pregnancy outcomes [45–49]. Bringing this procedure to the office setting decreases the cost and thus may make this more available to patients with infertility concerns who are found to have a uterine septum.

Lastly, retrieval of intrauterine foreign bodies such as retained or embedded interuterine devices can easily be retrieved with in-office operative hysteroscopy. If the IUD strings cannot be retrieved from the endocervix by conservative probing or manipulation, use of office hysteroscopy with graspers may be used to locate and remove the IUD, either by finding the wayward sting or by grasping the IUD itself (Fig. 9.9a, b). Also, at times embedded IUDs may be sufficiently embedded that grasping the IUD itself is not enough. Consideration of use of dissection of the endomyometrium surrounding the embedded portion of the IUD can be undertaken with the hysteroscopic graspers in order to loosen the tissue surrounding the IUD and facilitate removal.

Complications

Although office hysteroscopy is a safe procedure, there are still some potential complications, which if even cannot be completely avoided can be minimized. In a prospective multicenter trial of 13,600 procedures, Jansen et al. determined an overall complication rate of 0.95 % for operative and 0.13 % for diagnostic hysteroscopy [50].

The most common type of complication is of the mechanical and traumatic type. Perforation is the most common of these which can be mechanical or due to thermal energy sources. Perforation may occur during difficult dilation, when the uterus is excessively ante- or retroflexed, or because of a stenotic cervix. The ripening of the cervix prior to the procedure with 400 mcg of intravaginal misoprostol can decrease this complication rate [19]. Utilizing flexible plastic dilators are sometimes more useful for the stenotic cervix than small lacrimal dilators which can also be used in the stenotic cervix. Gently assessing the direction and location of the canal will prevent false tract formation or perforation, both of which result in need for termination of

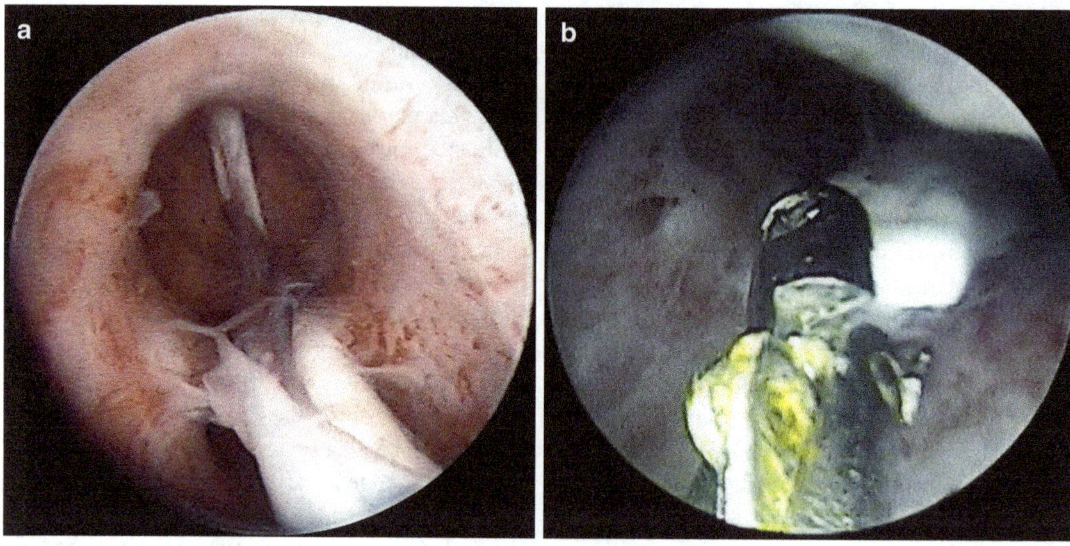

Fig. 9.9 (**a**) Embedded levonorgestrel IUD at uterine fundus with IUD strings seen adjacent and along the base of the IUD. (**b**) Use of hysteroscopic graspers to identify and remove an IUD

the procedure. In the office setting, a small 3 mm flexible hysteroscope can often be introduced to directly visualize the canal using hydrodissection with the normal saline inflow to help find and dilate the canal. Often in multiparous patients with prior misoprostol treatment, dilation is not necessary at all and office hysteroscope can be introduced directly. Traction on the anterior lip of the cervix with a tenaculum often straightens the canal allowing for easier introduction into the cavity.

After dilation and operative hysteroscopy is performed, instruments must be carefully introduced and kept in view at all times. Scissors can perforate the uterus during of polypectomy or transection of synechiae or a uterine septum. Fundal and posterior lower uterine segment locations are more frequently perforated. Most mechanical perforations don't need any further intervention. However, great concern should be taken with Electrosurgical perforations as bowel injuries can occur. This type of perforation thus requires laparoscopy to run and assess the bowel. This is one reason why resection of deeper myomas should not be attempted in the office setting.

Cervical lacerations are rare and cause minimal bleeding. Often pressure is adequate to stop bleeding from the laceration site. If bleeding persists, suturing, cauterization, or silver nitrate sticks can be used to control the bleeding. Excessive bleeding during hysteroscopy can result from injuries of cervical or low uterine segment vessels. If able to be visualized, directed cautery with biopolar coagulation energy can often control the bleeding. Balloon tamponade of the uterine cavity with Foley catheter with a 30-cc balloon [51] or packing the uterus with dilute vasopressin solution has also been described [52]. Treatment with GnRH or danazol before hysteroscopic myomectomy has also been described as a method to decrease blood loss during procedure [53].

Prolonged use of electrodes with high voltage can cause thermal injures of introitus and perineal skin. Whereas introduction of bipolar electrodes to office hysteroscopy decreases the energy spread and these related complications [7].

Frequency of complications from fluid overload secondary to absorption of distention media is much reduced with the use of saline solution instead of non-ionic distention media (like glycine, sorbitol, or mannitol), which is the main benefit of using bipolar energy for mechanical resection [7]. If it occurs, excess fluid absorption can cause dilutional hyponatremia and hypoosmolality. Therefore, diligent monitoring of fluid intake and output during hysteroscopic surgery is necessary to prevent these complications. There are many fluid management systems on the market which all serve the same function. Fluid deficit should be assessed with every bag of distention media that is used and reported to the surgeon by the nurse. In general, a fluid deficit of 750–1,000 mL is an alarm for quickening the procedure and a deficit greater than 1,500 mL indicates that a procedure may have to be terminated [54]. In order to reduce the fluid deficit in the office the smallest caliber hysteroscope needed should be used with the lowest pressure required to maintain adequate visualization of the cavity. Rarely, would the pressure have to be increased beyond about 70 mmHg. Management of inflow and outflow, reducing outflow to a rate just enough to maintain clearance of blood and debris will ensure minimal fluid usage and thus reduce the deficit.

Infection is a rare delayed complication of hysteroscopy. A retrospective cohort study of 1,028 office hysteroscopic procedures demonstrates an infection risk of 0.001 % [55]. Risk factors for infection include a prolonged procedure, cervicovaginal infections or history of pelvic inflammatory disease. In patients at risk, assessment of Gonorrhea or Chlamydia should be performed prior to scheduling the hysteroscopy. If positive, and appropriate treatment followed by a test of cure to document resolution of the infection should be performed. In general, antibiotic prophylaxis is not indicated for hysteroscopic procedures and thus utilization of preoperative or postoperative antibiotics is not commonly used.

Conclusion

Operative hysteroscopic procedures are now amenable to transition to the office setting due to advancements in hysteroscope technology with smaller diameter scopes as well as new instrumentation, both energy related and destructive. Removal of small endometrial polyps and submucosal myomas can be attempted in the office setting with use of local anesthesia and adjunct oral, intravenous or intramuscular medication. Removal of foreign objects and other endometrial pathology can now be attempted in the office with resultant savings in time and cost for all parties. Knowledge of equipment and selection of appropriate patients play a key role in developing this technique for office practice.

Acknowledgments Much thanks goes to Rahshanda Askanova MD, OB/GYN Resident, Trakya University, Edirne, Republic of Turkey for her assistance in collecting data and references was well as help in the draft of the chapter.

References

1. Bakour SH, Jones SE, Khan KS. Accuracy of diagnostic ambulatory hysteroscopy. Ambulatory hysteroscopy an evidence-based guide to diagnosis and therapy. 1st ed. London: Royal Society of Medicine Press; 2006.
2. Grimbizis GF, Tsolakidis D, Mikos T, Anagnostou E, Asimakopoulos E, Stamatopoulos P, Tarlatzis BC. A prospective comparison of transvaginal ultrasound, saline infusion sonohysterography, and diagnostic hysteroscopy in the evaluation of endometrial pathology. Fertil Steril. 2010;94(7):2720–5.
3. Litta P, Merlin F, Saccardi C, Pozzan C, Sacco G, Fracas M, Capobianco G, Dessole S. Role of hysteroscopy with endometrial biopsy to rule out endometrial cancer in postmenopausal women with abnormal uterine bleeding. Maturitas. 2005;50(2):117–23.
4. Epstein E, Ramirez A, Skoog L, et al. Dilation and curettage fails to detect most focal lesions in the uterine cavity in women with postmenopausal bleeding. Acta Obstet Gynecol Scand. 2001;80:1131–6.
5. Clark TJ, Voit D, Gupta JK, et al. Accuracy of hysteroscopy in the diagnosis of endometrial cancer and hyperplasia: a systematic quantitative review. JAMA. 2002;288(13):1610–21.
6. Porreca MR, Pansini N, Bettocchi S, Loverro G, Selvaggi L. Hysteroscopic polypectomy in the office without anesthesia. J Am Assoc Gynecol Laparosc. 1996;3(1):40.
7. Bettocchi S, Ceci O, Di Venere R, et al. Advanced operative office hysteroscopy without anaesthesia: analysis of 501 cases treated with a 5 Fr bipolar electrode. Hum Reprod. 2002;17:2435–8.
8. Bettocchi S, Nappi L, Ceci O, Selvaggi L. Office hysteroscopy. Obstet Gynecol Clin North Am. 2004;31:641–54.
9. Bettocchi S, Nappi L, Ceci O, Selvaggi L. What does 'diagnostic hysteroscopy' mean today? The role of the new techniques. Curr Opin Obstet Gynecol. 2003;15:303–8.

10. Haynes PJ, Hodgson H, Anderson AB, Turnbull AC. Measurement of menstrual blood loss in patients complaining of menorrhagia. Br J Obstet Gynaecol. 1977;84(10):763–8.
11. Prentice A. Medical management of menorrhagia. West J Med. 2000;172(4):253–5.
12. Kelecsi S, Kaya E, Alan M, Alan Y, Bilge U, Mollamahmutoglu L. Comparison of transvaginal sonography, saline infusion sonography, and office hysteroscopy in reproductive-aged women with or without abnormal uterine bleeding. Fertil Steril. 2005;84:682–6.
13. Marret H, Perrotin F, Body G, Berger C, Lansac J. Sonohysterography: a prospective survey of results and complications in 81 patients. Eur J Obstet Gynecol Reprod Biol. 2002;102:42–7.
14. Krampl E, Bourne T, Hurlen-Solbakken H, Istre O. Transvaginal ultrasonography sonohysterography and operative hysteroscopy for the evaluation of abnormal uterine bleeding. Acta Obstet Gynecol Scand. 2001;80:616–22.
15. Soares SR, Reis MM, Camargos AF. Diagnostic accuracy of sonohysterography, transvaginal sonography, and hysterosalpingography in patients with uterine cavity diseases. Fertil Steril. 2000; 73:406–11.
16. Cooper NA, Smith P, Khan KS, Clark TJ. Does cervical preparation before outpatient hysteroscopy reduce women's pain experience? A systematic review. BJOG. 2011;118(11):1292–301.
17. Esin S, Baser E, Okuyan E, Kucukozkan T. Comparison of sublingual misoprostol with lidocaine spray for pain relief in office hysteroscopy: a randomized, double-blind, placebo-controlled trial. J Minim Invasive Gynecol. 2013;20(4):499–504.
18. Valente EP, de Amorim MMR, Costa AAR, de Miranda DV. Vaginal misoprostol prior to diagnostic hysteroscopy in patients of reproductive age: a randomized clinical trial. J Minim Invasive Gynecol. 2008;15:452–8.
19. Singh N, Ghosh B, Naha M, Mittal S. Vaginal misoprostol for cervical priming prior to diagnostic hysteroscopy-efficacy, safety and patient satisfaction: a randomized controlled trial. Arch Gynecol Obstet. 2009;279:37–40.
20. Campo R, Molinas CR, Rombauts L, Mestdagh G, Lauwers M, Braekmans P, Brosens I, Van Belle Y, Gordts S. Prospective multicentre randomized controlled trial to evaluate factors influencing the success rate of office diagnostic hysteroscopy. Hum Reprod. 2005;20(1):258–63.
21. Jacobs VR, Paepke S, Schwarz-Boeger U, Fischer T, Pildner von Steinburg S, Plattner B, Schmalfeldt B, Schaaf H, Kiechle M. Development of a thinner and more flexible type of minihysteroscope with a controlled 90-degree bendable tip for vision-guided endometrium biopsy. J Minim Invasive Gynecol. 2005;12 (5):426–31.
22. Emanuel MH, Wamsteker K. The Intra Uterine Morcellator: a new hysteroscopic operating technique to remove intrauterine polyps and myomas. J Minim Invasive Gynecol. 2005;12:62–6.
23. van Dongen H, Emanuel MH, Wolterbeek R, et al. Hysteroscopic morcellator for removal of intrauterine polyps and myomas: a randomized controlled pilot study among residents in training. J Minim Invasive Gynecol. 2008;15:466–71.
24. Miller C, Glazerman L, Roy K, Lukes A. Clinical evaluation of a new hysteroscopic morcellator—retrospective case review. J Med. 2009;2:163–6.
25. Daniele A, Ferrero A, Maggiorotto F, Perrini G, Volpi E, Sismondi P. Suspecting malignancy in endometrial polyps: value of hysteroscopy. Tumori. 2013;99 (2):204–9.
26. Bettocchi S, Ceci O, Nappi L, Di Venere R, Masciopinto V, Pansini V, Pinto L, Santoro A, Cormio G. Operative office hysteroscopy without anesthesia: analysis of 4863 cases performed with mechanical instruments. J Am Assoc Gynecol Laparosc. 2004;11(1):59–61.
27. Puchalski A, Brodowska A, Bielewicz W. Bipolar hysteroscopic electrosurgery done with Versapoint system: comparison to operations done with monopolar electrodes, own experience. Ginekol Pol. 2000;71(9):1212–6.
28. Garuti G, Centinaio G, Luerti M. Outpatient hysteroscopic polypectomy in postmenopausal women: a comparison between mechanical and electrosurgical resection. J Minim Invasive Gynecol. 2008;15 (5):595–600.
29. Dealberti D, Riboni F, Prigione S, Pisani C, Rovetta E, Montella F, Garuti GM. New mini-resectoscope: analysis of preliminary quality results in outpatient hysteroscopic polypectomy. Arch Gynecol Obstet. 2013;288(2):349–53.
30. Wamsteker K, Emanuel MH, de Kruif JH. Transcervical hysteroscopic resection of submucous fibroids for abnormal uterine bleeding: results regarding the degree of intramural extension. Obstet Gynecol. 1993;82(5):736–40.
31. Laughlin SK, Stewart EA. Uterine leiomyomas. Individualizing the approach to a heterogeneous condition. Obstet Gynecol. 2011;117(2 Pt 1):396–403.
32. Valle RF, Sciarra JJ. Intrauterine adhesions: hysteroscopic diagnosis, classification, treatment, and reproductive outcome. Am J Obstet Gynecol. 1988;158:1459–70.
33. Pabuccu R, Atay V, Orhon E, Urman B, Ergun A. Hysteroscopic treatment of intrauterine adhesions is safe and effective in the restoration of normal menstruation and fertility. Fertil Steril. 1997;68:1141–3.
34. Guida M, Pellicano M, Zullo F, et al. Outpatient operative hysteroscopy with bipolar electrode: a prospective multicentre randomized study between local anaesthesia and conscious sedation. Hum Reprod. 2003;18:840–3.

35. Vilos GA. Intrauterine surgery using a new coaxial bipolar electrode in normal saline solution (Versapoint): a pilot study. Fertil Steril. 1999;72:740–3.
36. Schenker JG, Margalioth EJ. Intrauterine adhesions: an updated appraisal. Fertil Steril. 1982;37:593–610.
37. Orhue AA, Aziken ME, Igbefoh JO. A comparison of two adjunctive treatments for intrauterine adhesions following lysis. Int J Gynaecol Obstet. 2003;82:49–56.
38. Tsapanos VS, Stathopoulou LP, Papathanassopoulou VS, Tzingounis VA. The role of Sepralm bioresorbable membrane in the prevention and therapy of endometrial synechiae. J Biomed Mater Res. 2002;63:10–4.
39. Valle RF. Uterine septa. In: Bieber EJ, Loffer F, editors. Hysteroscopy, resectoscopy and endometrial ablation. Carnforth, UK: Parthenon; 2003. p. 75–86.
40. Buttram VC, Gibbons WE. Müllerian anomalies: a proposed classification (an analysis of 144 cases). Fertil Steril. 1979;32:40–6.
41. Homer HA, Li T-C, Cooke ID. The septate uterus: a review of management and reproductive outcome. Fertil Steril. 2000;73:1–14.
42. Acien P. Reproductive performance of women with uterine malformations. Hum Reprod. 1993;8:122–6.
43. Raga F, Bauset C, Remohi J, Bonilla-Musoles F, Simon C, Pellicer A. Reproductive impact of congenital Müllerian anomalies. Hum Reprod. 1997;12:2277–81.
44. Bettocchi S, Ceci O, Nappi L, Pontrelli G, Pinto L, Vicino M. Office hysteroscopic metroplasty: three "diagnostic criteria" to differentiate between septate and bicornuate uteri. J Minim Invasive Gynecol. 2007;14:324–8.
45. Grimbizis G, Camus M, Clasen K, Tournaye H, De Munck L, Devroey P. Hysteroscopic septum resection in patients with recurrent abortions or infertility. Hum Reprod. 1998;13:1188–93.
46. Fayez JA. Comparison between abdominal and hysteroscopic metroplasty. Obstet Gynecol. 1986; 68:399–403.
47. Vercellini P, Vendola N, Colombo A, Passadore C, Trespidi L, Fedele L. Hysteroscopic metroplasty with resectoscope or microscissors for the correction of septate uterus. Surg Gynecol Obstet. 1993; 176:439–42.
48. Fedele L, Bianchi S. Hysteroscopic metroplasty for septate uterus. Obstet Gynecol Clin North Am. 1995;22:473–89.
49. Pabuçcu R, Gomel V. Reproductive outcome after hysteroscopic metroplasty in women with septate uterus and otherwise unexplained infertility. Fertil Steril. 2004;81:1675–8.
50. Jansen FW, Vredevoogd CB, Van Ulzen K, et al. Complications of hysteroscopy: a prospective multicenter study. Obstet Gynecol. 2000;96:266–70.
51. Goldrath MH. Uterine tamponade for the control of acute uterine bleeding. Am J Obstet Gynecol. 1983;147:869–72.
52. Townsend DE. Vasopressin pack for treatment of bleeding after myoma resection. Am J Obstet Gynecol. 1991;165:1405–7.
53. Glasser MH. Endometrial ablation and hysteroscopic myomectomy by electrosurgical vaporization. J Am Assoc Gynecol Laparosc. 1997;4:369–74.
54. Loffer FD, Bradley LD, Brill AI, et al. Hysteroscopic fluid monitoring guidelines. J Am Assoc Gynecol Laparosc. 2000;7:438.
55. van Kerkvoorde TC, Veersema S, Timmermans A. Long term complications of office hysteroscopy: analysis of 1028 cases. J Minim Invasive Gynecol. 2012;19(4):494–7.

Office-Based Global Endometrial Ablation

10

Margaret L. McKenzie and Monique Yoder

Introduction

Abnormal uterine bleeding (AUB) is the all-encompassing term adopted to describe irregularities in the amount, frequency, and duration of uterine bleeding. The International Federation of Gynecology and Obstetrics introduced the PALM-COEIN classification system for uterine bleeding abnormalities in an effort to standardize nomenclature [1]. Along with the term AUB, descriptive terms to characterize the patterns of AUB were also adopted; the term menorrhagia was replaced with heavy menstrual bleeding (HMB) [2].

HMB is defined as menstrual blood loss of >80 mL per menstrual cycle. Asking pertinent questions may assist the healthcare provider to ascertain or quantify bleeding. Patients should be asked about the rate or frequency of sanitary product change. How often do they change sanitary products (tampons, pads) during heaviest flow or the total number of products used? Presence of blood clots with menstrual flow, and the size of clots (greater than 1 in. in diameter) should be documented. Basic laboratory tests including a complete blood count and ferritin level to assess for iron-deficiency anemia are also useful when combined with these questions to quantify the amount of menstrual blood loss [3]. However, the most practical and important quantification method to determine blood loss in the presence of HMB, is the individual patient's perception of excessive blood loss with menses, her distress, disruption of activities, and decreased quality of life she experienced due to HMB [4].

HMB is estimated to affect up to 30 % of reproductive-aged women [5] and has been reported to have a significant negative impact on patients' overall physical and psychological health, with disruption of work, family life, social activities, sexual function, and a decrease in global quality of life. HMB also has significant financial consequences, with estimated annual costs including physician visits, medical therapies, and surgical interventions ranging from 1 to 5 billion US dollars [5, 6].

Approximately 600,000 hysterectomies are performed in the United States annually and hysterectomy is the second most common surgery performed in reproductive age women in the United States, after cesarean section. The most common indications for hysterectomy are symptomatic uterine fibroids, followed by AUB and endometriosis. Costs associated with hysterectomy make up a significant proportion of the costs associated with treating AUB and HMB. Until the 1980s, treatment for HMB primarily consisted of expectant management, medical therapies, and surgical management including hysterectomy [3, 7, 8].

M.L. McKenzie, M.D. (✉) • M. Yoder, M.D.
Section of General Gynecology, Department of Obstetrics, Gynecology and Women's Health Institute, Cleveland Clinic, 9500 Euclid Avenue, Desk A-81, Cleveland, OH 44195, USA
e-mail: mckenzm@ccf.org; yoderb@ccf.org

J.D. Emery and M.F.R. Paraiso (eds.), *Office-Based Gynecologic Surgical Procedures*,
DOI 10.1007/978-1-4939-1414-2_10, © Springer Science+Business Media New York 2015

History of Global Endometrial Ablation

Surgical management of HMB is usually undertaken after medical therapy has failed. While hysterectomy is the definitive treatment for HMB with complete cessation of bleeding, it is also a major surgical procedure requiring general anesthesia with significant risk of intra and postoperative complications, increased recovery time, and associated costs [7].

Endometrial ablation as an alternative option for surgical management of HMB, became widely used in the late 1980s and 1990s. The first techniques used or "first-generation" methods of endometrial ablation, while effective, were all done in the operating room (OR) with hysteroscopic visualization of the uterine cavity and included laser endometrial ablation, rollerball ablation, transcervical resection/destruction of the endometrium (TCRE) with a resectoscope, or a combination of TCRE and rollerball ablation. These methods are considered the gold standard to which subsequently developed endometrial ablation techniques are compared [9–11].

While effective, the first-generation endometrial ablation procedures have limitations including the need for extensive training of the surgeon with a relatively high rate of associated complications in the inexperienced surgeon. Documented complications include uterine perforation, damage to abdominal and pelvic structures, cervical laceration, complications related to anesthesia, fluid overload and hemorrhage [11–13]. Due to these drawbacks with first-generation procedures, alternative global endometrial ablation (GEA) techniques have been developed that are safer, just as efficacious, and easier to perform with automated features necessitating less but appropriate training of the surgeon [9].

There are currently five devices which are approved by the United States Food and Drug Administration (FDA) for second-generation GEA: the Novasure® radiofrequency ablation device, the Hydro ThermAblator® (HTA) device, the Gynecare ThermaChoice® balloon ablation device, the Her Option® Cryoablation device, and the Microwave Endometrial Ablation (MEA) device. In addition each device has been used successfully in the office setting.

In-Office GEA Versus GEA in the OR

Second-generation GEA procedures are increasingly being performed in the office setting with local anesthesia (i.e., paracervical block) and minimal oral or IV sedation, rather than in the operating theater. In order to perform GEA successfully in the gynecology office, it is imperative that properly trained support personnel and appropriate facilities and equipment are in place (see Chap. 2). Basic emergency equipment and medications should be available per state and local regulations, and providers performing office procedures should develop protocols for preoperative and intraoperative anesthesia and analgesia. Patients who undergo office procedures involving sedation should be counseled regarding postoperative recovery and instructed to have a driver to take them home post-procedure [6, 8].

Furthermore, for a proceduralist or surgeon to be successful in performing office GEA procedures, patients must be thoroughly evaluated before the procedure. Underlying causes of AUB should be determined to determine the appropriateness of GEA as the most effective treatment option for her. Underlying causes of AUB such as polyps, adenomyosis, large (>3 mm) intracavitary leiomyoma, malignancy, coagulopathy, or ovulatory dysfunction should be ruled out with the pertinent imaging studies and treated before the procedure if necessary [1]. After underlying causes of AUB have been determined, patients with HMB have traditionally been managed medically. Hormonal therapy, tranexamic acid, nonsteroidal anti-inflammatory drugs (NSAIDs), and or the levonorgestrel-releasing intrauterine system (IUS) as first-line therapy and ideally a trial and failure of medical therapy should be documented prior to consideration of surgical intervention for treatment of HMB.

Patients who fail medical therapy or those considered as good candidates for office GEA should subsequently be evaluated for acceptability and tolerability of local anesthesia or sedation. The American Society of Anesthesiologists (ASA) classification, pain/procedural tolerance, and desire to undergo a minimally invasive procedure versus other options such as first-line GEA procedures or hysterectomy should be assessed (see Chap. 4). To determine a patient's suitability for office GEA, additional and specific considerations apply. Since FDA approval is based on completed childbearing, patients must be willing to use appropriate contraception as GEA does not prevent pregnancy and also because of the evidence that pregnancy outcomes after GEA are largely very poor [14, 15]. In addition, patients should be counseled on failure rates and risks of future hysterectomy due to the lost capacity to completely evaluate the uterine cavity in the future. The endometrial cavity and the uterus should be evaluated with either transvaginal ultrasound, saline infusion sonography (SIS), or office hysteroscopy. The length of the uterine cavity, thickness of the myometrium, and the presence of any structural anomalies should be documented. The uterine cavity should be evaluated for Mullerian anomalies, and intracavitary leiomyoma(s) >3 mm in size. Cesarean section scars should be evaluated and the thickness of the scar ascertained and documented. Depending on the length of the uterine cavity or the presence of uterine or intracavitary anomalies, certain GEA techniques, or GEA in general may be contraindicated. It is important that candidates for GEA be thoroughly counseled and be accepting of the fact that GEA usually does not guarantee amenorrhea, they should be informed that evidence shows significant lightening or normalization of menstrual bleeding [10, 11, 16].

Patient Selection for the Office

In general, healthy patients with anesthesia classification ASA II are good perspective candidates for office procedures like endometrial ablation. Our protocol for choosing patients for the office setting includes a thorough evaluation of the patient's capacity to tolerate an office procedure without intravenous (IV) sedation. Patients who fail to tolerate simple office procedures like endometrial biopsies, SIS, or office hysteroscopy are poor candidates for office endometrial ablations. Ultimately the patient must give informed consent (Chap. 3), which includes her receptiveness for performance in the office. For procedures that require concurrent ultrasound, such as cryoablation, body habitus, and the capacity for the patient to hold a full bladder to allow for adequate visualization during the procedure are other important considerations. In addition, the patient must be able to lie supine during procedures so any conditions, which prevent the supine position, should be considered (see Table 10.1) [10].

FDA-Approved GEA Methods

Some preoperative considerations before embarking on GEA include need for endometrial thinning, cervical dilation, prophylactic antibiotics, analgesia and/or sedation pre-procedure. Most of the FDA trials for the second-generation GEA devices used endometrial thinning pre-procedure with either a gonadotropin-releasing hormone (GnRH) agonist (i.e., goserelin) or dilation and curettage. The simplest option to ensure a thin endometrial lining pre-procedure is to schedule the procedure shortly after menstruation in the early proliferate phase of the menstrual cycle. Pharmacologic options for endometrial thinning include GnRH agonists; goserelin acetate (Zoladex®) being the most widely studied and associated with the best outcomes as well as FDA approval for this indication. Danazol, oral contraceptive pills (OCP) and medroxyprogesterone acetate injection may also be used to thin or stabilize the endometrium in the weeks prior to the procedure. Some form of endometrial thinning is advised pre-procedure, as it is associated with greater ease of procedure, fewer short-term complications, greater

Table 10.1 Patient selection criteria for global endometrial ablation devices

Global ablation device	ThermaChoice ($n = 137$)	Her Option ($n = 193$)	HTA ($n = 187$)	NovaSure ($n = 175$)	MEA ($n = 215$)
Protocol differences and exclusion criteria					
Maximum sound length (cm)	10	10	10.5	10	14
Inclusion of polyps	No	No	No	Yes (<2 cm)	Yes
Inclusion of submucosal fibroids	No	No	No	Yes (<2 cm)	Yes (<3 cm)
Inclusion of distorted cavities	No	No	No	No	Yes
Congenital malformations	No	No	No	No	Yes
Endometrial pretreatment	D&C	Lupron 3.75 mg	Lupron 7.5 mg	None	Lupron 3.75 mg
Gynecologic history					
Age (years)	40.4 (±4.8)	41.2 (±5.1)	40.7 (±5.2)	39.7 (±5.5)	40.5 (±4.6)
BMI	29.1 (±7.8)	29.3 (±8.4)	29.0 (±7.4)	27.6 (±6.3)	27.94 (±7.1)
Number of pregnancies	ND	2.5 (±1.2)	ND	2.7 (±1.3)	ND
Number of term deliveries	ND	2.4 (±1.2)	ND	2.2 (±1.1)	ND
Baseline diary score	552.5 (±712.2)	570 (±441)	596.55 (±787.6)	562 (±381)	451.8 (±356.6)
Uterine sounding length (cm)	8.5 (±1.3)	8.0 (±1.1)	8.3 (±1.3)	8.8 (±0.8)	8.09 (±1.0)

From: Bradley LD. Endometrial Ablation. In: Bradley LD, Falcone T (eds). *Hysteroscopy: Office Evaluation and Management of the Uterine Cavity*. Philadelphia, Mosby, 2009, with permission
BMI body mass index, *D&C* dilation and curettage, *HTA* Hydro ThermAblator, *MEA* microwave endometrial ablation, *ND* no data

endometrial atrophy, and better overall outcomes post-procedure [11, 17].

Cervical ripening with misoprostol, orally or vaginally, may also be advisable for selected patients with cervical stenosis or those who are nulliparous or perimenopausal. Administration of misoprostol may limit patient discomfort and decrease the incidence of cervical injury during the procedure, but these benefits should be weighed against potential side effects such as uterine cramping and bleeding. In addition, the potential for increased transcervcial leakage of fluid if the HTA system is used should be managed, and patients should be counseled accordingly. Prophylactic antibiotics are not recommended for GEA procedures and the rate of post-procedure endometritis is very low. It is therefore up to the clinician's judgment in using antibiotics if an individual patient is perceived to be at increased risk for infection (i.e., history of acute or chronic endometritis, vaginitis, gonoccocal or chlamydial infection) [9, 10, 16].

As part of the procedural analgesia and anesthesia protocol, patients are often pretreated with an oral analgesic and/or anxiolytic prior to the procedure. Detailed instructions include thorough pre-procedure counseling on what to expect, local anesthesia and analgesics, use of heating pads/warm packs and soothing background music. A dedicated support person is recommended for transportation post procedure.

The choice of the specific GEA modality to be used is based on many factors. Availability of different systems at a given facility, provider preference, and/or specific patient history and characteristics may make one modality superior over another (i.e., presence of intracavitary leiomyoma). The five currently FDA-approved second-generation GEA systems are as follows (see Table 10.2) [11].

Table 10.2 Non-resectoscopic endometrial ablation device comparisons

Method	Pretreatment	Outside diameter (mm)	Approximate treatment time (min)	Sounded uterine length (cm)[a]		Treatment in the presence of submucosal leiomyomata			
				Minimum	Maximum	Published evidence	Type	Diameter (cm)	US Food and Drug Administration Approval
ThermaChoice (thermal balloon)	Mechanical (suction aspiration)	5.5	8	4	10	Yes (Level I)	II	Smaller than or equal to 3	No
Her Option (cryotherapy)	Gonadotropin-releasing hormone agonist	4.5	10–18	Not specified	10	None	Not applicable	Not applicable	No
Hydro ThermAblator (heated free fluid)	Gonadotropin-releasing hormone agonist	7.8	14	4	10.5	Yes (Level II-3)	I[b], II	Not specified	No
Microwave endometrial ablation system (microwave energy)	Gonadotropin-releasing hormone agonist	8.5	2.5–4.5	6	14	Yes (Level I)	I[b], II	Smaller than or equal to 3	Yes
NovaSure (radiofrequency electricity)	None	7.2	1–2	6	10	Yes (Level II-2)	I, II	Smaller than or equal to 3	No

Reprinted from: American College of Obstetricians and Gynecologists. Endometrial ablation. ACOG Practice Bulletin No. 81. Obstet Gynecol 2007; 109:1233–48, with permission

[a]From device activation to withdrawal

[b]Selected

NovaSure®

The NovaSure endometrial ablation device is bipolar, single-use mesh electrode that utilizes radiofrequency energy to vaporize and coagulate the endometrium with simultaneous suction that pulls endometrial tissue into contact with the device while evacuating debris and steam generated by vaporization. Power delivery is calculated automatically based on measurements by the sounding device of the uterine cavity width and length, and the system includes an automatic safety feature based on carbon dioxide insufflation pressure that helps detect uterine perforation. The ablation portion of the procedure takes approximately 80–90 s. The NovaSure system has been used to perform office GEA throughout the United States with both IV and non-IV sedation with good outcomes [10, 16].

Gynecare ThermaChoice®

Several balloon endometrial ablation systems exist, however the ThermChoice® system is the only such device with FDA approval. The ThermaChoice® is a single-use device consisting of balloon tipped catheter containing a heating element. After insertion into the uterus the balloon is inflated with mixture of 5 % dextrose in water (D5W) to a predetermined pressure between 160 and 180 mmHg, and heated to approximately 87 °C for 8 min, ablating the endometrium by direct thermal effect. Because the system operates with high intrauterine pressures, there may be more issues with patient discomfort during the procedure, and the procedure is usually performed with IV sedation and analgesia. The ThermaChoice® system has been used in patients with small (<3 mm) intracavitary fibroids, as long as they do not obstruct deployment of the balloon [10, 16].

Hydro ThermAblator®

The HydroThermAblator® system employs a single-use sheath in combination with a rigid hysterscope to instill heated, free-flowing normal saline into the uterine cavity to achieve endometrial ablation. It is the only second-generation GEA modality that is performed under direct hysteroscopic visualization. After the sheath is inserted into the uterus, free-flowing saline is instilled at low pressures and after a diagnostic period of approximately 2 min, the saline is heated to 90 °C for approximately 3 min, allowed to circulate at that temperature for 10 min, then after a 1 min cooling period the device is removed. A new sheath has been designed with a cervical sealing mechanism to prevent leakage of fluid during the procedure, and the system's controller unit automates the processes of uterine distention, fluid heating, temperature monitoring, and maintenance of a closed system. Due to the use of a non-fixed system employing a free-flowing solution for thermal endometrial ablation, the ThermAblator is uniquely suited to treatment of uteri with intracavitary fibroids as long as they do not obstruct the cavity, and significant shrinkage of leiomyoma(s) has been observed with use of the system. In short-term follow-up studies, the ThermAblator system has shown similar outcomes to gold-standard roller ball ablation [10, 16].

Her Option® Cryoablation

The Her Option® Cryoablation system achieves endometrial ablation with cyrotherapy or freezing. The procedure is performed with ultrasound guidance and monitoring, under which a disposable probe is inserted into the uterine cavity and directed to the cornua. Once the probe is in place on one side, it is activated to produce an expanding freeze zone ("iceball") which is monitored by ultrasound, the endpoint being determined manually by the operator and ultrasound appearance. This is repeated at the opposite cornual area, and in certain cases, lower in the endometrial cavity. The overall procedure takes approximately 10 min. It should be noted that the failure rate of cyroablation increases significantly with an increased size of uterine cavity, up to 70 % with cavities measuring >11 cm [10, 16].

Microwave Endometrial Ablation® System

The MEA system utilizes microwave energy similar to that employed in commercial microwave ovens, which exerts a direct effect on tissue and on adjacent, deeper level tissue through thermal propagation. Either a disposable or reusable probe may be used for the procedure. That is inserted into the uterine cavity to the uterine fundus. Once at the fundus, when the tissue around the probe is heated to 30 ° C the probe is activated and moved from side-to-side down the uterine cavity to treat the entire endometrial surface. The probe must be in contact with the endometrium in order for the treatment to be effective. It should be noted that measurement of the myometrium with imaging is imperative pre-procedure, as burns to surrounding organs have been reported with MEA, to ensure that the myometrial thickness is consistently at least 8 mm, with a manufacturer recommendation of 10 mm for an increased safety margin. Clinicians should also be aware of any intracavitary anomalies, specifically leiomyoma, as though they are not a contraindication to using the system, they should increase concern for possible distortion or thinning of the endometrium and increased risk for burns [10, 16].

Outcomes of GEA

Approximately 20–25 % of women who undergo endometrial ablation as the initial surgical modality for treatment of HMB will have subsequent treatment, usually repeat ablation or hysterectomy, usually due to continued or recurrent problems with menstrual bleeding [18]. This fact may undermine much of the significant cost benefit associated with GEA versus hysterectomy as an initial surgical treatment option for HMB [11, 12, 19]. It has been found that age at the time of procedure may be a predictor of subsequent hysterectomy following GEA, specifically women under age 40 who undergo GEA have been found to be at significant risk [20].

Given these facts, it should be reiterated that thorough pre-procedure evaluation of patients including presentation, age, medical history, desired as well as expected outcomes and a careful, detailed characterization of uterine and intracavitary anatomy is of paramount importance in determining if a patient is an appropriate candidate for GEA, and which GEA modality should be used to assure the best possible outcomes (see Table 10.3) [10].

"Tips & Tricks"/Troubleshooting

In general, appropriate patient selection, adequate timing of the cycle for performance of the procedure, adequate cervical preparation, and proper pre-procedure endometrial cavity evaluation, predicts the success of the GEA procedures. All procedures, except for radiofrequency ablation, should be performed only after adequate preparation of the endometrium. It is important to wait after analgesia is administered (typically 5–10 min) and effective before starting the procedure as the patient's discomfort will sabotage any chances of success. The paracervical block should be used liberally in all patients and allowed to take effect before starting the procedure. In addition, preparing the cervix with misoprostol pre-procedure can help to minimize patient discomfort during the procedure.

Complications

Short-term or procedural complications can occur with office endometrial ablation. These include uterine perforation, injury to surrounding abdominal or pelvic structures, hemorrhage, cervical injury, infection, lower genitourinary (GU) tract thermal injury, and post-ablation tubal ligation syndrome with post-ablation pain (both early and late). There can also be complications related to anesthesia as well as intolerance and abandonment of the procedure with light sedation: the patient should be counseled that increased discomfort may be a sign to stop the procedure before completion. Although complications

Table 10.3 Patient satisfaction and amenorrhea rates associated with non-resectoscope endometrial ablation compared with resectoscopic ablation at 12 months[a]

	Non-resectoscopic/resectoscopic ablation (%)		
Device	Satisfaction rate	Amenorrhea rate[b]	Diary success (score: 75 or less)
ThermaChoice (thermal balloon)	96/99[c]	13.2/27.2	80.2/84.3
Hydro ThermAblator (heated free fluid)	___[d]	35.3/47.1	68.4/76.4
Her Option (cryotherapy)	86/88[e]	22.2/46.5	67.4/73.3
NovaSure (radiofrequency electricity)	92/93[c]	36/32.2	77.7/74.4
Microwave Endometrial Ablation System (microwave energy)	92/93[c]	55.3/45.8	87/83.2

Adapted from Sharp HT. Assessment of new technology in the treatment of idiopathic menorrhagia and uterine leiomyomata. Obstet Gynecol 2006; 108:990-1003

Reprinted from: American College of Obstetricians and Gynecologists. Endometrial ablation. ACOG Practice Bulletin No. 81. Obstet Gynecol 2007; 109:1233–48, with permission

[a]Based on US Food and Drug Administration pivotal trials

[b]Based on intent to treat

[c]Patients reported being satisfied or very satisfied

[d]Quality-of-life scores compared with baseline only

[e]Patients reported being very or extremely satisfied

Table 10.4 Percentages of postoperative adverse events occurring within 2 weeks of non-resectoscopic endometrial ablation surgery[a]

Complication	ThermaChoice (thermal balloon)	Hydro ThermAblator (heated free fluid)	Her Option (Cryotherapy)	NovaSure (radiofrequency electricity)	Microwave ablation system (microwave energy)
Urinary tract infection	0.8	2	3	0.6	0.5
Vaginal infection	0.8	0	1	0.6	2.3
Fever	0	0	0	0	1.4
Endometritis	2.1	1	0	0	2.8
Thermal injury[b]	0	1	0	0	0
Abdominal pain	0	2	4	0.6	3.2
Hematometra	0	0	0	0.6	0
Bacteremia	0	0	0	0	0.5

From: Sharp HT. Assessment of new technology in the treatment of idiopathic menorrhagia and uterine leiomyomata. Obstet Gynecol 2006; 108:990-1003

Reprinted from: American College of Obstetricians and Gynecologists. Endometrial ablation. ACOG Practice Bulletin No. 81. Obstet Gynecol 2007; 109:1233–48, with permission

[a]Reported during US Food and Drug Administration pivotal trials

[b]Involving an extremity

have been documented, the newer GEA techniques when chosen correctly, are popular with most women because the rates of major complications are low compared with the first-generation GEA methods, and satisfaction rate very high (see Table 10.4) [10].

As earlier stated, it is very important to counsel patients thoroughly evaluating them for appropriateness for the office setting, and to ensure adequate birth control is used concomitantly after GEA, as endometrial ablation does not preclude subsequent pregnancy, and pregnancy outcomes following GEA are uniformly poor [14, 15]. It should be noted that it is not recommended to perform sterilization with Essure® at the same time as a GEA procedure. Patients may choose to undergo sterilization with Essure® and confirmation of tubal occlusion with the required hysterosalpingogram (HSG) confirmation test, *prior* to GEA. Currently only three GEA modalities are approved by the FDA for use with Essure® microcoils in situ: ThermaChoice® balloon ablation, Novasure radiofrequency ablation and HTA hydrothermal ablation [21].

Conclusion

In-office GEA is a safe and reliable technique to treat heavy uterine bleeding that is refractory to medical or implant therapies. Patient evaluation and selection are critical to produce quality outcomes and a satisfactory patient experience, both during the procedure and after the procedure with improved menstrual function. Establishing office protocols for pre-procedure work-up, anesthesia, and analgesia during the procedure and patient preparation are also vitally important. Lastly, awareness of complications during and after the GEA procedure should be considered and managed accordingly. Selection of the appropriate GEA modality requires operator experience in order to achieve the best patient outcomes.

References

1. Munro MG, Critchley HO, Broder MS, Fraser IS, et al. FIGO classification system (PALM-COEIN) for causes of abnormal uterine bleeding in nongravid women of reproductive age. Int J Gynaecol Obstet. 2011;113(1):3–13.
2. Committee on Practice Bulletins-Gynecology. Practice bulletin no. 128: diagnosis of abnormal uterine bleeding in reproductive-aged women. Obstet Gynecol. 2012;120:197–206.
3. Warner PE, Critchley HO, Lumsden MA, Campbell-Brown M, Douglas A, Murray GD, Menorrhagia I. Measured blood loss, clinical features, and outcome in women with heavy periods: a survey with follow-up data. Am J Obstet Gynecol. 2004;190:1216–23.
4. Apgar BS, Kaufman AH, George-Nwogu U, Kittendorf A. Treatment of menorrhagia. Am Fam Physician. 2007;75:1813–9.
5. Liu Z, Doan QV, Blumenthal P, Dubois RW. A systematic review evaluating health-related quality of life, work impairment, and health-care costs and utilization in abnormal uterine bleeding. Value Health. 2007;10:183–94.
6. Munro MG, Dickersin K, Clark MA, et al. The surgical treatments outcomes project for dysfunctional uterine bleeding: summary of an Agency for Health Research and Quality-sponsored randomized trial of endometrial ablation versus hysterectomy for women with heavy menstrual bleeding. Menopause. 2011;18:445–52.
7. Merrill RM, Layman AB, Oderda G, Asche C. Risk estimates of hysterectomy and selected conditions commonly treated with hysterectomy. Ann Epidemiol. 2008;18:253–60.
8. Whiteman MK, Hillis SD, Jamieson DJ, et al. Inpatient hysterectomy surveillance in the United States, 2000-2004. Am J Obstet Gynecol. 2008;198:34.e1, 34.e7.
9. Lethaby A, Penninx J, Hickey M, Garry R, Marjoribanks J. Endometrial resection and ablation techniques for heavy menstrual bleeding. Cochrane Database Syst Rev. 2013;(8):CD001501.
10. American College of Obstetricians and Gynecologists. Endometrial ablation. ACOG Practice Bulletin No. 81. Obstet Gynecol. 2007;109:1233–48.
11. Bradley LD. Endometrial ablation. In: Bradley LD, Falcone T, editors. Hysteroscopy: office evaluation and management of the uterine cavity. Philadelphia: Mosby; 2009.
12. Daniels JP, Middleton LJ, Champaneria R, et al. Second generation endometrial ablation techniques for heavy menstrual bleeding: network meta-analysis. BMJ. 2012;344:e2564.
13. Overton C, Hargreaves J, Maresh M. A national survey of the complications of endometrial destruction for menstrual disorders: the MISTLETOE study. Minimally invasive surgical techniques–laser, endothermal or endoresection. Br J Obstet Gynaecol. 1997;104(12):1351–9.
14. Bowling MR, Ramsey PS. Spontaneous uterine rupture in pregnancy after endometrial ablation. Obstet Gynecol. 2010;115:405–6.
15. Roux I, Das M, Fernandez H, Deffieux X. Pregnancy after endometrial ablation. J Reprod Med. 2013;58:173–6.
16. Glasser MH. Practical tips for office hysteroscopy and second-generation "global" endometrial ablation. J Minim Invasive Gynecol. 2009;16(4):384–99.
17. Lethaby A, Hickey M. Endometrial destruction techniques for heavy menstrual bleeding. Cochrane Database Syst Rev. 2002;(2):CD001501. Review.

Update: Cochrane Database Syst Rev. 2005;(4): CD001501.

18. Dickerson K, Munro MG, Clark M, et al. Hysterectomy compared with endometrial ablation for dysfunctional uterine bleeding: a randomized controlled trial. Obstet Gynecol. 2007;110:1279–89.
19. El-Nashar SA, Hopkins MR, Creedon DJ, St Sauver JL, Weaver AL, McGree ME, et al. Prediction of treatment outcomes after global endometrial ablation. Obstet Gynecol. 2009;113:97–106.
20. Longinotti MK, Jacobson GF, Hung YY, Learman LA. Probability of hysterectomy after endometrial ablation. Obstet Gynecol. 2008;112(6):1214–20.
21. Aldape D, Chudnoff SG, Levie MD. Global endometrial ablation in the presence of EssureR microinserts. Rev Obstet Gynecol. 2013;6:80–8.

11 Cystoscopy

Audra Jolyn Hill and Marie Fidela R. Paraiso

Introduction

Office cystoscopy is a valuable tool in the evaluation of patients who present with lower urinary tract symptoms in adjunct with a complete physical examination. Cystoscopy allows for a minimally invasive view of the internal lower urinary tract with relatively low morbidity for female patients. Although routine cystoscopy is not recommended, it may be indicated if a patient presents with the following symptoms:

- Recurrent urinary tract infections
- Persistent irritative voiding symptoms (urgency, dysuria, etc.)
- Unexplained bladder pain
- Periurethral mass
- Urinary leakage of unknown etiology
- Hematuria (if indicated per American Urological Association guidelines) [1]

A.J. Hill, M.D. (✉)
Division of Urogynecology and Pelvic Reconstructive Surgery, Obstetrics, Gynecology & Women's Health Institute, Cleveland Clinic Foundation, 9500 Euclid Avenue, Desk A81, Cleveland, OH 44195, USA
e-mail: hilla8@ccf.org

M.F.R. Paraiso, M.D.
Cleveland Clinic Lerner College of Medicine at Case Western Reserve University, Cleveland, OH, USA

Center for Urogynecology and Reconstructive Pelvic Surgery, Obstetrics, Gynecology, and Women's Health Institute, Cleveland Clinic, Cleveland, OH, USA

Glickman Urological and Kidney Institute, Cleveland Clinic, Cleveland, OH, USA
e-mail: paraism@ccf.org

Historical Perspective

The concept of visualizing the bladder occurred as early as 1805 by Bozzini with the use of hollow funnels, candle light, and a mirror to assist with light deflection in a device called the *Leichleiter*. This was used to track bullet pathways in wounded soldiers via the pharynx, nasal cavities, and the urethra. Initially, the overall concept was rejected by the Faculty of Vienna. However despite this, the conceptual idea continued to be developed throughout the nineteenth century. Numerous instrument modifications occurred with the mirror eventually being replaced by a prism to assist with previous problematic inverted images and in 1879, the first cystoscope was created by Nitze and Leiter that added an adequate light source using tungsten wire that prevented "overheating" of the instrument. Unfortunately this required a complicated cooling system which only increased the complexity of design. This was remedied with the development of a small low-amperage light bulb, called a mignon bulb, initially created by two New York physicians in 1881, that was able to easily fit into the tip of the cystoscope which resolved the complicated lighting system previously used. This small advancement allowed for further device variations/developments and slightly decreased the cost of the cystoscope [2, 3]. In 1894, due to the significant cost of the instrument and overall complexity, Dr. Howard Kelly invented the use of

J.D. Emery and M.F.R. Paraiso (eds.), *Office-Based Gynecologic Surgical Procedures*, DOI 10.1007/978-1-4939-1414-2_11, © Springer Science+Business Media New York 2015

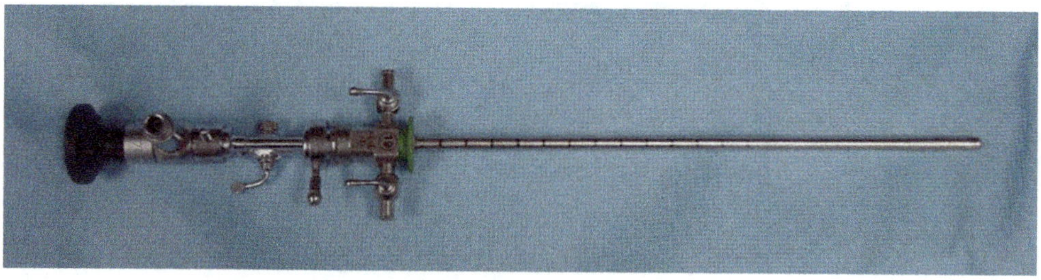

Fig. 11.1 Rigid cystoscope

an air cystoscope that required limited equipment, offered ease of use, and introduced techniques that allowed cystoscopy to be available for all physicians [4]. Continued device progression continued and in 1954, with the introduction of Hopkins' fiber optic telescope that allowed the operator the ability to alter viewing angles during the procedure and enhanced overall visualization; modern cystoscopy was born [2]. Multiple technological advancements ensued throughout the following years, most recently with the development of the flexible cystoscope in 1973 that has allowed for an even wider angle of view and the ability to visualize the bladder neck in its entirety [5].

With the progression of modern age cystoscopes, patients now have the ability to undergo an in-office procedure with minimal discomfort. With the increased awareness of cost effectiveness in the healthcare system and the large proportion of diagnostic cystoscopies that result in "normal findings," in-office cystoscopy has become the preferred modality over an outpatient surgical procedure. Benefits of office cystoscopy include avoidance of any anesthetic risk, overall decreased procedural cost, and if for diagnostic purposes alone, office cystoscopy provides a minimally invasive procedure that can provide a therapeutic effect if no abnormal findings are visualized. If abnormalities are noted, a patient can then undergo appropriate counseling and be provided with a referral to specialist if indicated.

Equipment

To properly perform office cystoscopy, one must have the minimal following equipment: (1) a cystoscope, (2) a light source, and (3) distending media.

Two types of cystoscopes are currently available: rigid or flexible. Rigid cystoscopes, as seen in Fig. 11.1, are composed of three separate pieces. The first component is the telescope which is usually 15 French in diameter. The lens of a telescope may come in 0, 30, 70, or 120° variations. A 30° or 70° cystoscope will usually suffice for the diagnostic evaluation of the bladder. The next component is the sheath which ranges in sizing from 15 to 28 French in diameter. The sheath allows the telescope and distending media to be introduced simultaneously into the bladder cavity and allows for passage of operative instruments if needed. The proximal end has two irrigating ports (inflow and outflow) with the distal end having fenestrations to permit passage of instruments if indicated. Larger sheaths are needed for operative cystoscopy, usually up to 22 French to allow passage of instruments measuring 4 French or less. Lastly, the bridge is needed to form a watertight seal between the sheath and the telescope. Figure 11.2 illustrates the separate pieces needed for assembly.

Flexible cystoscopes have the ability to combine the optical system along with irrigation capabilities into a single unit. The flexible tip of the cystoscope allows for a deflection of 290° and has a diameter ranging from 15 to 18 French. See Figs. 11.3, 11.4, and 11.5. Multiple investigations have been performed comparing rigid versus flexible cystoscopy, however some studies included male patients and other studies evaluated quality-of-life outcomes between patients who underwent office flexible cystoscopy compared to those who underwent a rigid

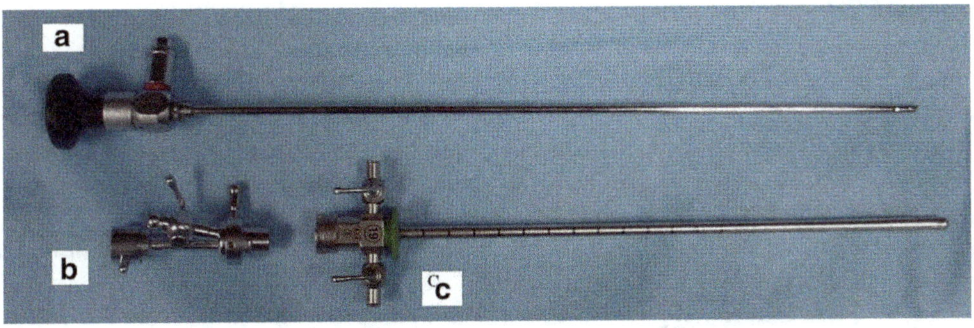

Fig. 11.2 Components of rigid cystoscope (**a**) telescope (**b**) bridge (**c**) sheath

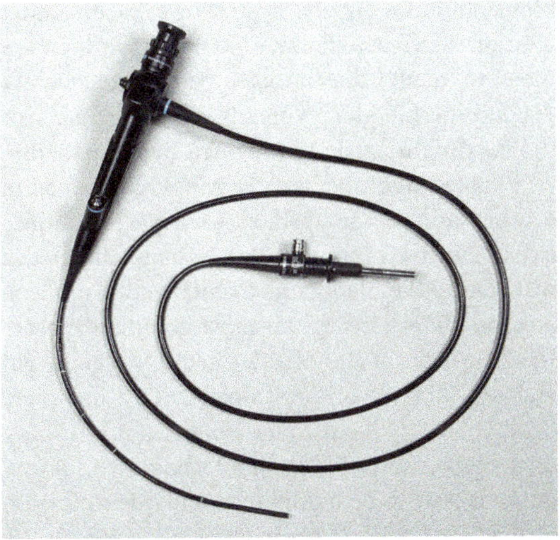

Fig. 11.3 Flexible cystoscope

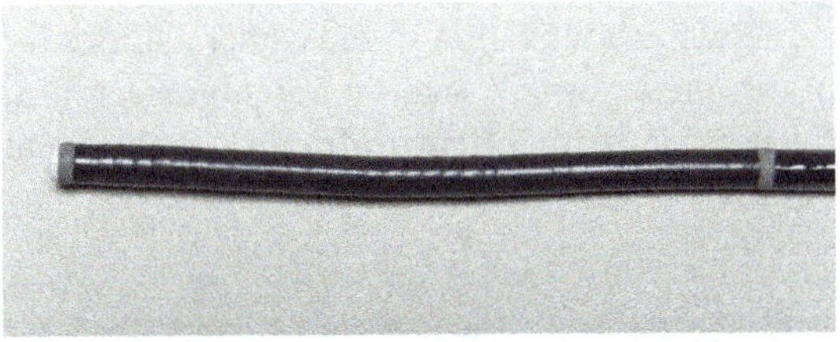

Fig. 11.4 Tip of flexible cystoscope

cystoscopy under general anesthesia [6]. More recently, studies by Gee et al. and Quinoz et al. comparing rigid and flexible in-office cystoscopy specifically in women, found no difference between either modality in regards to tolerance of the procedure and both techniques having equivalent morbidity [7, 8]. Also, flexible and

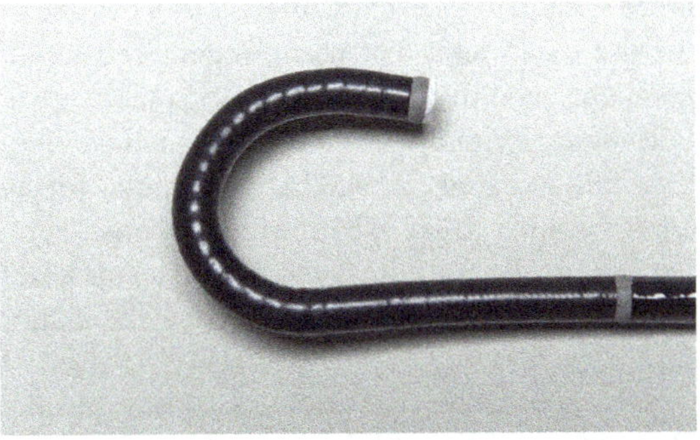

Fig. 11.5 Tip of flexible cystoscope with maximum curvature

rigid cystoscopes have been shown to be equally efficacious in their diagnostic capabilities [9]. Therefore, one should select the cystoscope that they are most comfortable with.

Illumination can be provided by either a halogen or xenon lamp along with fiberoptic or fluid-filled light cables that attach to the telescope at the eyepiece. A standard xenon 175-W lamp is the most commonly used given its immediate responsiveness once turned on and the ability to produce a high intensity illumination. Fluid-filled cables tend to have a longer shelf life, but fiberoptic cables are typically less expensive and are more susceptible to damage with routine use. Routine cystoscopy may also be performed looking through the telescope alone, but with the use of a camera and video monitoring system, patients and physicians are able to view the internal anatomy at the same time. This allows for enhanced teaching, image documentation, and potential patient distraction during the procedure [3]. Of note, complete systems are able to be purchased that routinely include a light source, camera, and video monitor.

Distending media may be either a conductive fluid (lactated ringers, normal saline), a nonconductive fluid (sterile water, 5 % glycine, 5 % mannitol, or 3 % sorbitol), or gas. Carbon dioxide and air were among the first agents used to distend the bladder during the early development of cystoscopy [4]. As technology progressed, with the potential concern of development of an "air embolism" accompanied by patient's tolerability of the procedure and the poor visualization noted with gas cystoscopy, there was a decline in the use of air as a distending media and liquid media became the current accepted practice [4]. Selection of either a conductive or nonconductive fluid is based on whether a potential for an energy source to be used during the procedure. For diagnostic purposes, most physicians elect for either isotonic normal saline or sterile water.

Procedure in Detail

Office cystoscopy for female patients is usually performed in the dorsal lithotomy position with the patient undressed from the waist down and covered in a sterile drape. Prior to this, the patient is instructed to void and a dip-stick urinalysis is performed to rule out an active urinary tract infection. Per the American Urological Association guidelines, routine antibiotic prophylaxis is not indicated for diagnostic cystoscopy unless the following risk factors are present and a negative urine culture is not documented prior to the procedure: immunocompromised state, known anatomic abnormalities of the urinary tract, active infection, chronic steroid use, or external catheter use [1]. Consent for cystoscopy is obtained and the urethra is cleansed with either a povidine–iodine solution or equivalent antimicrobial solution if an allergy exists. A disposable urinary catheter is inserted to obtain a post void residual if indicated and a topical analgesic may or may not be applied directly into the urethra from a tube or needleless syringe.

Under sterile technique, the equipment is assembled with the proper cystoscope, a light source, distending media, and imaging source if desired. If rigid cystoscopy is selected, a 30° or 70° cystoscope is routinely used along with a 17 French sheath. For rigid cystoscopy, ensure closure of all the appropriate ports to prevent leakage, turn on the light source and open the distending media flow to allow passage of a minimal amount of liquid media. For both flexible and rigid cystoscopy, gently guide the tip of the cystoscope into the distal urethra under direct visualization and follow the central opening past the urethrovesicular junction (UVJ) into the bladder cavity. Some physicians prefer the use of a blunt obturator for the cystoscopy sheath rather than direct visualization. One may then increase the flow of the distending media to adequately distend the bladder, typically around 300 cc, or the maximum capacity tolerated by the patient.

Evaluation of the bladder is best performed in a systematic routine fashion. Multiple techniques exist to ensure complete 360° visualization, with visualizing the bladder as a clock and inspection at each "hour" being the most commonly used. Identification of the bladder neck, trigone, right and left ureteral orifices along with a complete evaluation of the bladder epithelium, and any anatomic abnormalities should be noted. Orientation is able to be maintained with identification of the "air bubble" that is routinely found at the dome of the bladder. Cystoscopic images are seen in Figs. 11.6, 11.7, 11.8, and 11.9. If a rigid scope is used, rotation of the fiberoptic cable with stabilization of the camera allows for a complete survey with minimal discomfort. Of note, it is important to limit the movement of the tip of the cystoscope at the UVJ as this may

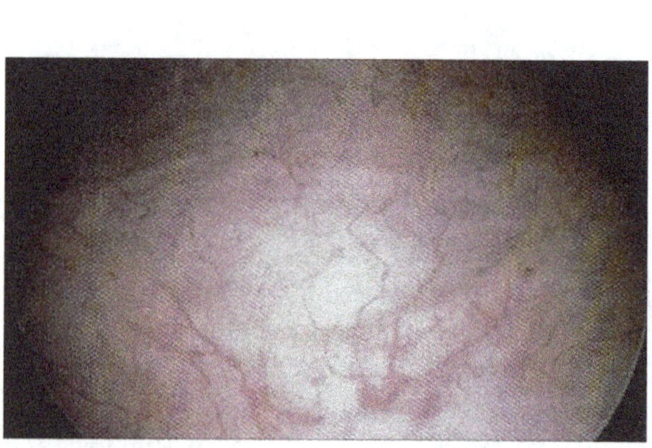

Fig. 11.6 View of bladder cystoscopically

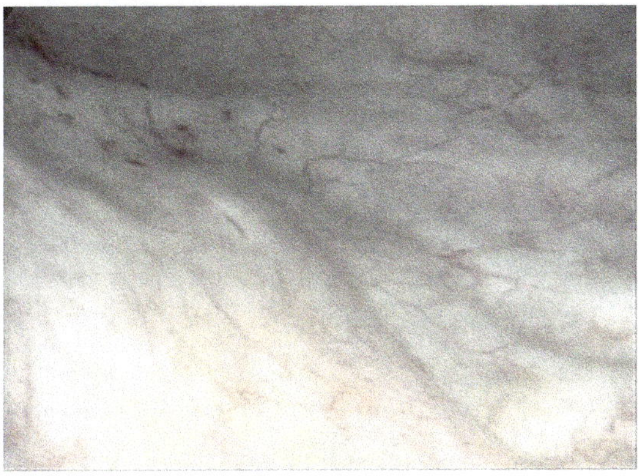

Fig. 11.7 Right ureteral orifice

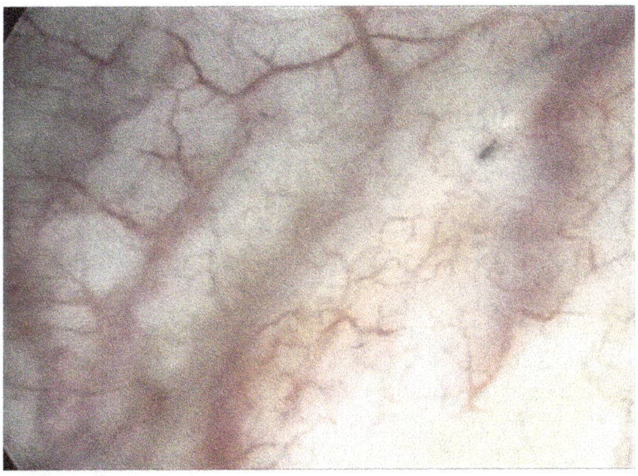

Fig. 11.8 Left ureteral orifice

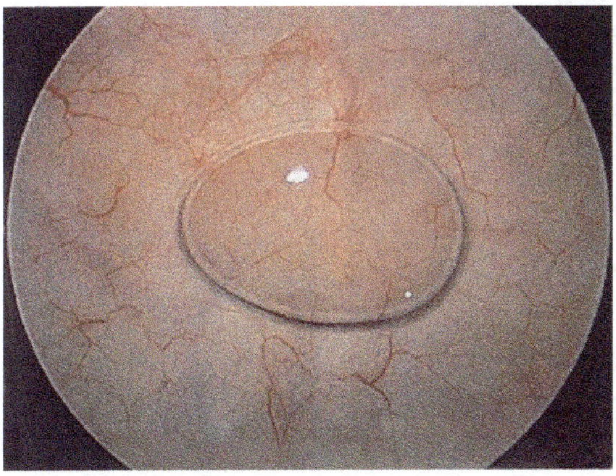

Fig. 11.9 Air bubble

cause significant patient discomfort. Upon completion of cystoscopy, evaluation of the urethra may be obtained by increasing the liquid media flow and slowly retracting the cystoscope while

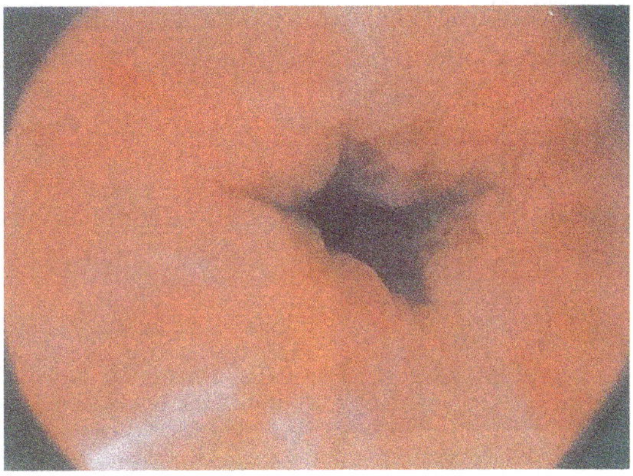

Fig. 11.10 Urethra

keeping the urethral opening in the center of the screen as seen in Fig. 11.10. This may require a slight downward or upward angle of the cystoscope depending on camera orientation. Ideally, if a detailed examination of the urethra is desired, use of a 0° telescope is recommended.

Troubleshooting

Need for urethral dilation if small sheath is not available:

1. If urethra appears atrophic and stenotic during office exam prior to scheduling the cystoscopy, consider pre-cystoscopic application of vaginal estrogen if not contraindicated.
2. Use of graduated urethral dilators and possible need of periurethral block with local anesthesia for dilation to a diameter that accommodates the intended cystoscopic sheath.

Potential device malfunctions are listed below:

1. Slow flow: Ensure proper ports are open and the distending media is elevated above patient's pubic bone.
2. Poor visualization: Focus the camera and if needed cleanse the scope and lens. Check all cable connections and evaluate the light intensity. Ensure the bladder is completely full. If debris or bleeding is noted, one may need to open the port opposite the inflow to allow bladder to drain followed by refilling.

3. No Picture: Check all cable attachments and recheck power on all components. Evaluate individual pieces for potential broken components. Check the camera, lamp, light cords, and video monitoring system. If light source is adequate, but there is no video transmitting, consider removing the camera and viewing through the eyepiece alone. Ultimately refer to the industry representative or manufacturing guidelines.

Post Procedural Complications

Symptoms that may be experienced following office cystoscopy are similar to a urinary tract infection. Patients may report increased urinary frequency, urgency, slight dysuria, and mild hematuria. These symptoms typically are mild in nature and usually resolve within 24–48 h [10] and last no longer than 7 days [8]. Patients should be instructed to call if they experience severe symptoms or if there is a concern for potential infection. Pre-procedure urine analysis is used to identify patients with an active urinary infection and to postpone the elective cystoscopy until a later date. All patients should be encouraged to ensure adequate fluid intake following the procedure.

References

1. Wolf Jr JS, Bennett CJ, Dmochowski RR, Hollenbeck BK, Pearle MS, Schaeffer AJ, et al. Best practice policy statement on urologic surgery antimicrobial prophylaxis. J Urol. 2008;179(4):1379–90.
2. Samplaski MK, Jones JS. Two centuries of cystoscopy: the development of imaging, instrumentation and synergistic technologies. BJU Int. 2009;103 (2):154–8.
3. Cundiff GW, Bent AE. Endoscopic diagnosis of the female lower urinary tract. 1st ed. London: Harcourt Brace and Company; 1999.
4. Schultheiss D, Machtens SA, Jonas U. Air cystoscopy: the history of an endoscopic technique from the late 19th century. BJU Int. 1999;83(6):571–7.
5. Tsuchida S, Sugawara H. A new flexible fibercystoscope for visualization of the bladder neck. J Urol. 1973;109(5):830–1.
6. Kavoussi LR, Clayman RV. Office flexible cystoscopy. Urol Clin North Am. 1988;15(4):601–8.
7. Gee JR, Waterman BJ, Jarrard DF, Hedican SP, Bruskewitz RC, Nakada SY. Flexible and rigid cystoscopy in women. JSLS. 2009;13(2):135–8.
8. Quiroz LH, Shobeiri SA, Nihira MA, Brady J, Wild RA. Randomized trial comparing office flexible to rigid cystoscopy in women. Int Urogynecol J. 2012;23(11):1625–30.
9. Walker L, Liston TG, LLoyd-Davies RW. Does flexible cystoscopy miss more tumours than rod-lens examination? Br J Urol. 1993;72(4):449–50.
10. Stav K, Leibovici D, Goren E, Livshitz A, Siegel YI, Lindner A, et al. Adverse effects of cystoscopy and its impact on patients' quality of life and sexual performance. Isr Med Assoc J. 2004;6(8):474–8.

Urodynamic Testing

12

Nathan Kow and Marie Fidela R. Paraiso

Introduction

Urodynamic testing is an office-based assessment that can be useful in evaluating the function of the lower urinary tract (LUT). It comprises of several distinct tests that aim to measure various aspects of urine storage and evacuation. The complexity of testing depends largely on the indications for urodynamics and the desired information that a clinician requires.

In order to understand and interpret urodynamic testing, it is important for the practitioner to understand the normal physiology of urine storage and evacuation. While a detailed discussion regarding normal bladder physiology is beyond the scope of this chapter, the basic assumptions are as follows: (1) the bladder has the ability to accommodate urine with a nearly constant low intravesical pressure; (2) the patient has the ability to suppress micturition at all bladder volumes; (3) the patient has the ability to voluntarily initiate the voiding reflex, including relaxation of the urethra and contraction of the detrusor muscle. These basic functions of urine storage and evacuation are evaluated through the various components of urodynamic testing.

Furthermore, urodynamic testing should be performed and recorded in a standardized fashion to allow for clear communication between the various health care practitioners who will be involved with the care of the patient. Recognizing this importance of clear communication, the International Continence Society (ICS) has published several reports with the goal of providing standardized terms and definitions for many of the parameters that are evaluated during urodynamic testing.

The aim of this chapter is to provide the reader an overview of the potential indications, basic interpretation, benefits, and limitations of what urodynamic testing can provide.

Indications

While urodynamic testing has been available to physicians for some time now, their indications remain controversial. There is currently no accepted list of indications for when to obtain urodynamic testing. When determining whether there is need for testing, several factors must be weighed including the cost of the urodynamic testing, patient history, clinical findings, and

N. Kow, M.D. (✉)
Division of Urogynecology and Pelvic Reconstructive Surgery, Department of Obstetrics, Gynecology & Women's Health Institute, Cleveland Clinic Foundation, 9500 Euclid Avenue, Desk A81, Cleveland, OH 44195, USA
e-mail: kown@ccf.org

M.F.R. Paraiso, M.D.
Cleveland Clinic Lerner College of Medicine at Case Western Reserve University, Cleveland, OH, USA

Center for Urogynecology and Reconstructive Pelvic Surgery, Obstetrics, Gynecology, and Women's Health Institute, Cleveland Clinic, Cleveland, OH, USA

Glickman Urological and Kidney Institute, Cleveland Clinic, Cleveland, OH, USA
e-mail: paraism@ccf.org

J.D. Emery and M.F.R. Paraiso (eds.), *Office-Based Gynecologic Surgical Procedures*,
DOI 10.1007/978-1-4939-1414-2_12,

Table 12.1

Indications for urodynamic testing
Complicated history
Stress incontinence before surgical correction
Urge incontinence not responsive to therapy
Recurrent urinary loss after previous surgery for stress incontinence
Frequency, urgency, and pain syndromes not responsive to therapy
Nocturnal enuresis not responsive to therapy
Lower urinary tract dysfunction after pelvic radiation or radical pelvic surgery
Neurologic disorders
Continuous leakage
Suspected voiding difficulties

Adapted from Walters MD, Karram MM, editors. Urogynecology and Reconstructive Pelvic Surgery. 3rd ed. Philadelphia: Mosby Elsevier; 2007

whether test findings would change treatment or management. A suggested list of indications is listed in Table 12.1 [1].

The most recent report by International Consultation on Incontinence (ICI) states that the role of urodynamic studies in clinical practice should be (1) to identify or to rule out factors contributing to the LUT dysfunction and assess their relative importance (2) to obtain information about other aspects of LUT dysfunction (3) to predict the consequences of LUT dysfunction for the upper urinary tract (4) to predict the outcome, including undesirable side effects, of a contemplated treatment (5) to confirm the effects of intervention or understand the mode of action of a particular type of treatment; especially a new one (6) to understand the reasons for failure of previous treatments for urinary incontinence, or for LUT dysfunction in general [2].

Components

Urodynamic testing comprises of five unique tests that can be performed individually or together, depending on the desired information. These tests are generally categorized by the specific bladder function they intend to assess. The components of urodynamic testing that evaluate bladder filling and storage include filling cystometry (single or multichannel). Bladder emptying or voiding is evaluated by uroflowmetry and pressure-flow studies (voiding cystometry). Finally, urethral function is evaluated by urethral pressure profilometry and leak point pressure.

Evaluation of Bladder Filling and Storage

Filling Cystometry

The normal bladder has the ability to accommodate significant amounts of volume while maintaining a low intravesical pressure. Cystometry is the component of urodynamic testing that evaluates the relationship between volume and pressure during the filling and storage phase. The aim is to assess bladder sensation, bladder capacity, detrusor activity, and bladder compliance [3]. It utilizes the basic principle of instilling a filling medium (normal saline or X-ray contrast solution for videourodynamics) while simultaneously measuring various pressures (abdominal, vesical, and/or urethral) in order to evaluate the function of the bladder during the filling/storage phase.

Several variations of filling cystometry are available, including simple cystometry, single-channel, or multichannel cystometry. Simple cystometry involves the placement of a catheter that is attached to a 60 cc syringe with the plunger removed placed approximately 15 cm above the level of the pubic symphysis. The bladder is filled with a standard amount of filling media. Finally, a cough stress test and evaluation of post-void residual can be performed at the conclusion of simple cystometry. Because a pressure catheter is not utilized, evaluation of filling pressures cannot be assessed. Despite this, evaluation of bladder sensation and the determination of detrusor contractions can be obtained using this simple test.

If more information is desired, filling cystometry can be performed using a single catheter in the bladder (single-channel cystometry) or multiple catheters (multichannel cystometry). While very few studies have compared single and multichannel cystometry, the latter has the potential to improve the specificity of cystometry by avoiding false-positive tests. Today, multichannel cystometry is performed routinely over single-channel cystometry.

The technical aspects of the procedure are discussed later in the chapter, but in brief, two catheters are placed in order to measure *vesical pressure* (P_{ves}) and *abdominal pressure* (P_{abd}). P_{det} is measured with a catheter placed in the bladder while P_{abd} is measured with a catheter placed in the rectum or vagina. *Detrusor pressure* (P_{det}) is estimated as a subtracted value ($P_{det} = P_{ves} - P_{abd}$). The bladder is filled with filling medium typically at a supraphysiologic filling rate while the patient is asked to report when various sensations are experienced: *first sensation of filling* (FSF), *first desire to void* (FDV), *strong desire to void* (SDV), symptoms of *urge*, and *pain*. The bladder is filled until *maximum cystometric capacity* (MCC) is reached. *Compliance*, which is a measure of the viscoelastic property of the bladder, is calculated by dividing the volume change by the change in P_{det}. Provocative measures can be performed throughout the test to simulate potential stresses on the bladder [3, 4].

Interpretation of multichannel cystometrics requires knowledge of the normal filling parameters. Several studies have been performed to determine normal values for the various filling cystometry variables [5–12]. While there is known to be significant intercenter and interpatient variability, the ICI recommends that in general the following guidelines be used for interpretation: FSF at 170–200 cc, FDV at 250 cc, SDV a 400 cc, MCC at 480 cc. Based on these parameters, *increased bladder sensation* is defined as sensations that occur at a lower bladder volume than what would normally be expected, while *reduced bladder sensation* is defined as sensations that occur at a higher bladder volume than what would normally be expected [2].

Additionally, the P_{det} during filling should remain low and constant. Rises in P_{det}, not associated with a detrusor contraction, indicate decreased compliance and must be noted. Evaluation of detrusor function is achieved by examining the tracing for the presence of detrusor contractions. Urodynamic detrusor contractions are defined as any significant rise in P_{det} during filling or provocation (Fig. 12.1). A normal or stable tracing should be absent of any detrusor contractions. The presence of detrusor contractions indicates an unstable detrusor that is referred to as *detrusor overactivity*.

As with all urodynamic tests, the results obtained from filling cystometry can be highly variable, depending on various technical aspects (i.e., type of catheters, type of media, filling rate, patient position) and differences in interpretation. Furthermore, the test provides only the results of a single filling cycle. Despite this, it continues to be a frequently utilized test to evaluate patients for stress, urge, or mixed incontinence.

Evaluation of Bladder Emptying or Voiding

Post-void Residual

The simplest evaluation of bladder emptying is to obtain a post-void residual either after passive or active filling of the bladder. Techniques for determining post-void residual (PVR) include ultrasonic techniques (transvaginal, abdominal, and Doppler planimetry) or catheterization. The choice of technique should be based on availability of equipment, diagnostic accuracy, and considerations of patient comfort. While ultrasonic techniques are the least invasive, they represent indirect measures of volume based on measurements on several axis that may introduce error. Direct measurement utilizing a catheter places the patient at some discomfort during the initial placement of catheter, but is generally well tolerated. It has a distinct advantage as it provides the most accurate measure of PVR.

Normal values for post-void residuals are often quoted as values less than 50–100 cc [13, 14]. An isolated finding of an elevated PVR should be interpreted with caution as variation in PVRs can be due to either patient or equipment factors. It is important to ensure that an abnormal PVR is found on repetitive testing. A high PVR often indicates incomplete voiding due to either

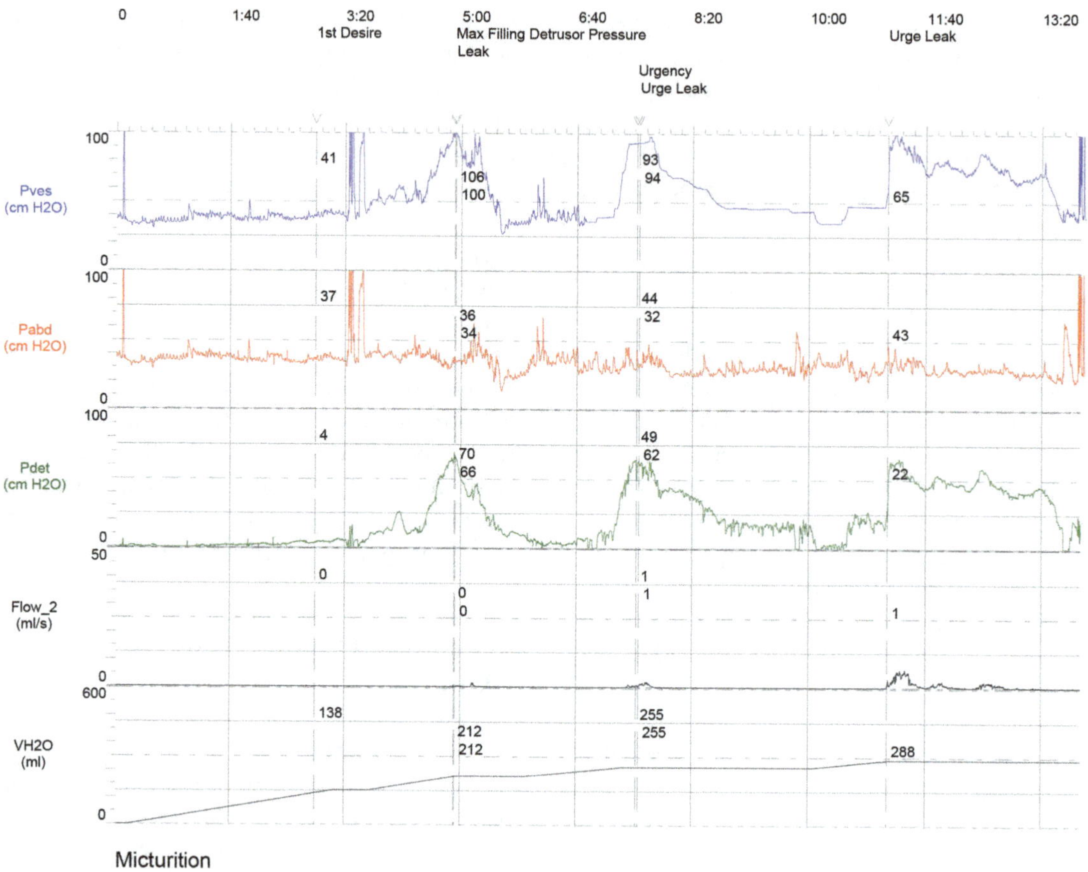

Fig. 12.1 Detrusor overactivity: multichannel cystometry showing detrusor overactivity

poor detrusor contractility or outlet obstruction and should prompt further investigation.

Noninvasive Uroflowmetry

Noninvasive uroflowmetry describes a test utilized to calculate the urine flow in relation to voided volume. Patients are asked to void into an electronic volume detector that measures weight changes over time. A graphical representation of the flow pattern is generated for the clinician to interpret. Urine flow is described as continuous or intermittent. Additionally, several objective values are calculated including, *flow rate* (volume expelled per unit of time), *maximum flowrate* (Q_{max}), and *total voided volume* [15].

In a normal uroflow, a flow curve generated should rise in amplitude until a high maximum flowrate is achieved and subsequently taper off as micturition is completed. The curve should appear smooth without rapid changes throughout the entire voiding phase (Fig. 12.2).

Clinical utility of noninvasive uroflowmetry has been debated, especially in the case of women. The advantage is the relative low cost of the test and potential use as a preliminary screening tool for voiding dysfunction. Interpretation of uroflowmetry is highly dependent on the voided volume. In general, experts agree that in order to properly assess a uroflow study, the patient must void at least 150 cc. Maximum flow rates in women vary with age, sex, and the starting urine volume. Several studies have established maximum urine flow rates to be greater than 12 mL/s [13, 16]. According to the most recent ICS guidelines, abnormally slow flow rates have been determined as under the tenth percentile of the Liverpool nomogram which takes into account the voided volume [17, 18].

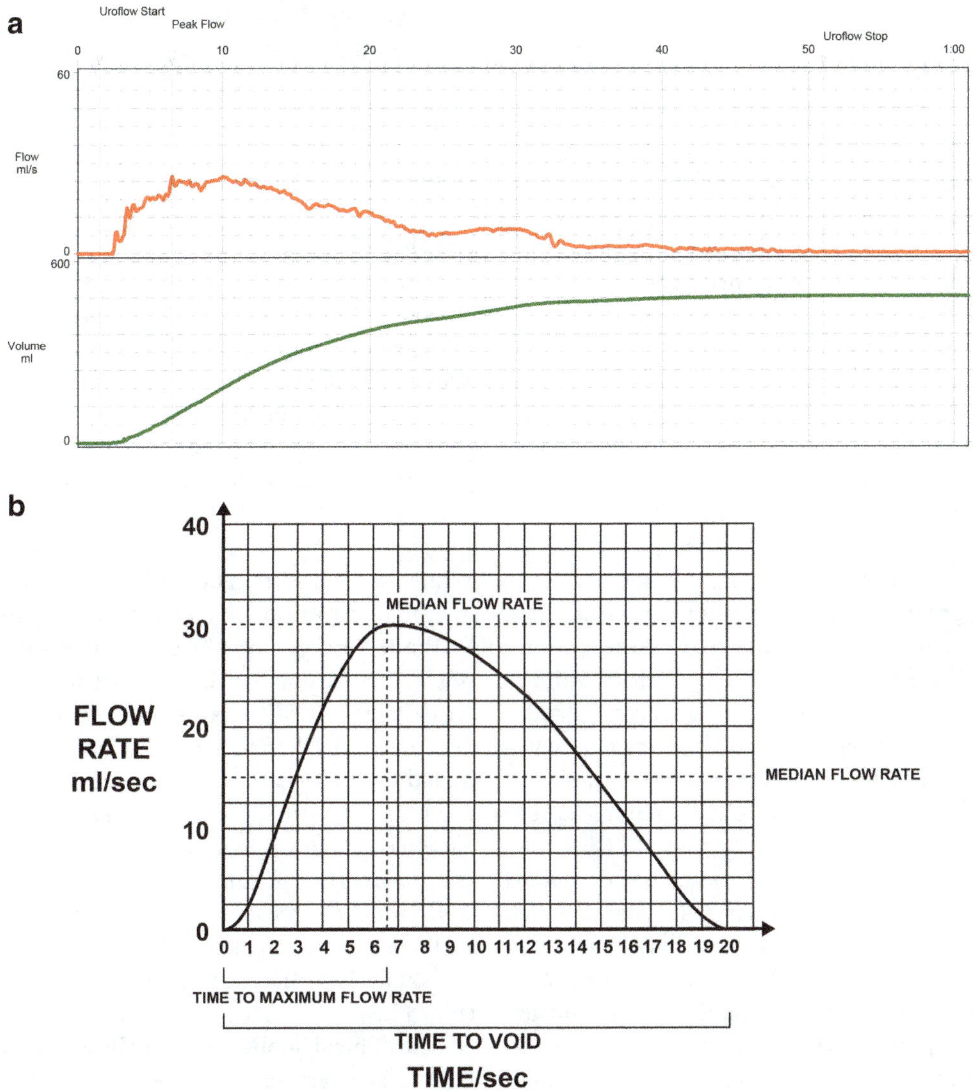

Fig. 12.2 Uroflow: (**a**) Actual uroflow showing a normal flow curve. (**b**) For ease of interpretation, a simplied tracing with variability removed is provided to illustrate how various measurements are obtained

Abnormalities in the flow pattern or rate can be due to various pathologies. While specific pathologies that may produce an abnormal uroflow are beyond the scope of this chapter, in general, factors that affect passive relaxation of the bladder neck (i.e., bladder neck obstruction), urethral resistance (i.e., urethral stricture), or detrusor contractility (i.e., neuropathic lesions, pharmacologic manipulation, etc.) will alter the uroflowmetric parameters.

Pressure-Flow Study

Pressure-flow study combines the basic principles of uroflowmetry with the addition of abdominal and bladder pressure measurements. This combination allows evaluation of the pressures that are being generated during the voiding phase, therefore allowing the clinician to examine the pressure volume relationship during micturition. The goal of interpreting a pressure-flow study is to assess whether the neurologic mechanism of micturition is intact. This includes the ability of the detrusor muscle to contract and generate an appropriate voiding pressure, the urethral sphincter to relax, and that the timing of these events are coordinated to provide a smooth continuous flow.

Measurements obtained during a pressure-flow study have been defined by ICS and include *premicturition pressure*, *opening time*, *opening pressure*, *maximum pressure*, *pressure at maximum flow*, *closing pressure*, *contraction pressure at maximum flow*, and *flow delay* [3]. While the definitions and interpretations of these measurements are beyond the scope of this chapter, it is important to realize that these additional measurements are possible due to the use of pressure catheters and allow the practitioner to objectively assess for voiding dysfunction.

In general, abnormalities in a pressure-flow study can be categorized into three general groups of pathologies including detrusor contractility issues (i.e., acontractile detrusor), bladder outlet obstructions (i.e., stricture), or neurophysiologic abnormalities (i.e., detrusor sphincter dyssynergia). Evaluation of the voiding P_{det} and flow rate can help the practioner delineate the potential cause. Abnormal pressure-flow studies fall under two general patterns: (1) low flow rate and an elevated P_{det}, suggestive of bladder outlet obstruction; (2) low flow rate and low P_{det}, suggesting potential contractility issue with the detrusor muscle. Several studies have looked to determine specific urodynamic criteria to diagnose bladder outlet obstruction. Furthermore, Blavais and Groutz created a nomogram based on several previous studies and defined bladder outlet obstruction as the presence of a free Q_{max} < 12 mL/s and P_{det} of > 20 cm H_2O in a pressure-flow study [19].

While the utility of pressure-flow studies in women have been debated, the most common indications for pressure-flow studies in women include evaluation of obstructed voiding or voiding dysfunction includes preoperative evaluation of patients with pelvic organ prolapse, patients who have undergone previous pelvic surgery, or postoperative patients who have new onset voiding dysfunction. Finally, while it can be performed as an individual test, most often it is combined with filling cystometric studies.

Urethral Function Testing

Urethral Pressure Profile

Urethral pressure profile (UPP) is a test that attempts to measure the urethral pressure throughout the length of the urethra during rest. Variations of the UPP include cough or stress pressure profiles in which the same procedure is performed while the patient coughs. It involves placement of a urethral pressure catheter that will measure the intraluminal pressure as the catheter is withdrawn at a constant rate of speed. While several different catheter types exist, microtransducers are the most commonly used.

While less commonly used today, the goal of UPP is to distinguish between intrinsic sphincter deficiency (ISD) from stress urinary incontinence (SUI). Several objective measurements including *maximum urethral pressure* (MUP), *urethral closure pressure profile* (UCPP), *maximum urethral closure pressure* (MUCP), *functional profile length*, and *pressure "transmission" ratio* are measured in order to assess the urethral closure mechanism. MUCP is calculated by taking the difference between MUP and P_{ves} (Fig. 12.3).

The clinical applicability of UPP is limited by lack of standardization of the procedure and in the interpretation of the test itself. Several authors have attempted to correlate lower MUCP with SUI. Other studies have sought to use MUCP to predict surgical success and failure. Several retrospective studies show higher postsurgical failure rates in women with low MUCP, often defined as ≤ 20 cm H_2O [20, 21]. However, a recent review of the role of urodynamic evaluation of SUI showed no clear benefit in improving case selection or surgical technique. The author concluded that urodynamic assessment (LLP and UPP) could not accurately predict the outcome of surgical management of SUI [22].

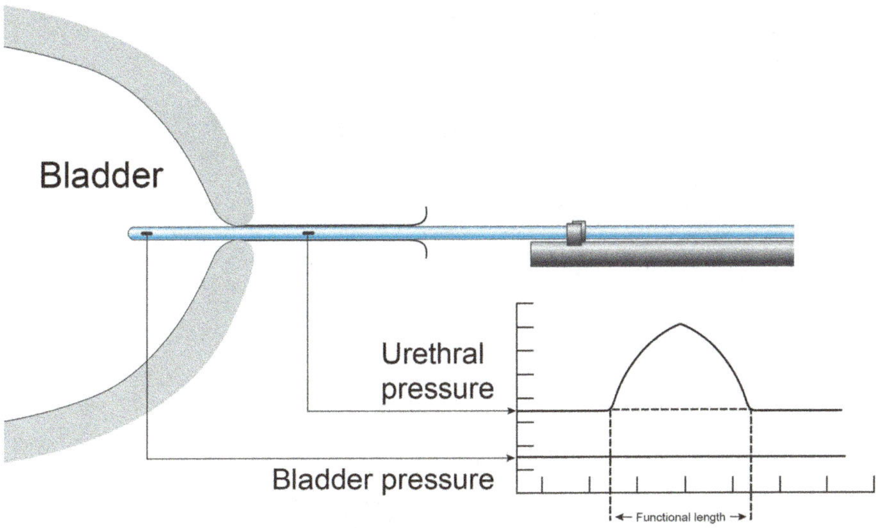

Fig. 12.3 Urethral pressure profile: Illustration showing a normal tracing

Leak Point Pressure

The ability of the urethra to prevent the involuntary leakage of urine can be evaluated by measuring the leak point pressure. Under normal physiologic and functional conditions, the urethral resistance should generate enough pressure to compensate for any abdominal or detrusor pressure that would be experienced through normal activities. Leak point pressure is defined as the lowest detrusor (P_{det}) or intravesical pressure (P_{ves}) at which involuntary expulsion of urine from the urethral meatus is observed.

It is important to understand the difference between detrusor leak point pressure (DLPP) and abdominal leak point pressure (ALPP). DLPP a static test that determines the lowest P_{det} at which leakage of urine occurs in the absence of a detrusor contraction or increased abdominal pressure. ALPP is a dynamic test that determines the lowest P_{ves} at which leakage occurs during an intentional increase in abdominal pressure (i.e., cough or valsava).

DLPP attempts to measure the ability of the urethra to resist increasing detrusor pressure. Unlike ALPP, DLPP is not used to evaluate SUI. Instead it is related to bladder compliance and outlet resistance. Much of our understanding of DLPP is based on work that was done by McGuire et al. who evaluated myledysplastic children and noted that patients that had a DLPP >40 cm H_2O developed upper-tract disease [23, 24].

ALPP on the other hand attempts to assess the ability of the urethra to resist increased abdominal pressure. As such it is most often utilized to evaluate SUI. Several studies have attempted to use ALPP to differentiate between SUI due to urethral hypermobility and SUI due to ISD. While there remains debate regarding how to interpret ALPPs, some practitioners suggest that a ALPP <60 cm H_2O is correlated with ISD. This is based on two studies that attempted to correlate ALPP with severity of SUI. McGuire's study of 125 women noted 81 % of patients with an ALPP <60 cm H_2O had ISD [25]. The second study by Nitti et al., looked at 64 women and noted that 50 % of women with ISD had an ALPP <60 cm H_2O [26].

ALPP is often further divided by the modality for which increased P_{abd} is obtained. ALPP obtained during coughing is performed by asking the patient to sequentially increase the intensity of cough in order to elicit leakage of urine. The lowest recorded pressure is recorded as the ALPP. An alternative to utilizing coughing as the provocative maneuver is to determine ALPP during a valsalva maneuver. ALPP measured during a valsalva maneuver may provide a more accurate

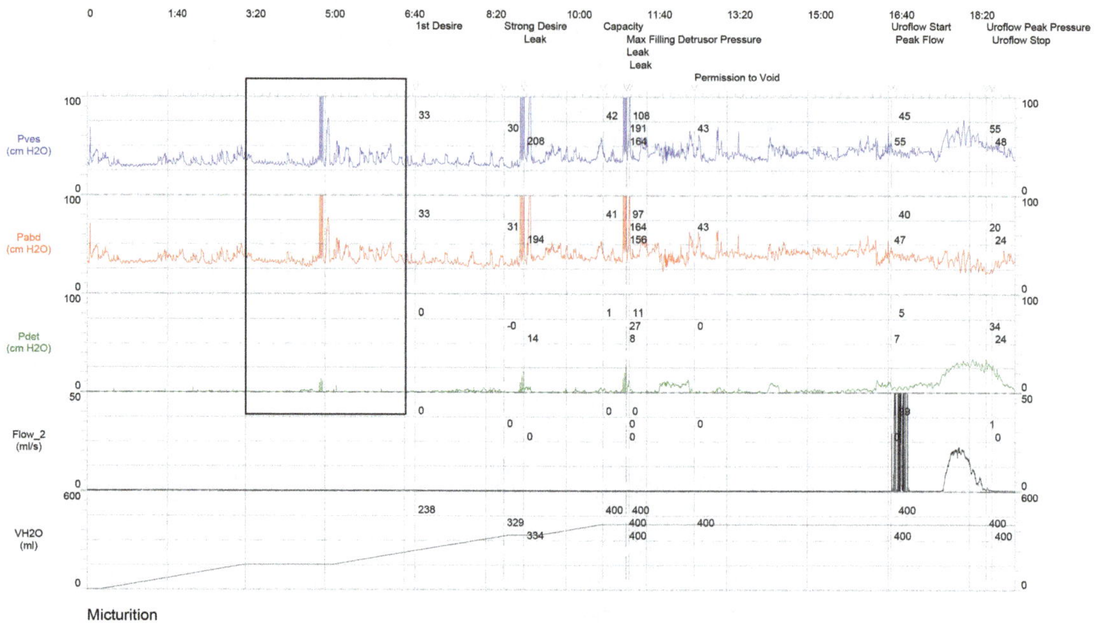

Fig. 12.4 Abdominal leap point pressure: multichannel cystometry showing leak point pressure determination

measure of ALPP as it provides a more controlled rise in P_{abd} as compared to the sharp rise in pressure obtained during coughing (Fig. 12.4).

While ALPP can be obtained as a single urodynamic test, the ICS recommends against this practice as several studies have show that isolated ALPPs are not helpful as predictors of success for suburethral sling procedures in patients with SUI [27]. Our practice obtains leak point pressures intermittently during cystometry, starting at a bladder volume of approximately 150 cc, and additionally at 50 cc intervals.

Diagnostic Effectiveness for Various Disease States

There are several urologic and urogynecologic conditions that the gynecologist should be familiar with in which urodynamic testing may be helpful

Stress Urinary Incontinence

SUI is a condition in which a patient has involuntary leakage of urine during an increase in intra-abdominal pressure in the absence of a detrusor contraction. While a diagnosis of SUI can be made by history and office evaluation (cough stress test), some physicians have utilized urodynamic testing to diagnose SUI. There continues to be debate regarding whether urodynamics is required in patients with uncomplicated demonstrable SUI. A recent trial of 630 women randomized to office evaluation (urethral hypermobility, cough or valsalva stress test, post-void residual) or urodynamic testing (noninstrumented uroflowmetry, filling cystometry with Valsalva leak-point pressures, and a pressure-flow study) for uncomplicated SUI demonstrated non-inferiority between the two preoperative evaluation strategies. Successful treatment was seen in 76.9 % of women undergoing urodynamic testing compared with 77.2 % of women undergoing office evaluation only [28]. These results are consistent with our practice and recommend that urodynamic testing is unnecessary in patients with uncomplicated SUI.

With regards to the utilization of urodynamic testing to determine if patients have occult SUI prior to surgical management of pelvic organ prolapse, the data has been unclear regarding the best course of action. Several studies have described techniques for prolapse reduction during urodynamic testing including manual reduction with fingers, large cotton swab, single speculum blade, ring forceps, or pessary. In one large study evaluating the various methods of prolapse reduction, similar sensitivities for detection of occult SUI were shown (17–39 %), with the exception of the pessary, which was less sensitive (5 %) [29]. In our practice we routinely perform prolapse reduction urodynamic testing in patients scheduled for surgical management of pelvic organ prolapse in order to detect occult SUI and aid in preoperative counseling.

Overactive Bladder/Urge Urinary Incontinence

Overactive bladder (OAB) is a condition that is characterized by symptoms of urgency (often accompanied by frequency and nocturia), with or without urgency urinary incontinence, in the absence of urinary tract infection or other obvious pathology [3]. It is important to understand that this definition does not require urodynamic testing in order to make a diagnosis. While the presence of detrusor overactivity (DO) on cystometry is often used interchangeably with OAB, the association with overactive bladder/urge urinary incontinence (OAB/UUI) and urodynamic detrusor overactivity is poor. In a large retrospective review of 4,500 women in which neurological disorders were excluded, the sensitivity and specificity of DO for OAB symptoms were 54 % and 68 %, respectively [30]. This study also demonstrated that there are a significant proportion of false-positive and false-negative symptoms. While urodynamic testing can provide objective data, it is important that both the clinician and patient understand a finding of DO does not predict therapeutic outcomes for UUI.

Equipment and Setup

The equipment required to perform urodynamic studies is dependent on the complexity of information required by the practitioner. It is important for the practitioner to determine their need before purchasing a more complex system as they can be very costly.

If simple urodynamic studies are all that is required for the physician, the equipment and set up is very inexpensive. As described in the previous section, simple office cystometry only requires a 60 cc syringe and a catheter. Other inexpensive studies include determination of PVR that can be achieved by a sterile disposable straight catheter. In many cases, this setup may be sufficient instead of more complex electronic systems.

If the practioner determines that additional information is required, then an electronic system can be purchased. There are a variety of systems that are available for the evaluation of the LUT with many that have the capability to evaluate other aspects of the pelvic floor such as anorectal function. While differences between the different available systems and their components are beyond the scope of this chapter, in general, the required setup includes a multichannel urodynamics system, uroflow, and multi-position chair for placing the patient that allows for easy patient positioning for pressure catheter placement and evaluation of incontinence (Fig. 12.5). Additionally, disposable items including instillation media, pressure catheters, EMG pads, and various types of tubing specific for the system is required.

Technique

While no standard order has been established for the different components of urodynamic testing, for patients undergoing evaluation we recommend a workflow: (1) noninvasive uroflowmetry; (2) multichannel cystometry with provocative maneuvers and determination of ALPPs; (3) pressure-flow study. With regards to urethral profilometry profile, we utilize a similar technique as suggested by Hilton and Stanton [31].

Noninvasive uroflowmetry

1. Patients present with a symptomatically full bladder and are asked to void spontaneously

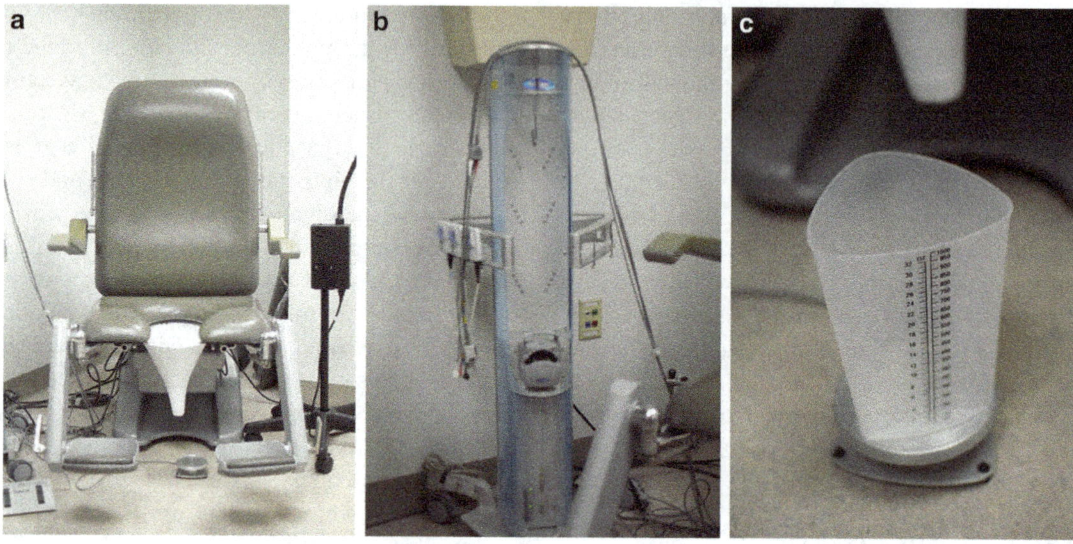

Fig. 12.5 Setup for multichannel urodynamic testing: (**a**) uroflow chair (**b**) multichannel urodynamic system (**c**) Uroflowmeter

in a uroflow chair. After the patient has completed voiding, a post-void residual is obtained using a sterile transurethral disposable catheter. A sample of the catheterized urine is tested for signs of a urinary tract infection prior to continuing with cystometry and pressure-flow studies.

Multichannel Cystometry

2. With the patient comfortably in the urodynamics chair, commercially available disposable microtransducer catheters are placed sequentially to measure vesical pressure and abdominal pressure. The vesical pressure catheter is placed into the bladder transurethrally and also serves as a filling port. The abdominal pressure catheter is placed either vaginally or rectally. Catheters are then secured to the inside of the leg in order to prevent catheter migration during testing.
3. Prior to connecting catheters to the urodynamics machine, the machine zeroed.
4. Catheters are connected to using the appropriate cables and the catheter tubing is connected to the vesical catheter filling port.
5. In order to ensure that the catheters are appropriately placed and functioning correctly, the patient is asked to cough in order to ensure cough-induced pressure spikes are detected by both the vesical and abdominal pressure catheters. If there is failure of an appropriate spike, repositioning of the catheters may be required.
6. Begin filling the bladder.
7. Throughout the filling phase, several points should be recorded including first sensation, FDV, SDV, and any symptoms of urge. Periodically, filling is interrupted in order to perform provocative activities (cough and valsalva) to evaluate for SUI. Leak point pressures should be obtained if incontinence is recorded.
8. Based on when the patient indicates maximum filling, additional evaluation of provocative maneuvers can be performed by asking the patient to stand and squat, walk in place, or heel bounce.
9. At the conclusion of the filling phase the patient is given "permission to void" in order to perform a pressure-flow study

Pressure-Flow study

10. Patients are asked to void with the catheters in place in order to evaluate the vesical, abdominal, and subtracted detrusor pressures during the voiding phase. In addition to evaluating the pressures during voiding, any

abnormalities in the voiding flow should be noted. If the patient is unable to void, the catheters may need to be removed and the pressure-flow study aborted. At this point uroflowmetry may be performed if previously inadequate. Additionally, provocative measures may be repeated if stress incontinence has not been diagnosed if the condition is suspected.

Urethral Pressure Profilometry

1. After filling the bladder to MCC, the catheter is secured to a mechanical puller
2. The proximal transducer is pulled through the urethra at a constant speed in order to measure static urethral pressure. Urethral closure pressure is recorded on a separate channel.
3. If a cough or stress pressure profile is desired, the same procedure is repeated while the patient is asked to cough repetitively at a consistent intensity, every 2–3 s.

Complications

Complications related to urodynamic testing are very uncommon and are generally related to preprocedural anxiety, procedural or postprocedural discomfort or infection.

Several studies have investigated the procedural anxiety related to urodynamic testing. In one study of 100 women undergoing urodynamic testing, anticipated preprocedural pain as evaluated by a visual analogue scale was significantly higher than experienced postprocedural pain [32]. Additionally, a qualitative study regarding patient satisfaction related to urodynamics identified themes of anxiety and embarrassment [33]. These factors should be taken into account during counseling and during the procedure by both the ordering physician and the practitioner performing the urodynamic tests that are ordered.

Risk of developing a urinary tract infection related to urodynamic testing has been reported to be between 3 and 20 % [34–36]. The risk is related to the placement of urethral and bladder pressure catheter or if active filling is utilized for urodynamic studies. Several studies have suggested the use of pre or post-procedural antibiotic prophylaxis. A recent meta-analysis identified eight randomized controlled trials with a total of 995 patients. They reported a 40 % reduction in the risk of significant bacteriuria with the use of prophylactic antibiotics (OR 0.39; 95 % CI 0.24–0.61) [37]. However, before deciding whether to utilize antibiotic prophylaxis when performing urodynamics, a thorough consideration of the costs and benefits must be entertained. A decision analysis model performed by Lowder et al. showed that prophylactic antibiotics after urodynamic testing was beneficial if the baseline rate of UTI was greater than 10 % [38]. In our clinic, we do not routinely administer antibiotic prophylaxis for urodynamic testing.

Associated Studies

Videourodynamics

Videourodynamics is a variation of multichannel filling cystometry and pressure-flow studies that utilize a radiographic filling media and fluoroscopy in order to provide real-time imaging of the bladder and urethra during both the filling and voiding phase. The advantages of this modification are that it may provide visualization of anatomic bladder and urethral pathology that would otherwise not be identified with conventional urodynamic testing. Several considerations with regards to videourodynamics are the additional costs, equipment, training and personnel, and the radiologic exposure to the patients since it requires fluoroscopy.

Conclusion

While controversy remains regarding the clinical applicability of some components of urodynamic testing, office-based evaluation using urodynamic testing can provide valuable information regarding bladder function. While not appropriate with all patients, those with complex medical histories, unclear symptoms, or refractory urogynecologic conditions may benefit from testing. Understanding which particular aspects of bladder function that are being investigated will ultimately yield the most helpful information with regards to diagnosis and potential treatment options. Additionally, practitioners should understand the limitations of these studies.

References

1. Walters MD, Karram MM, editors. Urogynecology and reconstructive pelvic surgery. 3rd ed. Philadelphia: Mosby Elsevier; 2007.
2. Abrams P, Cardoza L, Khoury S, Wein A, editors. Incontinence. 5th ed. Paris: ICUD-EAU; 2013.
3. Haylen BT, de Ridder D, Freeman RM, Swift SE, Berghmans B, Lee J, et al. An International Urogynecological Association (IUGA)/International Continence Society (ICS) joint report on the terminology for female pelvic floor dysfunction. Int Urogynecol J. 2010;21(1):5–26.
4. Abrams P, Blaivas JG, Stanton SL, Andersen JT. The standardisation of terminology of lower urinary tract function. The International Continence Society Committee on Standardisation of Terminology. Scand J Urol Nephrol Suppl. 1988;114:5–19.
5. Brostrom S, Jennum P, Lose G. Short-term reproducibility of cystometry and pressure-flow micturition studies in healthy women. Neurourol Urodyn. 2002;21(5):457–60.
6. Wyndaele JJ, De Wachter S. Cystometrical sensory data from a normal population: comparison of two groups of young healthy volunteers examined with 5 years interval. Eur Urol. 2002;42(1):34–8.
7. van Waalwijk van Doorn ES, Remmers A, Janknegt RA. Conventional and extramural ambulatory urodynamic testing of the lower urinary tract in female volunteers. J Urol. 1992;147(5):1319–25; discussion 1326.
8. Robertson AS, Griffiths CJ, Ramsden PD, Neal DE. Bladder function in healthy volunteers: ambulatory monitoring and conventional urodynamic studies. Br J Urol. 1994;73(3):242–9.
9. Sorensen S. Urodynamic investigations and their reproducibility in healthy postmenopausal females. Scand J Urol Nephrol Suppl. 1988;114:42–7.
10. Sorensen S, Knudsen UB, Kirkeby HJ, Djurhuus JC. Urodynamic investigations in healthy fertile females during the menstrual cycle. Scand J Urol Nephrol Suppl. 1988;114:28–34.
11. Heslington K, Hilton P. Ambulatory monitoring and conventional cystometry in asymptomatic female volunteers. Br J Obstet Gynaecol. 1996;103(5):434–41.
12. Walter S, Olesen KP, Nordling J, Hald T. Bladder function in urologically normal middle aged females. A urodynamic and radiological investigation. Scand J Urol Nephrol. 1979;13(3):249–58.
13. Costantini E, Mearini E, Pajoncini C, Biscotto S, Bini V, Porena M. Uroflowmetry in female voiding disturbances. Neurourol Urodyn. 2003;22(6):569–73.
14. Haylen BT, Lee J, Logan V, Husselbee S, Zhou J, Law M. Immediate postvoid residual volumes in women with symptoms of pelvic floor dysfunction. Obstet Gynecol. 2008;111(6):1305–12.
15. Schafer W, Abrams P, Liao L, Mattiasson A, Pesce F, Spangberg A, et al. Good urodynamic practices: uroflowmetry, filling cystometry, and pressure-flow studies. Neurourol Urodyn. 2002;21(3):261–74.
16. Nager CW, Albo ME, Fitzgerald MP, McDermott S, Wruck L, Kraus S, et al. Reference urodynamic values for stress incontinent women. Neurourol Urodyn. 2007;26(3):333–40.
17. Haylen BT, Yang V, Logan V. Uroflowmetry: its current clinical utility for women. Int Urogynecol J Pelvic Floor Dysfunct. 2008;19(7):899–903.
18. Haylen BT, Ashby D, Sutherst JR, Frazer MI, West CR. Maximum and average urine flow rates in normal male and female populations–the Liverpool nomograms. Br J Urol. 1989;64(1):30–8.
19. Blaivas JG, Groutz A. Bladder outlet obstruction nomogram for women with lower urinary tract symptomatology. Neurourol Urodyn. 2000;19(5):553–64.
20. Miller JJ, Botros SM, Akl MN, Aschkenazi SO, Beaumont JL, Goldberg RP, et al. Is transobturator tape as effective as tension-free vaginal tape in patients with borderline maximum urethral closure pressure? Am J Obstet Gynecol. 2006;195(6):1799–804.
21. Guerette NL, Bena JF, Davila GW. Transobturator slings for stress incontinence: using urodynamic parameters to predict outcomes. Int Urogynecol J Pelvic Floor Dysfunct. 2008;19(1):97–102.
22. Lemack GE. Urodynamic assessment of patients with stress incontinence: how effective are urethral pressure profilometry and abdominal leak point pressures at case selection and predicting outcome? Curr Opin Urol. 2004;14(6):307–11.
23. McGuire EJ, Woodside JR, Borden TA, Weiss RM. Prognostic value of urodynamic testing in myelodysplastic patients. J Urol. 1981;126(2):205–9.
24. McGuire EJ, Woodside JR, Borden TA, Weiss RM. Prognostic value of urodynamic testing in myelodysplastic patients. 1981. J Urol. 2002;167(2 Pt 2):1049–53; discussion 1054.
25. McGuire EJ, Fitzpatrick CC, Wan J, Bloom D, Sanvordenker J, Ritchey M, et al. Clinical assessment of urethral sphincter function. J Urol. 1993;150(5 Pt 1):1452–4.
26. Nitti VW, Combs AJ. Correlation of Valsalva leak point pressure with subjective degree of stress urinary incontinence in women. J Urol. 1996;155(1):281–5.
27. Rodriguez LV, de Almeida F, Dorey F, Raz S. Does Valsalva leak point pressure predict outcome after the distal urethral polypropylene sling? Role of urodynamics in the sling era. J Urol. 2004;172(1):210–4.
28. Nager CW, Brubaker L, Litman HJ, Zyczynski HM, Varner RE, Amundsen C, et al. A randomized trial of

urodynamic testing before stress-incontinence surgery. N Engl J Med. 2012;366(21):1987–97.
29. Visco AG, Brubaker L, Nygaard I, Richter HE, Cundiff G, Fine P, et al. The role of preoperative urodynamic testing in stress-continent women undergoing sacrocolpopexy: the Colpopexy and Urinary Reduction Efforts (CARE) randomized surgical trial. Int Urogynecol J Pelvic Floor Dysfunct. 2008;19 (5):607–14.
30. Digesu GA, Khullar V, Cardozo L, Salvatore S. Overactive bladder symptoms: do we need urodynamics? Neurourol Urodyn. 2003;22(2):105–8.
31. Hilton P, Stanton SL. A clinical and urodynamic assessment of the Burch colposuspension for genuine stress incontinence. Br J Obstet Gynaecol. 1983;90 (10):934–9.
32. Ellerkmann RM, McBride AW, Dunn JS, Bent AE, Blomquist JL, Kummer LG, et al. A comparison of anticipatory and postprocedure pain perception in patients who undergo urodynamic procedures. Am J Obstet Gynecol. 2004;190(4):1034–8.
33. Shaw C, Williams K, Assassa PR, Jackson C. Patient satisfaction with urodynamics: a qualitative study. J Adv Nurs. 2000;32(6):1356–63.
34. Cundiff GW, McLennan MT, Bent AE. Randomized trial of antibiotic prophylaxis for combined urodynamics and cystourethroscopy. Obstet Gynecol. 1999;93(5 Pt 1):749–52.
35. Okorocha I, Cumming G, Gould I. Female urodynamics and lower urinary tract infection. BJU Int. 2002;89(9):863–7.
36. Sabanathan K, Duffin HM, Castleden CM. Urinary tract infection after cystometry. Age Ageing. 1985;14(5):291–5.
37. Latthe PM, Foon R, Toozs-Hobson P. Prophylactic antibiotics in urodynamics: a systematic review of effectiveness and safety. Neurourol Urodyn. 2008;27 (3):167–73.
38. Lowder JL, Burrows LJ, Howden NL, Weber AM. Prophylactic antibiotics after urodynamics in women: a decision analysis. Int Urogynecol J Pelvic Floor Dysfunct. 2007;18(2):159–64.

Peri-urethral Injections

13

Megan E. Tarr

Abbreviations

PBA Peri-urethral bulking agent
SUI Stress urinary incontinence

Introduction

Urinary incontinence is a common and distressing problem with an overall prevalence of 15 % that rises steadily in later life [46]. Given the aging population, it is likely that the estimated 103,000 surgical procedures currently performed annually for the treatment of stress urinary incontinence (SUI) in the USA will increase [47, 62]. Several minimally invasive surgical options have been developed over the last several decades in an attempt to provide a safe and efficacious method for the surgical treatment of SUI. One such minimally invasive treatment is the injection of peri-urethral bulking agents (PBA). This chapter discusses the history of PBA, indications and contraindications for their use, injection techniques, success, and complication data for the currently available peri-urethral bulking procedures.

M.E. Tarr, M.D., M.S. (✉)
Urogynecology and Pelvic Reconstructive Surgery, Department of Obstetrics and Gynecology, Cleveland Clinic, 9500 Euclid Avenue, A-81, Cleveland, OH 44195, USA
e-mail: tarrm@ccf.org

Mechanism of Action

Urethral coaptation at rest is provided by the urethral mucosa, submucosal vascular cushions, and smooth muscle elements. Submucosal bulking agents are believed to act by creating artificial urethral cushions that can improve urethral coaptation, resulting in urinary continence [31]. In a small study investigating the mechanism of action of bulking agents, Klarskov et al. injected 15 subjects with polyacrylamide gel and measured change in opening urethral pressure by urethral pressure reflexometry [30] 100 days postinjection. He noted that patients who exhibited improvement in their stress incontinence symptoms had significantly higher squeezing opening pressure than the group without an effect. From this data, he concluded that certain agents may increase the strength of the sphincter by providing a central filler that increases the length of muscle fibers and the power of the urethral sphincter.

Ideal Bulking Agent

Many experts who perform urethral bulking believe that the ideal urethral bulking agent is one that is non-immunogenic and biocompatible, creating minimal inflammatory and fibrotic response. The bulking agent's particle size needs to be a sufficient size to prevent migration from the injection site. Migration is thought to occur due to macrophage phagocytosis of

J.D. Emery and M.F.R. Paraiso (eds.), *Office-Based Gynecologic Surgical Procedures*, DOI 10.1007/978-1-4939-1414-2_13, © Springer Science+Business Media New York 2015

particles smaller than 80 μm; an agent that is >110 μm avoids macrophage phagocytosis and migration [42, 55]. Ideally, one should also utilize a low pressure injection system to prevent vascular introduction of the bulking agent.

History

Since 1938, a variety of materials have been injected into and around the urethra to treat SUI. Murless was the first to discuss the use of the sclerosing agent sodium morrhuate into the anterior vaginal wall and around the urethra [45]. In 1955, Quackels used paraffin wax in the perineum [51]. In 1973, Berg described injecting polytetrafluoroethylene paste (Poltef™), produced by the pyrolysis of Teflon™, into the urethral sphincter [8]. This was further popularized by Politano in 1974, and these treatments initially showed promise as simple, minimally invasive treatments for SUI [50]. The paucity of long-term outcome data for polytetrafluoroethylene and the reports of adverse events associated with local extrusion and distant particle migration to the liver, lung, and spleen minimized the support for and popularity of the procedure [42]. Gonzales de Garibay et al. described the use of autologous fat as a PBA in 1989 [19]. Although economical and readily available, subsequent studies have shown that there can be issues with injecting the agent into the correct location, rare complications with pulmonary fat embolus, and the long-term outcomes of fat as a PBA are poor [36].

Peri-urethral injections of cross-linked bovine collagen came to prominence in the 1990s after the successful use of collagen for cosmetic surgery and the treatment of vesicoureteric reflux were described [24]. Since the 1990s, use of glutaraldehyde cross-linked (GAX) bovine collagen (marketed as Contigen, C.R. Bard, Inc., Covington, GA) as a PBA gained universal acceptance. Immediate and delayed hypersensitivity to cross-linked bovine collagen necessitated skin testing several weeks prior to injection. Although considered to have a relatively low risk profile, more serious complications, such as osteitis pubis, arthralgias, and pulmonary embolism (resulting from intravascular injection), have been reported. The manufacturing of collagen by its parent company, however, ceased in 2011, and it is no longer available as a bulking agent. When compared with retropubic colposuspension, pubovaginal sling, and synthetic midurethral sling, urethral bulking with collagen has had less long-term success [1, 13, 52]. This has prompted the search for and development of newer agents.

Another synthetic agent, ethylene vinyl alcohol copolymer (marketed initially as Uryx and then later as Tegress, CR Bard, Covington, Georgia), was initially FDA approved in 2004 and found to have better long-term success than collagen in trials for FDA approval. This product, however, was found to be associated with high rates of urethral and vaginal extrusion and, consequently, was discontinued in 2007 [17, 28]. Another agent that had been used for pediatric vesicoureteral reflux, a combination of hydrophilic dextran polymer in a non-animal stabilized hyaluronic acid vehicle (Ziudex™) underwent initial FDA trials in the USA in 2003 and 2006, but was not FDA approved due to the high incidence (10–15 %) of pseudo-abscess [39, 40].

The PBA that are currently available in the USA for the treatment of SUI are carbon-coated zirconium oxide beads suspended in a water-based gel (Durasphere EXP®, Coloplast, Inc., Minneapolis, MN), calcium hydroxylapatite (Coaptite®, Boston Scientific Corp., Natick, MA), and silicon microimplants (Macroplastique®, Uroplasty, Inc., Minnetonka, MN), and were FDA approved for use in peri-urethral bulking in 1999, 2005, and 2006, respectively. Other agents that are still being studied for use as PBA are autologous cartilage [6, 7], human collagen [61], autologous primary myoblasts [54], and autologous muscle-derived stem cells [11].

Currently Used Bulking Agents: Success and Complications

Although the production of cross-linked bovine collagen was discontinued in 2011, most comparative studies of newer bulking agents use bovine collagen as the control bulking agent. The 2012 Cochrane Review on urethral injection therapy for SUI in women identified 14 trials including 2004 women that met inclusion for analysis [29]. The included trials were small, moderate quality, with limited long-term follow-up data and found to be unsuitable for meta-analysis. Their conclusions stated that currently available evidence remains insufficient to guide practice. The summary of the Cochrane Review follows.

One randomized trial compared peri-urethral injection (Macroplastique) agents to home-based pelvic floor exercises. At 3 months of follow-up, the group receiving the peri-urethral injections showed greater subjective "cure" or "marked improvement" 62.5 % versus 19 %, $p = .002$) [60]. The two trials comparing injectable agents with surgical interventions [Macroplastique versus pubovaginal sling [41]; collagen versus open Burch, open sling, open bladder neck suspension [13] found significantly better objective cure in the surgical groups.

Finally, only three trials included in the Cochrane Review compared routes of bulking agent injection [33, 40, 53]. The trial by Lightner looked at midurethral versus proximal urethral injection but utilized different bulking agents at each site; therefore, a comparison of outcomes was confounded by this variable [40]. Schulz et al. compared peri-urethral and transurethral methods of collagen injection and noted that both methods had similar subjective and objective outcomes at 1, 3, 6, and 12 months, but showed a higher rate of early postprocedural urinary retention in the peri-urethral injection group (30 % versus 5 %, $p < .05$) [53]. Kuhn et al. [33] found that midurethral and bladder neck injection seems to result in similar postprocedural continence levels.

The eight trials included in the Cochrane Review that compared different agents had wide confidence intervals. Overall, the currently available bulking agents were not shown to be more or less efficacious than collagen [29]. The efficacy and complication outcomes of pertinent trials included in the Cochrane Review are discussed in the sections that follow.

Carbon Beads (Durasphere, Durasphere EXP)

Durasphere, pyrolytic carbon-coated zirconium oxide beads, is suspended in an absorbable 2.8 % glycan polysaccharide carrier gel. Prior to its use in urethral bulking, this material had been used in several medical devices, such as replacement heart valves [4]. This material is radio-opaque and can be identified in radiographs and appears as dense as cortical bone on CT [49, 10]. On MRI, it appears hypodense on T1 and T2 weighted images and fails to enhance after gadolinium [10]. The initial carbon bead product (Durasphere) was found to be difficult to inject due to a large particle size of 200–550 μm, which resulted in injection needle obstruction. Consequently, a newer version of the product was developed, utilizing particles of 95–200 μm (Durasphere EXP®, Coloplast, Inc., Minneapolis, MN). Durasphere EXP is the only form of Durasphere available in the USA market and is the only currently available bulking material that is FDA approved for either transurethral or peri-urethral injection. Additionally, this is the only available bulking material that is not contraindicated for patients with a "fragile urethra," due to past radiation or past urethral surgery.

In a multicenter, double-blind randomized controlled trial of transurethral bladder neck injection of Durasphere compared with bovine collagen for treatment of intrinsic sphincter deficiency (aLPP <90 cm H_2O), Lightner et al. [38] found the two materials to be equivalent with respect to postprocedure continence grade and pad weight testing, with 66.1 % (76/115) in the Durasphere group and 65.8 % (79/120) in the bovine collagen group, reporting improvement in one or more Stamey continence grades ($p = 1.00$) (Table 13.1). A smaller volume of Durasphere was needed to obtain comparable clinical results (4.83 mL versus 6.23 mL, $p < .001$). Side effects of the agents were similar, but there was a higher incidence of postprocedure urinary urgency and acute retention in the Durasphere group (24.7 % and 16.9 %, respectively) compared with the bovine collagen

Table 13.1 Success outcomes for bulking agents from randomized controlled trials (RCT)[a]

Agent (author)	RCT design (N)	Follow-up (years)	Volume injected (mL)[b]	Dry/improved[c]	Subjects requiring multiple treatments
Durasphere [38]	Multicenter				
	Agent (176)	1	Agent: 4.83****	–/66 %	35 %
	Control (188)		Control: 6.23****	–/66 %	36 %
Durasphere [3]	Agent (25)	2.6	Agent: 4.5	40 %/80 %	
	Control (21)	2.8	Control: 4.2	14 %/62 %	
Coaptite [43]	Multicenter				
	Agent (131)	1	Agent: 2.15****	39 %/63.4 %	62 %†
	Control (100)		Control: 3.39****	37 %/57 %	74 %†
Macroplastique [20]	Multicenter				
	Agent (122)	1	Agent: 4.6	37 %†/62 %****	52 %
	Control (125)		Control: 4.6	25 %†/48 %****	58 %

[a]Comparison in all trials was transurethral bovine collagen
[b]Volume injected: mean volume of bulking agent injected at initial bulking treatment session
[c]Dry: Stamey grade 0 [4 level scale, with range from 0 = continent-dry to 3 = total incontinence regardless of activity [57]]
Improved: improvement of ≥1 Stamey Urinary Incontinence Scale grade
****$p < .001$ †$p < .05$

group (11.9 % and 3.4 %, respectively, $p = .001$). At 12 months of follow-up, urinary urgency resolved in a greater proportion of the Durasphere subjects (90 %) compared with the bovine collagen subjects (65 %, $p = .021$). Retention in all subjects resolved in 7 days following the procedure.

In a randomized, controlled, double-blind trial comparing Durasphere to bovine collagen, Andersen [3] found there was no difference in the percentage of patients with an improvement of one or more Stamey Continence Grades between the Durasphere group (80 %) and the bovine collagen group (61.9 %, $p = .205$) at an average of 2.6 and 2.8 years of follow-up, respectively (Table 13.1). At this long-term follow-up, 40 % (10/25) of the Durasphere subjects and 14.3 % (3/21) of the bovine collagen subjects reported that they were dry ($p = .099$). Complications rates were not reported in this trial.

Although Lighter et al. reported on radiologic stability of Durasphere, with no evidence of spread beyond local confines of the pelvis at 1- and 2-year follow-up [38], there have been reports of local migration into areas lateral to the urethra and along regional lymphatic chains [49]. Foreign body reactions with associated urethral prolapse and delayed presentation of a pseudoabscess 5 years postprocedure have been reported [9].

Calcium Hydroxylapatite (Coaptite)

Coaptite is composed of spherical calcium hydroxylapatite particles, ranging from 75 to 125 mm in diameter, in a carboxymethylcellulose gel carrier [16, 43]. The gel carrier degrades over several months, and the patient's fibroblasts infiltrate amongst the particles. Calcium hydroxylapatite is a constituent of human bone and teeth and has been used for 25 years in dental and orthopedic procedures [44]. It is radio-opaque and can be easily identified with plain film radiography and ultrasound after injection [16]. Calcium hydroxylapatite is neither immunogenic nor inflammatory and remains pliable after injection into soft tissues, lending itself to use in augmentation of the vocal cords and facial structures [5, 37]. Initial studies of its endoscopic use in the treatment of vesicoureteral reflux in pediatric subjects have shown it to be both durable and efficacious [44].

In a multicenter, prospective, randomized, single-blind trial of 296 women with SUI secondary to intrinsic sphincter deficiency, subjective improvement in urinary incontinence symptoms, as graded by the Stamey Urinary Incontinence Scale, were similar at 12-month follow-up for patients who received Coaptite compared to those who received bovine collagen (63.4 % versus 57 %, respectively, $p = 0.34$) ([43], Table 13.1). The cure rate (Stamey grade 0) at 12 months was also similar for both groups (39 % for Coaptite versus 37 % for Contigen, $p = 0.34$). A greater number of patients receiving Coaptite injections required only one injection over the first 6 months of the study (38.0 % versus 26.1 %, $p = 0.034$); however, most subjects required two to three injections in either group. There was no difference in the percentage of patients with transient urinary retention (41 % Coaptite versus 33 % bovine collagen), and there was less postprocedural urge incontinence in the Coaptite group (5.7 % versus 12 %, $p < .05$). There was one vaginal wall erosion in the Coaptite group, and one patient with dissection of the Coaptite beneath the trigonal mucosa, resulting in difficulty with visualization of one ureteral orifice cystoscopically. This patient, however, had no abnormal lab or radiographic abnormalities and had no urinary incontinence.

Serious adverse events related to Coaptite are rare. Palma et al. reported on a patient presenting with a 3 cm urethral prolapse containing macrophages surrounding the Coaptite particles 3 months after initial peri-urethral bulking with a total of 2.5 mL of Coaptite [48]. Coaptite has also been used in the pediatric population for vesicoureteral reflux and has been found to be quite safe in multicenter prospective trials [44].

Silicone (Macroplastique)

Macroplastique, a hydrogel-suspended cross-linked polydimethyl-siloxane elastomer, has been approved by the FDA as a urethral bulking agent since 2006 for the treatment of SUI secondary to intrinsic sphincter deficiency [37]. This bulking agent is composed of relatively large silicone particles measuring 100 μm to 450 μm in diameter (mean diameter approximately 180 μm) suspended in a non-silicone carrier gel that is excreted unchanged in the urine [16, 25, 56]. The silicone particles quickly become encapsulated in fibrin with minimal inflammation [16, 26]. Studies of this material in rat and canine models show that Macroplastique is not readily phagocytized by macrophages, and fibroblasts do not readily adhere to Macroplastique [56].

In a multicenter, randomized, controlled trial comparing transurethral Macroplastique to bovine collagen for treatment of intrinsic sphincter deficiency, a greater proportion 61.5 % (75/122) of the patients receiving Macroplastique had an improvement of at least one Stamey Grade compared with 48 % (60/125) receiving bovine collagen ($p < .001$) at 12-month follow-up [20]. Additionally, a greater proportion of the patients receiving Macroplastique were dry (Stamey grade 0) compared with those receiving bovine collagen (36.9 % versus 24.8 %, $p < .05$). The total number of subjects who underwent two treatments in the 12-month follow-up was the same for both groups (Macroplastique 52.5 % and bovine collagen 58.4 %, $p = .35$), and the treatment volumes were not significantly different between the Macroplastique and bovine collagen groups. Additionally, Incontinence Quality of Life scores (I-QOL) improved in a similar magnitude from baseline between the Macroplastique and bovine collagen groups. Overall, adverse effects were similar between the two treatment groups (59 % and 54.5 %) with urinary tract infection (23.8 % versus 24.8 %), dysuria (9 % versus 8 %), urgency (9 % versus 7.2 %), frequency (8.2 % versus 9.6 %), and urinary retention (6.6 % versus 3.2 %) being the most frequently reported in the Macroplastique and bovine collagen groups, respectively. Only one serious adverse event (pyelonephritis) was reported in the bovine collagen group.

Ghoniem et al. reported 2-year follow-up data on the above cohort of patients who had received Macroplastique [21]. Of the 67 patients included in this 2-year follow-up, 67 % were dry (Stamey grade 0). Of the 38 patients who were dry at 12 months, 33 (87 %) of these remained dry at

2 years. Overall and subscale I-QOL scores at 24 months were also improved significantly over baseline for the 2-year follow-up group ($p < .001$). The conclusions from this ancillary study are limited, as they only followed the Macroplastique patients for the additional 1 year, and only reported on 55 % (67/122) of the original Macroplastique cohort.

Bulking Procedure

Patient Characteristics, Indications, and Contraindications

In general, most patients are thought to be ideal candidates for urethral bulking if they have SUI associated with intrinsic sphincter deficiency, defined as a valsalva leak point pressure (VLPP) <60 cm H_2O or maximum urethral closure pressure <20–25 cm H_2O, with at least 150 mL bladder fill, and an immobile urethra. There is evidence, however, that bulking agents are effective in cases of SUI associated with higher VLPP or in cases where SUI occurs with bladder neck hypermobility [6, 7, 58]. Currently, Medicare requires a LPP $\leq$ 100 cm H_2O for procedural coverage. Other patients for whom bulking agents are considered are those who are medically compromised and cannot undergo a midurethral sling or have failed a prior surgery for stress incontinence [18, 32, 35]. In general, patients who are not considered to be optimal candidates for urethral bulking are those with urinary tract infections, urethral diverticula, poor urethral blood supply, high baseline post void residual urine volumes, severe detrusor overactivity, and reduced bladder capacity (<250 mL).

Necessary Equipment

The exact equipment required for a bulking procedure varies according to which agent you are utilizing for the procedure. In general, one needs a sterile prep solution for the vagina and peri-urethral tissues, 2 % lidocaine hydrochloride jelly (Uro-jet), 1 % lidocaine for peri-urethral blockade (if desired), sterile water, irrigation tubing with stopcock, camera, light cord, and cystoscopy tower. The type and size of endoscope utilized for peri-urethral bulking varies according to the bulking product.

Procedural Overview

The patient has a urinalysis upon arrival on the day of the procedure to assure there is no underlying urinary tract infection, and the procedure is cancelled if urinalysis suggests an existing urinary tract infection. According to the 2013 American Urological Association (AUA) Guidelines for urologic surgery antimicrobial prophylaxis, a prophylactic antibiotic (either a fluoroquinolone or trimethoprim-sulfamethoxazole) is given (http://www.auanet.org/common/pdf/education/clinical-guidance/Antimicrobial-Prophylaxis-PocketTable.pdf) [2]. Alternative antimicrobials include an aminoglycoside with ampicillin, first or second generation cephalosporin, or amoxicillin/clavulanate.

After informed consent and procedural time out are performed, the patient is placed in the dorsal lithotomy position, and betadine is used to perform a sterile preparation of the peri-urethral region and perineum. Local anesthetic, typically one 2 % lidocaine Uro-jet, is administered to the urethral lumen. Onset of anesthesia is typically 3–5 min. Additionally, a peri-urethral blockade with injectable local anesthetic, such as 1 % lidocaine, can be preformed. If this is done, injection at 3–4 o'clock and 8–9 o'clock is recommended, with approximately 4 mL of lidocaine used on each side [12].

Using a 30° operative cystoscope (lens degree can vary), the bulking agent is injected into the submucosa at two or more sites at the same level of the proximal urethra. Bulking agents can be injected just distal to the bladder neck or at the midurethra, although there is little data to support either approach. The efficacy of midurethral and bladder neck placement of urethral bulking agents has been compared in a small ($N = 30$), randomized study utilizing

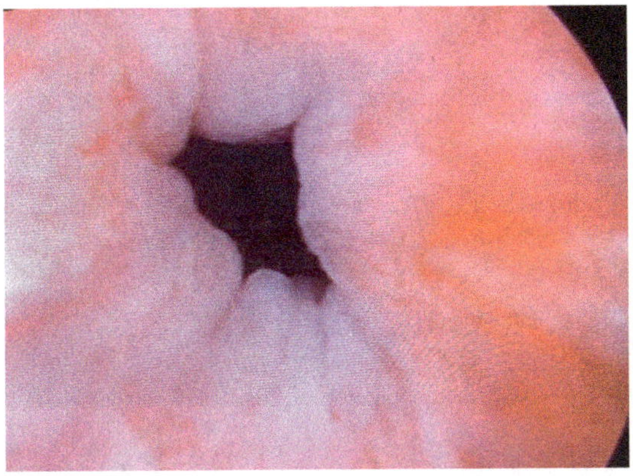

Fig. 13.1 Urethra prior to urethral bulking (Image courtesy of Drs. Mark Walters and Cecile Unger)

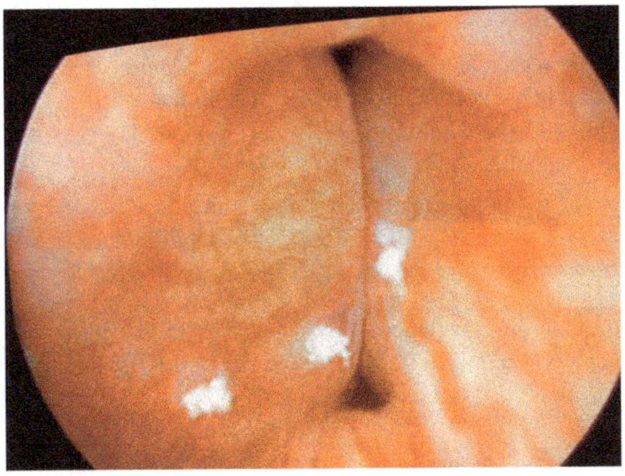

Fig. 13.2 Urethral coaptation after urethral bulking (Image courtesy of Drs. Mark Walters and Cecile Unger)

transurethral collagen [33]. At 10 months postoperatively, patients' satisfaction on a visual analog scale did not significantly differ, and the proportion with negative cough stress tests did not differ between the bladder neck and midurethral groups (60 % versus 66 %, respectively). Bulking agents can also be injected peri-urethrally through the perineum, while viewing the bulking effect simultaneously with a cystoscope. The procedure for peri-urethral injections is discussed in the Procedural section for Durasphere EXP below. Most clinicians, however, seem to feel more comfortable with transurethral injections.

After the clinician has delivered what is perceived to be an adequate volume of the bulking material so that the urethral lumen coapts (Figs. 13.1 and 13.2), the patient is asked to cough. If transurethral urine loss is witnessed, additional bulking material may be administered. Once the bulking procedure is finished, the patient is asked to void. If she cannot void spontaneously, intermittent self-catheterization with a small diameter (8–12 French) catheter is taught. Clinicians may also prefer to teach intermittent self-catheterization prior to the procedure. Patients are typically given home-going instructions and precautions by the nursing staff and treating physician. Follow-up is typically arranged at 1–3 months, and patients are encouraged to call with any concerns.

Tips and Tricks for Specific Bulking Agents

Each urethral bulking agent and injection system has its own unique features and challenges. Please refer to Table 13.2 for a summary of currently available bulking agents and their corresponding supplies. The following text summarizes instructions pertinent to each specific agent.

Durasphere (Durasphere EXP® Office Procedure Guide) [15]

Transurethral Injection

Preparation

- Hold needle by its wings, and align the arrow on the 1 mL syringe tip with the dark bar located on the needle hub
- Turn the syringe to connect the needle to the hub
- Move the hand on the syringe back to finish tightening the syringe to the needle with a 360° rotation, until the arrow is aligned with the dark bar located on the needle
- Prime the needle

Needle Placement

- Chose a position between 4 and 8 o'clock
- At the level of the midurethra, position the needle bevel toward the urethral lumen
- Puncture the tissue at a 45° angle, do not insert past the needle bevel

Table 13.2 Currently FDA-approved agents for peri-urethral bulking

Bulking agent (FDA approval)	Trade name (manufacturer)	Gauge needle	Syringe for agent	Injection locations (typical total volume)
Glutaraldehyde cross-linked bovine collagen (1993)	Contigen™ (Bard, Inc.)[a]	22–23 g	2.5 mL	(2.5–5 mL)
Pyrolytic carbon coated graphite beads (carbon) (1999)	Durasphere EXP™ (Coloplast, Inc.)	Transurethral 18/20 g 15 in. Peri-urethral 18/20 g 1.5 in.	Transurethral 1.0 mL Peri-urethral 3.0 mL	Between 4 o'clock 8 o'clock At 3 and 9 o'clock (2–4 mL)
Calcium hydroxylapatite (CaHA) (2005)	Coaptite™ (Boston Scientific)	21 g[b]	1.0 mL	4 o'clock 8 o'clock (2–4 mL)
Polydimethylsiloxane particles (silicone) (2006)	Macroplastique™ (Uroplasty)	18/20 g	2.5 mL	6 o'clock 2 o'clock[c] 10 o'clock[c] (5.5 mL)

[a]Production of Contigen ceased in 2011
[b]End injection and Sidekick needle available
[c]May deliver 1.25 mL rather than 2.5 mL at these locations

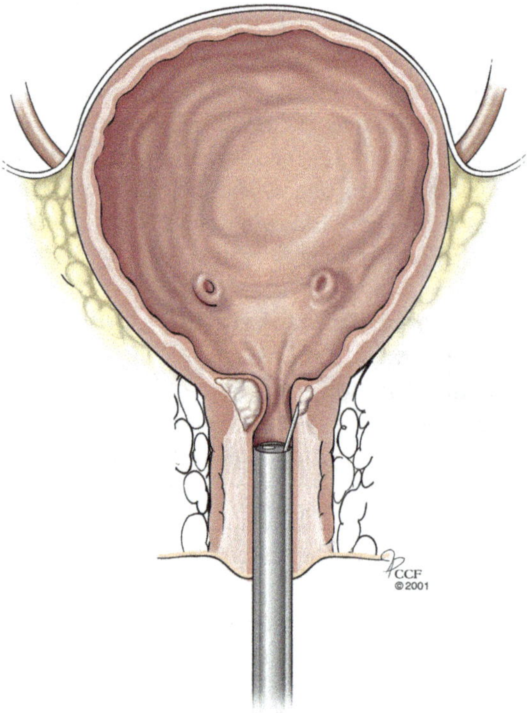

Fig. 13.3 Transurethral injection of bulking agent

- Re-angle the scope to an orientation parallel to the urethra (Fig. 13.3)
- Tunnel the needle toward the bladder neck for 1–2 cm, using needle markings as a guide

Injection
- Use consistent, moderate thumb pressure on the plunger to inject evenly
- The submucosa should distend toward the urethral lumen
- You can also rotate the orientation of the needle bevel superiorly and inferiorly, to facilitate flow of the agent
- Choose an opposing site for the second injection, and repeat the above procedures until the bladder neck coapts
- Most procedures will require 4 or more 1 mL syringes of the bulking agent

Peri-urethral Injection

Preparation
- Attach the 1.5 in., bent pencil point tip needle to a 3 mL syringe filled with sterile saline
- The needle has a 15° bend to facilitate submucosal injection between the lamina propria and the muscularis

Needle Placement
- Insert the 30° cystoscope into the urethra, with the scope lens oriented toward the side of the urethra where the injection is planned
- Note the two peri-urethral dimples at 3 and 9 o'clock
- Position the needle tip at the dimple with the needle hub parallel to the scope. The proximal

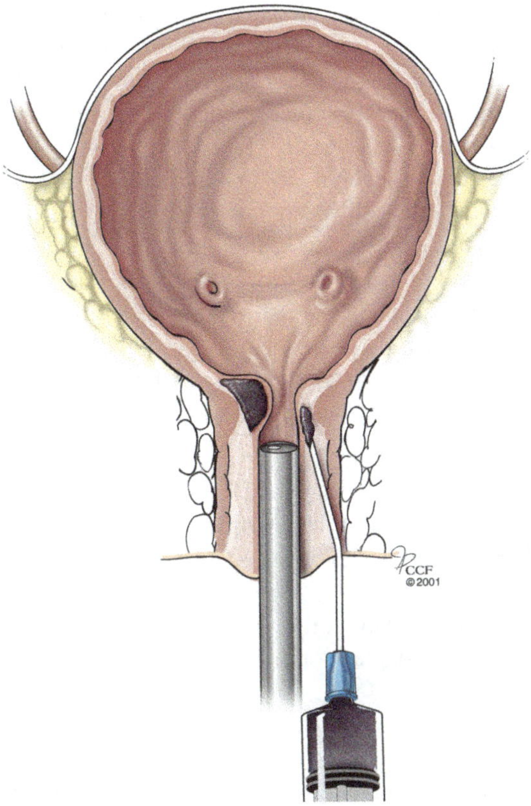

Fig. 13.4 Peri-urethral injection of bulking agent

half of the needle will be angled away from the scope

- Penetrate the tissue and continue to advance the needle approximately 3 cm, keeping the needle hub parallel with the scope. Once advanced, the needle tip should be in the proximal urethra (Fig. 13.4)
- Verify needle tip placement in the submucosal plane gently wiggling the distal hub of the needle while looking through the cystoscope
- To assure correct needle placement, hydrodissect by injecting some fluid into the site. Temporary bulking of the tissue should occur if the needle is in the correct location. If no bulking occurs, reposition the needle more superficially

Injection

- Attach the 3 mL syringe containing the bulking agent to the needle

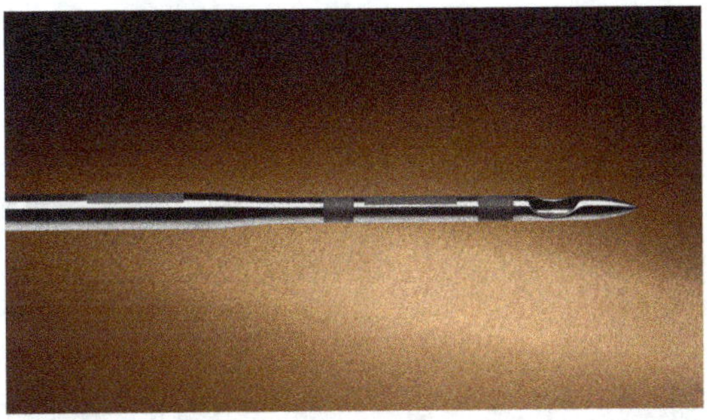

Fig. 13.5 Sidekick needle used for Coaptite (Images courtesy of Boston Scientific Corporation. Opinions expressed are those of the author alone and not Boston Scientific)

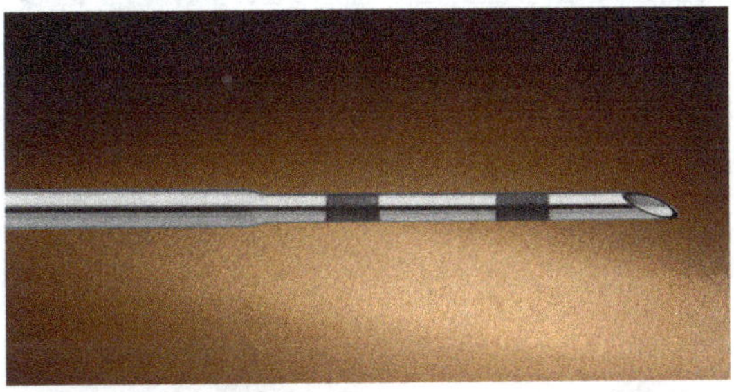

Fig. 13.6 End injection needle used for Coaptite (Images courtesy of Boston Scientific Corporation. Opinions expressed are those of the author alone and not Boston Scientific)

- Inject with slow, consistent pressure while observing the bulking effect
- If circumferential distribution of the material is occurring, keep injecting until complete coaptation is achieved
- If the product is not flowing circumferentially, continue to inject into the site until the bulge has crossed the urethral midline, then reposition the needle on the opposite side and continue the injection protocol, as above
- Most procedures require at least 4 mL of bulking agent

Coaptite (Coaptite® Injectable Implant Procedure Guide) [14]

Preparation

- Choose either the Sidekick (Fig. 13.5) or End injection (Fig. 13.6) needle

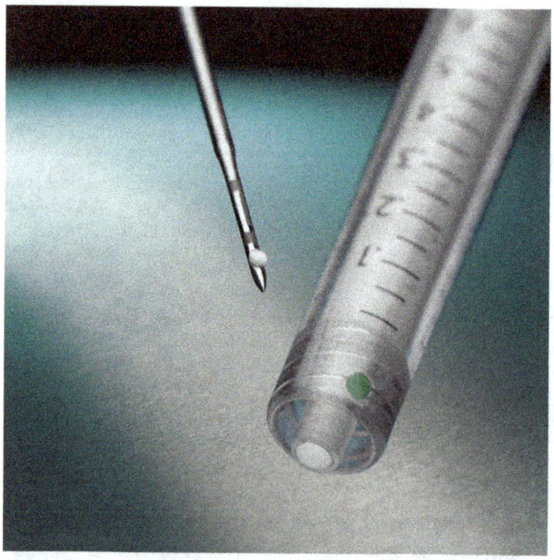

Fig. 13.7 Coaptite needle is attached to the injection syringe by aligning the green dot and securing it with 1.5 turns (Images courtesy of Boston Scientific Corporation. Opinions expressed are those of the author alone and not Boston Scientific)

- When connecting 1 mL syringe to needle, make sure that you line up the green dot on the syringe to the green circular hole on the needle hub (Fig. 13.7)
- Then, turn syringe to screw it onto needle hub (about one-and-a-half times) (Fig. 13.7)
- It should feel tight, you will probably hear a click or two, and you will see one of the green dots now through the circular hole on the needle hub
- When priming, the bulking agent should flow easily
- After priming, insert primed needle into the scope

Needle Placement
- At the midurethra, insert needle at 4 o'clock position into tissue at a 45° angle with the open bevel facing toward the urethral lumen until you get to the first black marking
- Adjust needle parallel to urethral lumen and advance needle somewhere between the first and second black marking, approximately 1 cm toward bladder neck

Injection
- Slowly inject
- If you feel resistance, resist pushing through it, as the aqueous carrier will only be placed
- Pull back on needle and/or rotate needle slightly to adjust placement where the bulking material flows easily (Fig. 13.3)
- After injection to a particular site is concluded, slowly remove needle part way
- When you start to see the first black marking coming out of the injection site, pause for a few seconds (~10) before removing it completely
- This will help limit any extravasation
- Repeat injection a 8 o'clock position

Macroplastique (Macroplastique® Procedure Guide) [63]

Preparation
- Slide adapter over syringe (Fig. 13.8)
- Lock adapter onto administration device (Fig. 13.9)
- Remove plastic cap from syringe containing product
- Attach winged needle hub and turn 2–2.5 times to tighten needle onto syringe (Figs. 13.10 and 13.11)
- Remove plastic needle sheath
- Prime needle by squeezing lever of administration device (Fig. 13.12)
- When product flows from needle tip, depress release mechanism to stop flow

Needle Placement
- Use the black needle hash marks to guide the depth of the needle prior to releasing the bulking agent.
- Tilt the scope at a 30–40° angle in relation to the urethral lumen to advance the needle into the tissue to level of the first mark on the needle at the 6 o'clock position on the urethra.
- Once the first mark is passed, reduce the needle angle to close to 0° to the urethral lumen and advance the needle to the second hash mark.
- The bulking agent should then be released in the midurethra.

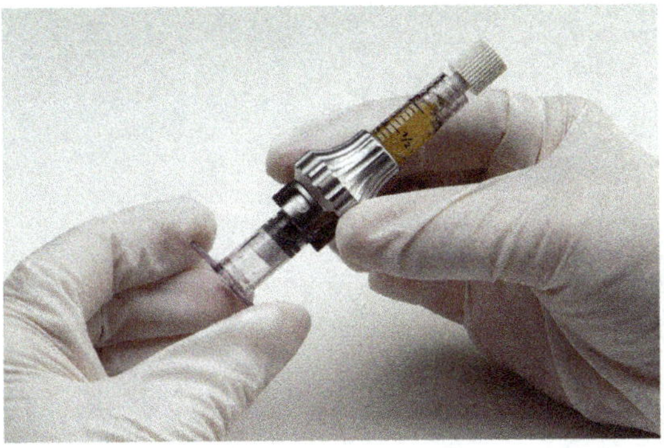

Fig. 13.8 Sliding metal adapter over syringe containing Macroplastique (Images courtesy of ©Uroplasty, Inc. All rights reserved)

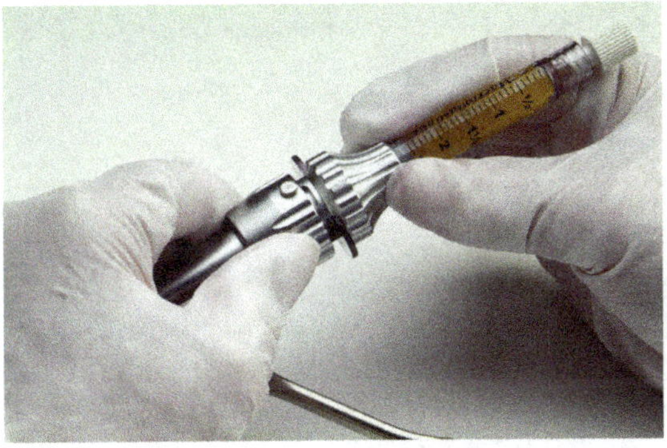

Fig. 13.9 Locking adapter onto administration device for Macroplastique (Images courtesy of ©Uroplasty, Inc. All rights reserved)

- If the patient has a short urethra, the site will be just passing the first hash mark on the needle.
- The black arrows on the needle indicate needle bevel and orientation. The needle bevel should face toward the urethral lumen when injecting.

Injection

- Allow 1.5 min to release the entire 2.5 mL syringe at the 6 o'clock position, and use a slow, consistent injecting technique.
- If you do not see an immediate bleb, you are likely too deep and need to pull needle back slightly.
- Once the agent is injected, wait 30 s before withdrawing the needle.
- If you see product extruding at the incision site, you are either injecting too quickly or you didn't tunnel the needle far enough into the tissue.
- The administration device rotates 360° for precise placement.
- Typically administer 1.25 mL of the agent at 10 and 2 o'clock after injecting at the 6 o'clock position.

Short- and Long-Term Complications

Most complications related to urethral bulking agents are urinary tract infections (10–25 %), transient urinary retention (3–40 %), dysuria (8–10 %), urinary urgency (7–11 %), and localized pain [20, 38, 43]. Rates specific to each agent are discussed in the above sections. More rare localized complications, such as urethral erosions [27, 28], sterile abscess [9, 59], urethral abscess [23], urethral prolapse [22, 48], and urethral diverticulum [34], have been reported. In addition, complications due to distant particle migration, such as pulmonary embolus [59] and deposition in local and distant lymph nodes and organs [49], have been reported. Bovine collagen causes a systemic immunogenic response in 2–5 % of patients.

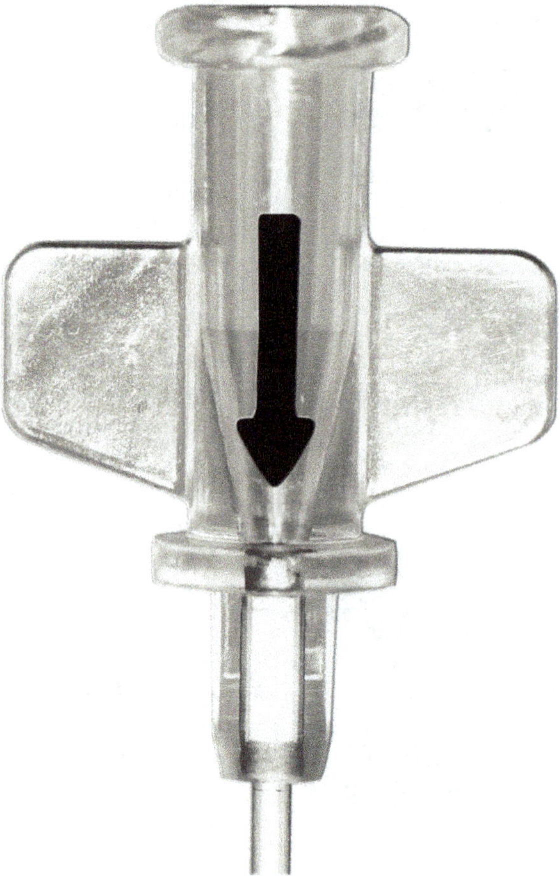

Fig. 13.10 Use of wings to attach needle to syringe containing Macroplastique (Images courtesy of ©Uroplasty, Inc. All rights reserved)

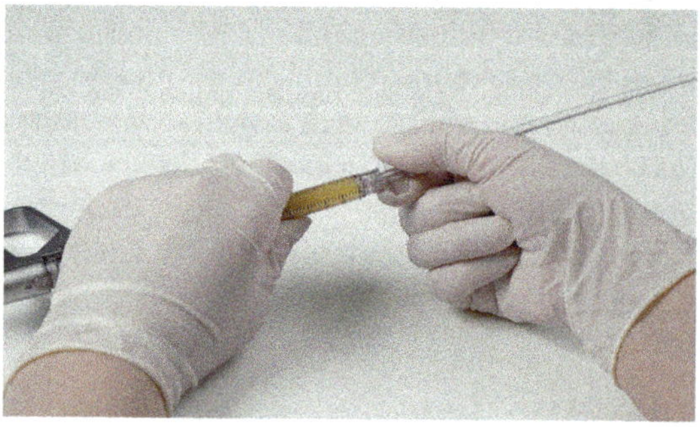

Fig. 13.11 Attaching winged needle hub and syringe of Macroplastique (Images courtesy of ©Uroplasty, Inc. All rights reserved)

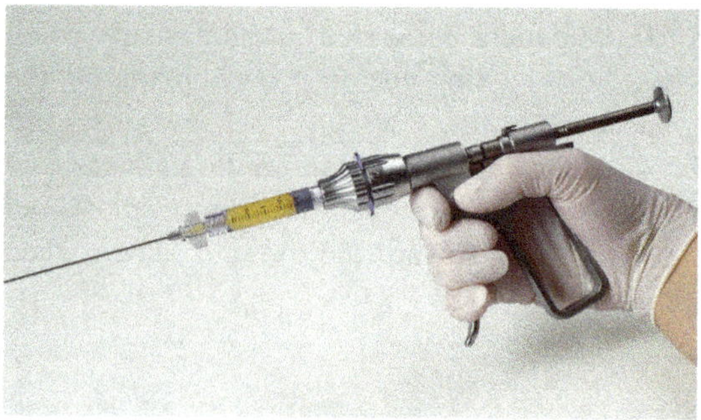

Fig. 13.12 Priming needle by squeezing the level of the administration device (Images courtesy of ©Uroplasty, Inc. All rights reserved)

Conclusions

Despite their variable short- and long-term success rates, PBA are a viable treatment option for SUI. Although many agents have not stood the test of time, prospective, randomized trials of the three currently available bulking agents in the USA offer hopeful data concerning improvement in continence at 1–2 years. Overall, these agents are well tolerated in women of various ages, varying comorbid conditions, and varying histories of past continence surgeries.

References

1. Albo ME, Litman HJ, Richter HE, Lemack GE, Sirls LT, Chai TC, et al. Treatment success of retropubic and transobturator mid urethral slings at 24 months. J Urol. 2012;188:2281–7.
2. American Urologic Association Pocket Guide May 15, 2013 for Urologic Surgery Antimicrobial Prophylaxis. http://www.auanet.org/common/pdf/education/clinical-guidance/Antimicrobial-Prophylaxis-PocketTable.pdf. Accessed 6 Oct 2013.
3. Andersen RCM. Long-term follow-up comparison of Durasphere and Contigen in the treatment of stress urinary incontinence. J Low Genit Tract Dis. 2002;6:239–43.
4. Cao H. Mechanical performance of pyrolytic carbon in prosthetic heart valve applications. J Heart Valve Dis. 1996;5(1):S32–49.
5. Belafsky PC, Postma GN. Vocal cord augmentation with calcium hydroxylapatite. Otolaryngol Head Neck Surg. 2004;131(4):351–4.
6. Bent AE, Foote J, Siegel S, Faerber G, Chaos R, Gormley EA. Collagen implant for treating stress urinary incontinence in women with urethral hypermobility. J Urol. 2001;166:1354–7.
7. Bent AE, Tutrone RT, McLennan MT, Lloyd LK, Kennelly MJ, Badlani G. Treatment of intrinsic sphincter deficiency using autologous ear chondrocytes as a bulking agent. Neurourol Urodyn. 2001;20:157–65.
8. Berg S. Polytef augmentation urethroplasty. Arch Surg. 1973;201:379–81.
9. Berger MB, Morgan DM. Delayed presentation of pseudoabscess secondary to injections of pyrolytic carbon-coated beads bulking agent. Female Pelvic Med Reconstr Surg. 2012;18:303–5.
10. Bridges MD, Petrou SP, Lightner DJ. Urethral bulking agents: imaging review. AJR Am J Roentgenol. 2005;185:257–64.
11. Carr LK, Steele D, Steele S, Wagner D, Pruchnic R, Jankowski R, Erickson J, Huard J, Chancellor MB. 1-year follow-up of autologous muscle derived stem cell injection pilot study to treat stress urinary incontinence. Int Urogynecol J. 2008;19:881–3.
12. Cerruto MA, Zattoni F. Bulking agents: anesthesia techniques. Urologia. 2009;76:45–8.
13. Corcos J, Collet JP, Shapiro S, Herschorn S, Radomski SB, Schick E, et al. Multicenter randomized clinical trial comparing surgery and collagen injections for treatment of female stress urinary incontinence. Urology. 2005;65:898–904.
14. Coaptite® injectable implant procedure guide. www.bostonscientific.com/gynecology, Accessed 10 Oct 2013.
15. Durasphere EXP® office procedure guide. www.us.coloplast.com, Accessed 10 Oct 2013.
16. Dmochowski RR, Appell RA. Injectible agents in the treatment of stress urinary incontinence in women: where are we now? Urology. 2000;56(S6A):32–40.
17. Erekson EA, Sung VW, Rardin CR, Myers DL. Ethylene vinyl alcohol copolymer erosion after use as a urethral bulking agent. Obstet Gynecol. 2007;109:490–2.
18. Faerber GJ. Endoscopic collagen injection therapy in elderly women with type I stress urinary incontinence. J Urol. 1996;155:512–4.
19. de Garibay AS G, Castillo-JImenco JM, York M, Gomez P, Sebastian-Borruel JL. Endoscopic autotransplantation of fat tissues in the treatment of urinary incontinence in the female. J Urol (Paris). 1989;95:363.
20. Ghoniem G, Corcos J, Comiter C, Bernhard P, Westney OL, Herschorn S. Cross-linked polymethylsiloxane injection for female stress urinary incontinence: results of a multicenter, randomized, controlled single-blind study. J Urol. 2009;181:204–10.
21. Ghoniem G, Corcos J, Comiter C, Bernhard P, Westney OL, Herschorn S. Durability of urethral bulking agent injection for female stress urinary incontinence: 2 year multicenter study results. J Urol. 2010;183:1444–9.
22. Ghoniem GM, Khater U. Urethral prolapse after durasphere injection. Int Urogynecol J. 2006;17:297–8.
23. Gopinath D, Smith AR, Reid FM. Periurethral abscess following polyacrylamide hydrogel (Bulkamid) for stress urinary incontinence. Int Urogynecol J. 2012;23:1645–48.
24. Haab F, Zimmern PE, Leach GE. Urinary stress incontinence due to intrinsic sphincteric deficiency: experience with fat and collagen periurethral injections. J Urol. 1997;157:1283–6.
25. Harriss DR, Iacovou JW, Lemberger RJ. Peri-urethral silicone microimplants (Macroplastique) for the treatment of genuine stress incontinence. Br J Urol. 1996;78:722–8.
26. Henley DR, Barrett DM, Weiland TL, O'Connor MK, Malizia AA, Wein AJ. Particulate silicone for use in periurethral injections: local tissue effects and search for migration. J Urol. 1995;153(6):2039–43.

27. Hurtado EA, Appell RA. Complications of Tegress injections. Int Urogynecol J. 2009;20:127.
28. Hurtado E, McCrery R, Appell R. The safety and efficacy of ethylene vinyl alcohol copolymer as an intra-urethral bulking agent in women with intrinsic urethral deficiency. In Urogynecol J. 2007;18:869–73.
29. Kirchin V, Page T, Keegan PE, Atiemo K, Cody JD, Mc Clinton S. Urethral injection therapy for urinary incontinence in women. Cochrane Database Syst Rev. 2012;(2):Art No.:CD003881. doi:10.1002/14651858. CD003881.pub3.
30. Klarsov N. Urethral pressure reflexometry. Dan Med. 2012;59(3):B4412.
31. Klarsov N, Lose G. Urethral injection therapy: what is the mechanism of action? Neurourol Urodyn. 2008;27:789–92.
32. Koski ME, Enemchukwu EA, Padmanabhan P, Kaufman MR, Scarpero HM, Dmochowski RR. Safety and efficacy of sling for persistent stress urinary incontinence after bulking injection. Urology. 2011;77:1076–80.
33. Kuhn A, Stadlmayr W, Lengsfeld D, Mueller MD. Where should bulking agents for female urodnamic stress incontinence be injected? Int Urogynecol J. 2008;19:817–21.
34. Kumar D, Kaufman MR, Dmochowski RR. Case reports: periurethral bulking agents and presumed urethral diverticula. Int Urogynecol J. 2011;22:1039–43.
35. Lee HM, Lee YS, Han JY, Jeong JY, Choo MS, Lee KS. Transurethral injection of bulking agent for treatment of failed mid-urethral sling procedures. Int Urogynecol J. 2010;21:1479–83.
36. Lee PE, Kung RC, Druta HP. Periurethral autologous fat injections as treatment for female stress urinary incontinence: a randomized double-blind controlled trial. J Urol. 2001;165:153–8.
37. Lightner DJ. Review of the available urethral bulking agents. Curr Opin Urol. 2002;12:333–8.
38. Lightner DJ, Calvosa C, Andersen R, Klimberg I, Brito CG, Snyder J, et al. A new injectable bulking agent for treatment of stress urinary incontinence: results of a multicenter, randomized controlled, double-blind study of Dursphere. Urology. 2001;58:12–5.
39. Lightner DJ, Fox J, Klingele C. Cystoscopic injections of dextranomer hyaluronic acid into proximal urethra for urethral incompetence: efficacy and adverse outcomes. Urology. 2010;75:1310–4.
40. Lightner DJ, Rovner E, Corcos J, Payne C, Brubaker L, Druta H, et al. Randomized controlled multisite trial of injected bulking agents for women with intrinsic sphincter deficiency: mid-urethral injection of Zuidex via the Implacer versus proximal urethral injection of Contigen cystoscopically. Urology. 2009;74:771–77.
41. Maher CF, O'Reilly BA, Dwyer PL, Carey MP, Cornish A, Schluter P. Pubovaginal sling versus transurethral Macroplastique for stress urinary incontinence and intrinsic sphincter deficiency: a prospective randomized controlled trial. BJOG. 2005;112:797–801.
42. Malizia AM, Reiman HM, Myers RP. Migration and granulomatous reaction after periurethral injection of Polytef (Teflon). JAMA. 1984;251:3277–81.
43. Mayer RD, Dmochowski RR, Appell RA, Sand PK, Klimberg IW, Jacoby K, Graham CW, Snyder JA, Nitti VW, Winters JC. Multicenter prospective randomized 52-week trial of calcium hydroxylapatite versus bovine dermal collagen for treatment of stress urinary incontinence. Urology. 2007;69:876–80.
44. Mevorach RA, Hulbert WC, Rabinowitz R, Kennedy A, Kogan BA, Kryger JV, Caldamone A, Clark WR, Kaplan GW, Durkee CT, Elder JS. Results of a 2-year multicenter trial of endoscopic treatment of vesicoureteral reflux with synthetic calcium hydroxyapatite. J Urol. 2006;175:288–91.
45. Murless BC. The injection treatment of stress incontinence. J Obstet Gynaecol Br Emp. 1938;45:521.
46. Nygaard I, Barber MD, Burgio KL, Kenton K, Meikle S, Schaffer J, et al. Prevalence of symptomatic pelvic floor disorders in US women. JAMA. 2008;300:1311–6.
47. Oliphant SS, Wang L, Bunker CH, Lowder JL. Trends in stress urinary incontinence inpatient procedures in the United States, 1979-2004. Am J Obstet Gynecol. 2009;200(5):521.e1–6.
48. Palma PCR, Riccetto CLZ, Martins MHT, Herrmann V, de Fraga R, Billis A, et al. Massive prolapse of the urethral mucosa following injection of calcium hydroxylapatitie for stress urinary incontinence. Int Urogynecol J. 2006;17:670–1.
49. Pannek J, Brands FH, Senge T. Particle migration after transurethral injections of carbon coated beads for stress urinary incontinence. J Urol. 2001;166:1350–3.
50. Politano VA, Small MP, Harper JM, Lynne CM. Periurethral Teflon injection for urinary incontinence. J Urol. 1974;111:180.
51. Quackels R. Two cases of incontinence after adenomectomy cured by paraffine injection into the perineum. Acta Urol Belg. 1955;23(3):259–62 [in French].
52. Richter HE, Albo ME, Zyczynski HM, Kenton K, Norton PA, Sirls LT, et al. Retropubic versus transobturator midurethral slings for stress incontinence. N Engl J Med. 2010;362:2066–76.
53. Schulz JA, Nager CW, Stanton SL, Baessler K. Bulking agents for stress urinary incontinence: short-term results and complications in a randomized comparison of peri-urethral and transurethral injections. Int Urogynecol J. 2004;15:261–5.
54. Sebe P, Doucet C, Cornu J, Ciofu C, Costa P, de Medina SGD, et al. Intrasphincteric injections of autologous muscular cells in women with refractory stress urinary incontinence: a prospective study. Int Urogynecol J. 2011;22:183–9.
55. Smith DP, Kaplan WE, Oyasu R. Evaluation of polymethylsiloxane as an alternative in the endoscopic treatment of vesicoureteral reflux. J Urol. 1994;152:1221–4.

56. Solomon LZ, Birch BR, Cooper AJ, Davies CL, Holmes SAV. Nonhomologous bioinjectable materials in urology: 'size matters'? BJU Int. 2000;85:641–5.
57. Stamey TA. Urinary incontinence in the female: stress urinary incontinence. In: Harrison JH, Gittes RF, Ad P, editors. Campbells' urology. 4th ed. Philadelphia: WB Saunders; 1979. p. 2272–93.
58. Steele AC, Kohli N, Karram MM. Peri-urethral collagen injection for stress incontinence with and without urethral hypermobility. Obstet Gynecol. 2000;95:327.
59. Sweat SD, Lightner DJ. Complications of sterile abscess formation and pulmonary embolism following periurethral bulking agents. J Urol. 1999;161:93–6.
60. ter Meulen PH, Berghmans LC, Neiman FH, van Kerrebroeck PE. Effects of Macroplastique implantation system for stress urinary incontinence and urethral hypermobility in women. Int Urogynecol J. 2009;20:177–83.
61. Van Veggel L, Morrell M, Harris C, Dormans-Linssen M. A new devise for the treatment of female stress urinary incontinence. Proc Inst Mech Eng H. 2003;217(4):317–21.
62. Wu JM, Hundley AF, Fulton RG, Myers ER. Forecasting the prevalence of pelvic floor disorders in U.S. women 2010-2050. Obstet Gynecol. 2009;114:1278–83.
63. Macroplastique® Implants Instructions for Use. http://www.uroplasty.com/files/pdf/4226.pdf, Accessed 10 Oct 2013.

14 Trigger Point Injections for Pelvic Pain

Jeannine M. Miranne and Amy J. Park

Introduction

Chronic pelvic pain is one of the most challenging problems gynecologists encounter in clinical practice. This condition is common, affecting up to 15–20 % of women aged 18–50 [1, 2]. It is often multifactorial in etiology, necessitating a multimodal approach to treatment. Potential sources of chronic pelvic pain include not only the reproductive system, but also the gastrointestinal, urologic, and musculoskeletal systems. In addition, neurologic disease and psychological disorders may also cause or exacerbate chronic pelvic pain. Correct diagnosis and treatment of its underlying etiology(ies) requires a detailed history and thorough physical exam.

Although management of chronic pelvic pain often involves a combination of medical, physical, cognitive, and behavioral therapies, trigger point injections offer an additional option for treatment in a subset of patients. This office-based procedure has been used to improve pain associated with vaginismus, levator ani hypertonicity, vulvodynia, pudendal and ilioinguinal/iliohypogastric neuralgia. In this textbook chapter we review various injections used to treat pelvic pain, summarize the evidence for their use, and describe their role in treatment.

J.M. Miranne, M.D. (✉) • A.J. Park, M.D.
Section of Female Pelvic Medicine and Reconstructive Surgery, MedStar Washington Hospital Center/Georgetown University School of Medicine, Washington, DC 20010, USA
e-mail: Jeannine.M.Miranne@medstar.net; Amy.J.Park@medstar.net

Trigger Point Injections: A Historical Perspective

Trigger points refer to discrete areas of the body that are exquisitely tender to touch [3]. These hypersensitive areas are often nodular and usually represent taut bands of muscle [4, 5]. Trigger points that occur within skeletal muscle are also known as myofascial trigger points. If present within the levator ani or abdominal wall, trigger points can cause or exacerbate pelvic pain. Although the factors that contribute to their formation are unclear, one possible mechanism involves muscle strain with resultant nerve sensitization [3]. The presence of local ischemia may result in high concentrations of inflammatory mediators and neurotransmitters which stimulate local nociceptors resulting in pain [5]. Traditionally, trigger point injections involve infiltrating these tender areas with local anesthetic agents and/or steroids. Injection with local anesthetics often results in immediate pain relief [3, 4].

There are several theories which may explain why trigger point injections are effective in relieving pain [3–5]. Mechanical disruption of abnormal contractile elements may lead to resolution of muscle tautness [3, 4]. Fluid injection may dilute nerve-sensitized substances or may cause muscle fiber trauma and release of

J.D. Emery and M.F.R. Paraiso (eds.), *Office-Based Gynecologic Surgical Procedures*, DOI 10.1007/978-1-4939-1414-2_14, © Springer Science+Business Media New York 2015

intracellular potassium, resulting in a depolarizing nerve block [3–5]. Vasodilation induced by local anesthetics may increase uptake of excess metabolites [3, 5]. Other mechanisms that may explain efficacy include endorphin release [4] or release of additional inflammatory mediators which alter the local biochemical milieu, interrupting the positive feedback loops that perpetuate pain [5].

Although trigger point injections historically have involved the administration of local anesthetic agents such as lidocaine or bupivacaine, off-label use of botulinum toxin has come to play an increasingly important role in treatment over the past 10 years. Botulinum toxin is a potent neurotoxin produced by the anaerobic gram-positive bacterium *Clostridium botulinum*. When injected for therapeutic purposes, botulinum toxin binds to peripheral nerve endings and prevents acetylcholine release into the synaptic cleft at the neuromuscular junction, resulting in muscle paralysis [6]. There are seven distinct subtypes of botulinum toxin. Subtypes A and B are the only ones that are commercially available.

Botulinum toxin decreases muscle resting tone and contraction strength which presumably improves pain. In addition, animal studies [7, 8] suggest that it may also inhibit release of pain mediators and potentially decrease inflammation. This analgesic benefit is independent from the paralytic effect botulinum toxin has on muscles. Although botulinum toxin has been used for trigger point injections, it also offers an option for treatment in women with generalized levator ani spasm, vaginismus, and vulvodynia. Use of botulinum toxin to treat these conditions will be discussed later in this chapter.

Technique of Trigger Point Injections

The risks, benefits, potential complications, and alternatives of trigger point injections must be discussed prior to administration. Patients should be counseled that they may not experience maximum improvement in pain after one injection and that increased pain at the injection site may occur although this is usually self-limited, resolving within 24 to 48 h post-procedure [6]. Informed consent should be obtained and documented.

No standardized technique for injection has been established. A variety of approaches using different local anesthetics and needle types have been reported in the literature. The most commonly used anesthetic agents include 1 or 2 % lidocaine, 0.5 % bupivacaine, and 0.5 % ropivacaine [5] (Table 14.1). Epinephrine-containing anesthetics are generally avoided given vasoconstriction may induce local ischemia which potentially promotes trigger point formation [9]. While some authors [3] advocate use of a larger gauge needle to help penetrate and mechanically disrupt trigger points, others recommend a 25 or 27-gauge needle to decrease patient discomfort and the risk of bleeding. Needle length should be determined based on the planned depth of penetration. We generally use smaller gauge needles (22–25 gauge) if possible, although the pudendal nerve block kit is packaged with a 20-gauge needle. An Iowa trumpet may be used as a guide to facilitate injection (Fig. 14.1).

Trigger point injections should be performed using sterile technique. When injecting myofascial trigger points present in the levator ani, the patient should be placed in the dorsal lithotomy position, prepped, and draped. A vaginal exam is performed to confirm the location of the trigger points and the planned site(s) of injection. We tend to first perform a bilateral pudendal nerve block just medial to the ischial spines to achieve analgesia before administering trigger point injections throughout the levator ani. Injections can be performed transvaginally, transperineally, or subgluteally. In the latter approach, the needle is inserted inferior and medial to the ischial tuberosities and is guided towards a finger placed transvaginally or transrectally [5].

Table 14.1 Comparison of local anesthetic agents commonly used for trigger point injections

Agent	Onset of action (min)	Duration of effect (min)	Maximum total dose (mg)
Lidocaine	2–5	30–120	300
Bupivacaine	5–10	120–240	175
Ropivacaine	3–15	120–360	200

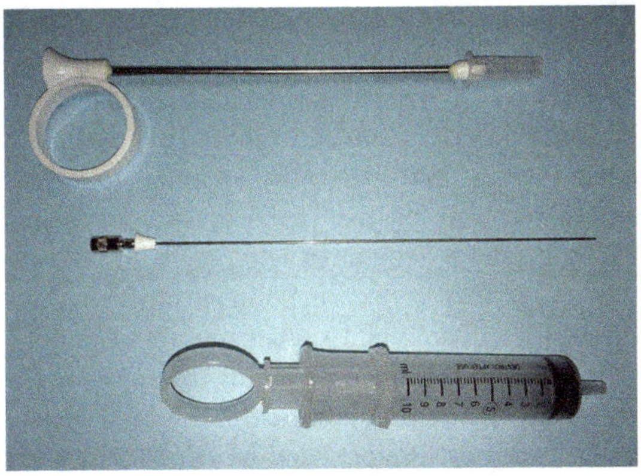

Fig. 14.1 Iowa trumpet needle guide, 20-gauge spinal needle with spacer, and 10 cc syringe

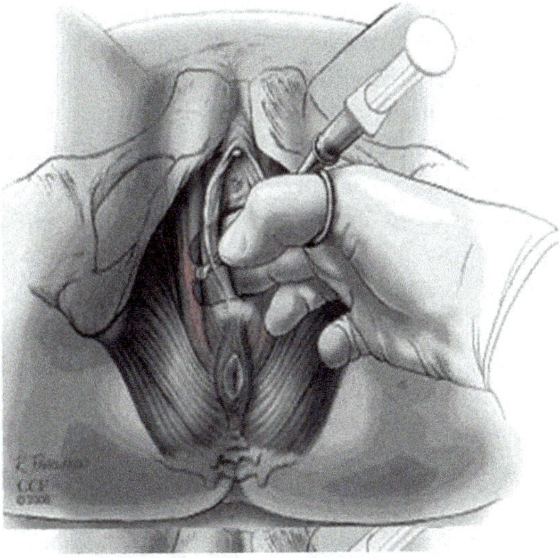

Fig. 14.2 Trigger point injection using a transvaginal approach. From Langford CF, Udvari NS, Ghoniem GM. Levator ani trigger point injections: an underutilized treatment for chronic pelvic pain. Neurourol Urodyn 2007;26(1):59-62

Transperineal injections can be performed for trigger points located in the perineal muscles or puborectalis, while the transvaginal approach offers access to trigger points located in the obturator internus muscles. The authors prefer either a transperineal or transvaginal approach (Fig. 14.2) given the proximity of the injection site to the trigger point and the relative ease of injection.

After identifying the location of the trigger points, the needle is inserted which may elicit a local twitch response [4, 5]. The syringe should be aspirated to avoid intravascular injection. Local anesthetic is then injected into the trigger point. We use 1 % lidocaine initially, and if a therapeutic effect is achieved, we then inject 9 cc of 0.5 % bupivacaine mixed with 1 cc of 40 mg of triamcinolone for longer lasting pain relief at a subsequent visit. Injections may be accomplished while slowly withdrawing the needle [4]. The needle may also need to be redirected to adequately infiltrate the entire trigger point. The number of injections performed depends on how many trigger points are identified on exam. Although we administer a steroid agent in addition to a local anesthetic, some authors [5] caution against use of steroid agents for myofascial trigger point injections because of the theoretical concern of muscle wasting with repeated use.

Botulinum neurotoxin has also been used for the treatment of trigger points. It is administered using the same technique of injection employed for injection of local anesthetic and steroid agents. The typical dose of botulinum toxin varies in the literature and most of the evidence supporting its efficacy is derived from treatment of conditions involving generalized levator ani spasm [6, 10–15]. Doses between 20 and 400 units diluted in sterile normal saline have been used [15]. The clinical effects of toxin injection may not become apparent until 24 to 72 h post-procedure [11] and have been reported to last between 2 and 6 months [10, 11]. Because botulinum toxin is a heat-labile protein, it may be prudent to instruct patients to avoid hot baths, Jacuzzis, steam rooms, and saunas for the first 2 weeks following injection [5].

Complications of Trigger Point Injections

Prior to the procedure clinicians must confirm the patient does not have an allergy to the agent that will be injected. They must also be aware of the possible risks of injection including infection, hematoma formation, and the potential for syncopal or presyncopal episodes. Toxicity from local anesthetic use can occur with intravascular

Table 14.2 Potential complications of trigger point injections

Potential complications	
Local anesthetics	Botulinum toxin
• Allergic reaction	• Allergic reaction
• Infection	• Infection
• Hematoma	• Hematoma
• Syncopal episode	• Syncopal episode
• Intravascular injection	• Intravascular injection
• Systemic toxicity	• Paralysis of nearby muscles
– Metallic taste	• Bowel/bladder dysfunction
– Perioral numbness	
– Tinnitus	
– Slurred speech and blurred vision	
– Altered consciousness	
– Convulsions	
– Cardiac arrhythmias	
– Cardiac arrest	

injection or by exceeding the maximum recommended dosage. Potential cardiovascular effects that may occur include cardiac arrhythmias and cardiac arrest. Symptoms of central nervous system toxicity include metallic taste, perioral numbness, and tinnitus (Table 14.2).

Side effects of botulinum toxin injection include spread of paralysis beyond the injection site, potential bowel or bladder dysfunction, and flu-like symptoms. In the only randomized controlled trial of botulinum toxin injections for pelvic pain [13], there was no statistically significant difference in reported side effects between the botulinum toxin and placebo groups. However, two women in the botulinum toxin group did develop intermittent pelvic floor dysfunction that was self-limited [13]. Botulinum toxin should be used with caution in patients using other medications that affect neuromuscular transmission such as muscle relaxants and anticholinergic agents and in those with an underlying neuromuscular disorder [16].

Vaginismus and Pelvic Floor Muscle Spasm

Vaginismus is defined as recurrent or persistent involuntary contraction of the musculature surrounding the distal third of the vagina [17]. This condition usually interferes with sexual intercourse. In addition to pain, vaginismus can cause psychological distress and interpersonal difficulties, which is why it is classified as a sexual pain disorder [18]. Vaginismus can involve spasm of the perineal and/or levator ani muscles. Treatment of vaginismus and generalized levator spasm includes physical therapy, biofeedback, and use of muscle relaxants. There is also a growing body of evidence which suggests that botulinum toxin injections may offer another viable option for treatment (Table 14.3).

The off-label use of botulinum toxin to treat levator spasm was first reported in 2004. Jarvis and colleagues [10] treated 12 women with a long-standing history of chronic pelvic pain and objective evidence of pelvic floor muscle hypertonicity with botulinum toxin type A (BOTOX, Allergan) injections. A total of 40 units were injected into 4 sites in the puborectalis and pubococcygeous under conscious sedation. At 3 months follow-up women experienced significant improvement in dyspareunia and dysmenorrhea. Pelvic floor resting pressures were also significantly reduced after injection. Although the maximum reduction in pressure was observed at 1 month post-injection, the mean resting pressure remained 25 % lower than baseline at 3 months post-injection.

Other authors [11–13] have also successfully managed pelvic floor muscle spasm using botulinum toxin. Romito and colleagues [11] treated two women with vestibulodynia and associated generalized levator spasm with botulinum toxin injections. Doses ranging between 40 and 80 units were injected into two sites in the levator ani under electromyography (EMG) guidance. Symptoms resolved in both cases. Patients remained symptom-free 3 months after injection with benefits persisting up to 6 months. In another study [12], botulinum toxin was administered to 39 patients with vaginismus resulting from vestibulodynia. A lower dose of 20 units was injected into the levator ani again under EMG guidance. Thirty-three patients completed follow-up. Although the majority needed repeat injections, almost two-thirds experienced resolution of their symptoms by the end

Table 14.3 Summary of the evidence for botulinum toxin use in gynecology

Authors	Study design	# of participants	Indication for use	Dose & type of botulinum toxin	Injection sites	Results
Jarvis et al. [10]	Prospective cohort	12	Chronic pelvic pain, Pelvic floor spasm	10 units botulinum toxin A injected at 4 sites; 40 units total	Puborectalis and pubococcygeous	Reduction in dyspareunia, dysmenorrhea, and pelvic floor pressures at 3 months
Romito et al. [11]	Case series	2	Vestibulodynia, Pelvic floor spasm	40–80 units, botulinum toxin A	Levator ani under EMG guidance	Symptom resolution at 3 months; benefits persisting up to 6 months
Bertolasi et al. [12]	Prospective cohort	39	Vestibulodynia, Vaginismus	20 units, botulinum toxin A	Levator ani under EMG guidance	Majority of patients needed repeat injections; symptom resolution in 63 % by 3 years after first injection
Ghazizadeh and Nikzad [23]	Prospective cohort	23	Vaginismus	150–400 units botulinum toxin A	Puborectalis, 3 injections on each side, total of 6 injections	Resolution of vaginismus on exam at 1 week post-injection in 96 % of patients. No recurrence at 12 months follow-up.
Abbott et al. [13]	RCT[a]	60	Chronic pelvic pain, Pelvic floor muscle spasm	20 units botulinum toxin A injected at 4 sites; 80 units total	Puborectalis and pubococcygeous	Reduction in dyspareunia pain scores from baseline for both botulinum toxin and placebo groups. Reduction in nonmenstrual pelvic pain for botulinum toxin group only.
Dykstra and Presthus [19]	Prospective cohort	12	Vestibulodynia	35 or 50 units of botulinum toxin A	Vestibule	Significant decrease in mean pain scores; duration of effect longer with higher dose
Yoon et al. [20]	Prospective cohort	7	Refractory chronic pelvic pain, Vulvodynia	20 units botulinum toxin A	Various sites in vestibule, levator ani, and perineal body	Significant improvement in pain scores. 5/7 patients required repeat injection. No recurrence at mean follow-up of ~1 year.
Petersen et al. [21]	RCT[a]	64	Vestibulodynia	20 units botulinum toxin A	Bulbospongiosis	Significant reduction in pain scores from baseline for both the botulinum toxin and placebo groups at 6 months post-injection. No significant difference between groups.

[a]Randomized, double-blinded, placebo-controlled

of follow-up, more than 3 years after the initial injection.

One study [13] provides level I evidence for botulinum toxin use in the treatment of levator ani spasm. In this double-blinded, placebo-controlled trial, 60 women with chronic pelvic pain and levator hypertonicity were randomized to receive 80 units of botulinum toxin type A

(Botox, Allergan Westport, Ireland) or saline injections. Both the Botox and the placebo group experienced a significant reduction in pain scores for dyspareunia from baseline after injection, but there was no statistically significant difference between groups. In addition, women in the Botox group also experienced a significant improvement in nonmenstrual pelvic pain. Although the results of this study are promising, the significant improvement in the placebo group suggests that the actual injection rather than the use of botulinum toxin may play a greater role in pain relief.

Vulvodynia

Off-label use of botulinum toxin in the treatment of vulvodynia has also been reported in the literature, although data regarding its efficacy are mixed. In a pilot study [19], 12 patients with vestibulodynia received subepithelial botulinum toxin injections in the vestibule. Doses of 35 or 50 units were used. All patients experienced a significant decrease in mean pain scores although the duration of effect was longer for patients who received the higher dose. In another small study of 7 patients who failed multiple forms of therapy [20], 20 units of botulinum toxin were injected into various sites in the vestibule, levator ani, and perineal body. Injection sites were determined after eliciting pain with gentle tactile stimuli. Only 2 of the 7 women in this study had levator spasm on exam. All 7 patients experienced resolution or reduction in pain post-injection. Five of the 7 required repeat injection to achieve adequate pain control. At mean follow-up of almost 1 year, no patient experienced recurrent pain. Despite these results, a randomized, double-blinded, placebo-controlled trial of 64 women with vestibulodynia [21] demonstrated no difference in post-injection pain scores between women who received botulinum toxin and women who received placebo at 6 month follow-up. In this study 20 units were injected into the vestibule. Patients in both the botulinum toxin and placebo groups experienced significant improvement in pain, and there was no statistically significant difference between groups. Again these data support the notion that injections and not necessarily botulinum toxin may aid in pain relief.

Repeat Botulinum Toxin Injections

Little is known about the effects of repeat botulinum toxin injections for pelvic pain. Because botulinum toxin is a protein, repetitive use can lead to the development of neutralizing antibodies which may prevent a clinical response with subsequent treatments. Higher doses and re-injection intervals less than 3 months may increase the risk of antibody formation [22]. Although doses up to 400 units have been effective in providing pain relief with little side effects [23], it seems prudent to use a lower dose based on these data. Additionally, animal studies have demonstrated muscle fiber wasting and reduced contractility following repeat botulinum toxin injections [24]. Nesbitt-Hawes and colleagues [25] demonstrated similar reductions in nonmenstrual pelvic pain, dyspareunia, and levator hypertonicity among women receiving single versus repeat botulinum toxin injections at 6 months post-procedure. However, these authors also found that women in the repeat injection group had lower maximum levator ani contraction pressures which persisted for the duration of the study. This finding underscores the need for larger studies with longer follow-up to determine long-term safety with repeated botulinum toxin use for pelvic pain relief.

Pudendal Nerve Injections

Pudendal neuralgia is another cause of chronic pelvic pain which can be treated with the use of injections. It commonly presents as pain in the vulva or perineum which is aggravated by sitting and relieved by standing or lying down. Nerve injections for this condition are usually both diagnostic and therapeutic.

The pudendal nerve is derived from the second, third, and fourth sacral nerve roots. It exits and then re-enters the pelvis through the greater and lesser sciatic foramina, passing between the sacrospinous and sacrotuberous ligaments at the level of the ischial spine. The nerve then courses anteriorly along the lateral wall of the ischiorectal fossa through Alcock's canal. After exiting Alcock's canal, it divides into three terminal branches: the dorsal nerve of the clitoris, the perineal nerve, and the inferior rectal nerve. Pudendal neuralgia may present as pain in the distribution of one or all of these terminal branches.

Potential etiologies of pudendal neuralgia include nerve compression and inflammation, with the former being more likely given the anatomic course of the nerve. The pudendal nerve is prone to compression and possible entrapment at the level of the ischial spine as it passes between the sacrospinous and sacrotuberous ligaments and again as it traverses Alcock's canal.

Pudendal nerve injections can be performed in the office using a traditional vaginal approach. After obtaining informed consent, the patient is placed in the dorsal lithotomy position and prepped and draped in the normal sterile fashion. Typically, a combination of a local anesthetic and steroid agent is used for injection. Although different preparations have been reported in the literature, we use 9 cc of 1 % lidocaine and 1 cc of 40 mg of triamcinolone for initial diagnosis. If a therapeutic effect is observed, bupivacaine is used instead of lidocaine.

To perform an injection on the patient's right side, the operator's right index and middle fingers are used to palpate the ischial spine on this side. Using the left hand, a 20-gauge spinal needle, Iowa trumpet needle guide, and syringe are introduced. The tip of the needle guide is advanced 1 cm medial and posterior to the ischial spine. When the needle guide is properly positioned, the needle tip is pushed past the guide through the vaginal epithelium and sacrospinous ligament. Aspiration is performed to ensure absence of intravascular location and the anesthetic–steroid combination is placed. This procedure is usually repeated on the contralateral side. Most patients experience immediate pain relief after injection.

A posterior approach can also be used to perform pudendal nerve injections in the office. In this approach patients are placed in the prone position and the needle is inserted medial to the sacrotuberous ligament at the level of the midanus. It is advanced into the ischiorectal fossa toward the ipsilateral ischial spine often using EMG. With this approach it is important to monitor for muscle contractions in the ipsilateral leg to avoid injection in the region of the sciatic nerve [26].

Pudendal nerve injections have also been performed under computed tomography or ultrasound guidance [27–29]. Proponents of image-guided needle placement argue that it provides for more accurate delivery of medication. Image-guided pudendal nerve injections are usually performed in the prone position and have been found to be effective in alleviating pain in some studies [27, 28].

Ilioinguinal/Iliohypogastric Nerve Injections

Neuralgias involving the ilioinguinal and iliohypogastric nerves can result in lower abdominal and/or groin pain. These nerves are at risk of injury during gynecologic surgery. Pfannenstiel and lower quadrant laparoscopic trocar incisions can result in potential nerve transection or entrapment. Pain is typically sharp or burning in quality and may be associated with parethesias. Like in the case of pudendal neuralgia, nerve injections may aid in both diagnosis and treatment.

The ilioinguinal and iliohypogastric nerves arise from the anterior rami of L1 and emerge from the lateral border of the psoas. They run anterior to quadratus lumborum before entering the anterior abdominal wall. Both nerves pierce the internal oblique muscle near the anterior superior iliac spine. They continue to travel in parallel between the internal and external oblique muscles. The iliohypogastric nerve, located more cephalad, terminates in the midline about 3 cm above the superficial inguinal ring, while the ilioinguinal nerve enters the inguinal canal and emerges from the superficial inguinal ring.

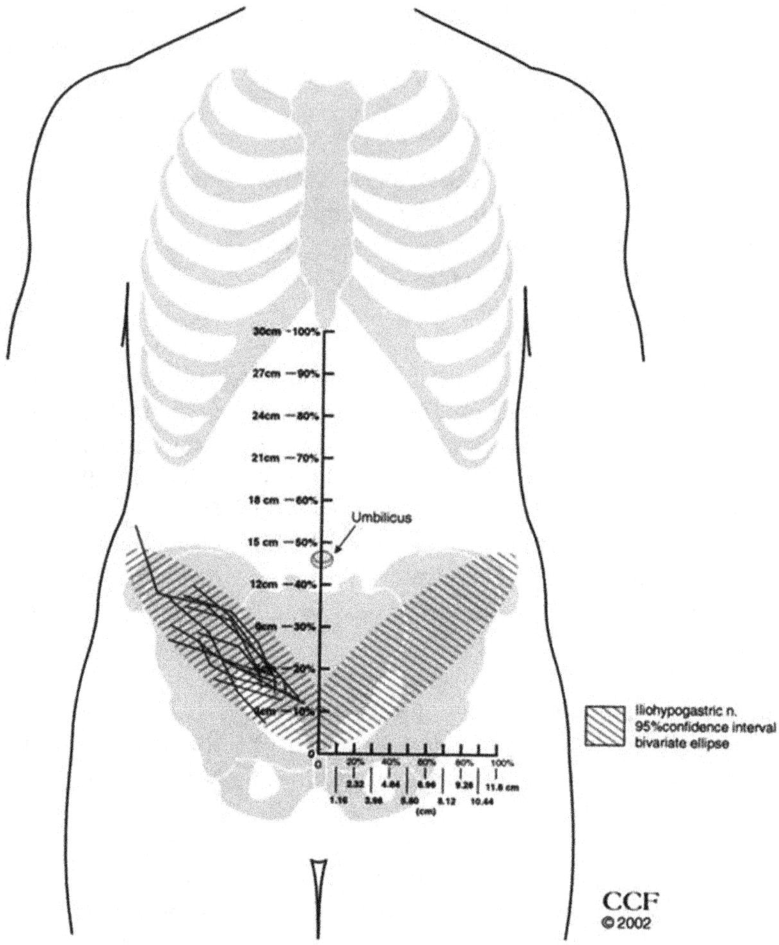

Fig. 14.3 Course of iliohypogastric nerve in 13 individuals. Solid lines represent the nerve while ellipses consisting of diagonal lines represent 95 % confidence intervals. The distances from the pubic symphysis to the xyphoid (*y*-axis) and from the pubic symphysis to the anterior superior iliac spine (*x*-axis) are displayed in centimeters and percent distance scales. *From Whiteside JL, Barber MD, Walters MD, Falcone T. Anatomy of ilioinguinal and iliohypogastric nerves in relation to trocar placement and low transverse incisions. Am J Obstet Gynecol 2003;189:1574–1578*

Cadaver dissections have shown that the iliohypogastric nerve enters the abdominal wall 2.1 cm medial and 0.9 cm inferior to the anterior superior iliac spine and terminates 3.7 cm lateral to the midline and 5.2 cm superior to the pubic symphysis (Fig. 14.3) [30]. Similarly, the ilioinguinal nerve was found to enter the abdominal wall 3.1 cm medial and 3.7 cm inferior to the anterior superior iliac spine, terminating 2.7 cm lateral to the midline and 1.7 cm superior to the pubic symphysis (Fig. 14.4).

The anterior superior iliac spine serves as an important anatomical landmark during ilioinguinal and iliohypogastric nerve injections. Techniques for injection have not been standardized [29] and there is a paucity of data in the gynecologic literature regarding this modality of treatment. One approach [31] involves inserting a blunt tip needle 2 cm medial and superior to the anterior superior iliac spine. Although use of this needle may provide for easier identification of the fascia and avoid injury to peripheral nerve endings [31, 32], a 20 or 22-gauge spinal needle can also be used. The needle is advanced until the fascia of the external oblique muscle is penetrated, which can be felt when there is a slight resistance to the needle. The area between the external and internal oblique muscles is then infiltrated. After this area is injected, the needle is further advanced, piercing the fascia of the internal oblique. A second injection is performed between the internal oblique and transverse abdominus muscles. The needle is then withdrawn to the dermis and redirected. Additional injections are administered between the oblique muscles and internal oblique and transverse abdominus muscles 15° medial and

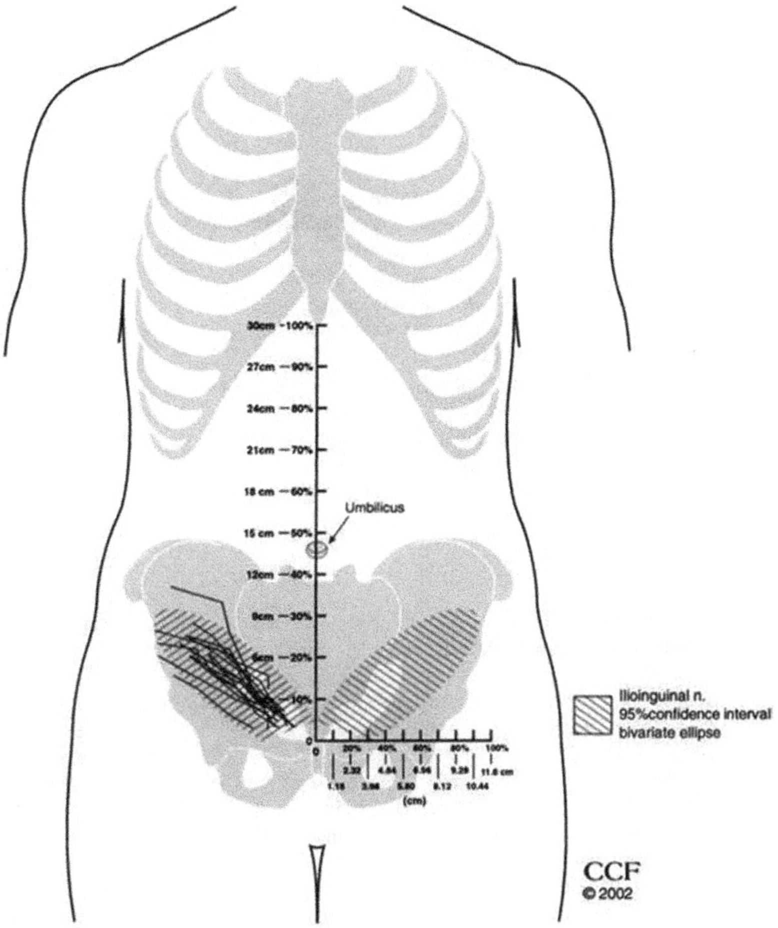

Fig. 14.4 Course of ilioinguinal nerve in 16 individuals. Solid lines represent the nerve while ellipses consisting of diagonal lines represent 95 % confidence intervals. The distances from the pubic symphysis to the xyphoid (y-axis) and from the pubic symphysis to the anterior superior iliac spine (x-axis) are displayed in centimeters and percent distance scales. *From Whiteside JL, Barber MD, Walters MD, Falcone T. Anatomy of ilioinguinal and iliohypogastric nerves in relation to trocar placement and low transverse incisions. Am J Obstet Gynecol 2003;189:1574-1578*

15° lateral to the original insertion point. Other techniques for injection involve inserting the needle 2–3 cm medial and inferior to the anterior superior iliac spine and infiltrating as the needle is withdrawn, repeating injections at steeper angles to penetrate all three muscle layers of the abdominal wall, and injecting towards the pubic symphysis in a fanlike fashion [29]. Although both local anesthetic agents and steroids have anecdotally been used for injection, most of the current literature describes the use of anesthetic agents to perform nerve blocks.

Summary

Chronic pelvic pain is a prevalent problem affecting up to 20 % of women ages 18 to 50. Successful management requires correct diagnosis and treatment of its underlying etiologies. Although the approach to treatment is often multimodal, injections may offer an option in certain conditions including levator ani trigger points, vaginismus, vulvodynia, and neuralgia of the pudendal, ilioinguinal or iliohypogastric nerves. Current evidence supporting the use of injections to treat these conditions remains limited. Future studies are needed to more clearly define the role of this office-based procedure in the treatment of pelvic pain.

References

1. Mathias SD, Kuppermann M, Liberman RF, Lipschutz RC, Steege JF. Chronic pelvic pain: prevalence, health-related quality of life, and economic correlates. Obstet Gynecol. 1996;87:321–7.

2. Jamieson DJ, Steege JF. The prevalence of dysmenorrhea, dyspareunia, pelvic pain, and irritable bowel syndrome in primary care practices. Obstet Gynecol. 1996;87:55–8.
3. Ling FW, Slocumb JC. Use of trigger point injections in chronic pelvic pain. Obstet Gynecol Clin North Am. 1993;20(4):809–15.
4. Langford CF, Udvari NS, Ghoniem GM. Levator ani trigger point injections: an underutilized treatment for chronic pelvic pain. Neurourol Urodyn. 2007;26 (1):59–62.
5. Moldwin RM, Fariello JY. Myofascial trigger points of the pelvic floor: associations with urological pain syndromes and treatment strategies including injection therapy. Curr Urol Rep. 2013;14(5):409–17. doi:10.1007/s11934-013-0360-7.
6. Abbott JA. The use of botulinum toxin in the pelvic floor for women with chronic pelvic pain—a new answer to old problems? J Minim Invasive Gynecol. 2009;16(2):130–5.
7. Jabbari B. Botulinum neurotoxins in the treatment of refractory pain. Nat Clin Pract Neurol. 2008;4 (12):676–85.
8. Cui K, Khanijou S, Rubino J, Aoki KR. Subcutaneous administration of botulinum toxin A reduces formalin-induced pain. Pain. 2004;107:125–33.
9. Criscuolo CM. Interventional approaches to the management of myofascial pain syndrome. Curr Pain Headache Rep. 2001;5:407–11.
10. Jarvis SK, Abbott JA, Lenart MB, Steensma A, Vancaille TG. Pilot study of botulinum toxin type A in the treatment of chronic pelvic pain associated with spasm of the levator ani muscles. Aust N Z J Obstet Gynaecol. 2004;44:46–50.
11. Romito S, Bottanelli M, Pellegrini M, Vicentini S, Rizzuto N, Bertolasi L. Botulinum toxin for the treatment of genital pain syndromes. Gynecol Obstet Invest. 2004;58:164–7.
12. Bertolasi L, Frasson E, Cappelletti JY, Vicentini S, Bordignon M, Graziottin A. Botulinum neurotoxin type a injections for vaginismus secondary to vulvar vestibulitis syndrome. Obstet Gynecol. 2009;114 (5):1008–16.
13. Abbott JA, Jarvis SK, Lyons SD, Thomson A, Vancaille TG. Botulinum toxin type A for chronic pain and pelvic floor spasm in women. Obstet Gynecol. 2006;108(4):915–22.
14. Park AJ, Paraiso MFR. Successful use of botulinum toxin type A in the treatment of refractory postoperative dyspareunia. Obstet Gynecol. 2009;114:484–7.
15. Abbott J. Gynecological indications for the use of botulinum toxin in women with chronic pelvic pain. Toxicon. 2009;54:647–53.
16. Allergan, Inc 2013. Highlights of prescribing information. Accessed from: http://www.allergan.com/assets/pdf/botox_pi.pdf
17. The American College of Obstetricians and Gynecologists. Practice bulletin #119: Female sexual dysfunction. 2011. http://www.acog.org/ Resources-And-Publications/Practice-Bulletins/Committee-on-Practice-Bulletins-Gynecology/Female-Sexual-Dysfunction
18. American Psychiatric Association. Diagnostic and statistical manual of mental disorders. 4th ed (Text rev). Washington, DC: APA; 2000.
19. Dykstra DD, Presthus J. Botulinum toxin type A for the treatment of provoked vestibulodynia: an open-label, pilot study. J Reprod Med. 2006;51 (6):467–70.
20. Yoon H, Chung WS, Shim BS. Botulinum toxin A for the management of vulvodynia. Int J Impot Res. 2007;19:84–7.
21. Petersen CD, Giraldi A, Lundvall L, Kristensen E. Botulinum toxin type A—a novel treatment for provoked vestibulodynia? Results from a randomized, placebo controlled, double-blinded study. J Sex Med. 2009;6(9):2523–37.
22. Lange O, Bigalke H, Dengler R, Wegner F, deGroot M, Wohlfarth K. Neutralizing antibodies and secondary therapy failure after treatment with botulinum toxin type A: much ado about nothing? Clin Neuropharmacol. 2009;32:213–8.
23. Ghazizadeh S, Nikzad M. Botulinum toxin in the treatment of refractory vaginismus. Obstet Gynecol. 2004;104:922–5.
24. Fortuna R, Vaz MA, Youssef AR, Longino D, Herzog W. Changes in contractile properties of muscles receiving repeat injections of botulinum toxin. J Biomech. 2011;44:39–44.
25. Nesbitt-Haws EM, Won H, Jarvis SK, Lyons SD, Vancaillie TG, Abbott JA. Improvement in pelvic pain with botulinum toxin type A—single vs. repeat injections. Toxicon. 2013;63:83–7.
26. Benson JT, Griffis K. Pudendal neuralgia, a severe pain syndrome. Am J Obstet Gynecol. 2005;192:1663–8.
27. McDonald JS, Spigos DG. Computed tomography-guided pudendal block for treatment of pelvic pain due to pudendal neuropathy. Obstet Gynecol. 2000;95:306–9.
28. Hough DM, Wittenberg KH, Pawline W, Mause TP, King BF, Vrtiska TJ, Farrell MA, Antolak SJ. Chronic perineal pain caused by pudendal nerve entrapment: anatomy and CT-guided perineural injection technique. AJR Am J Roentgenol. 2003;181 (2):561–7.
29. Peng PW, Tumber PS. Ultrasound-guided interventional procedures for patients with chronic pelvic pain—a description of techniques and review of the literature. Pain Physician. 2008;11(2):214–24.
30. Whiteside JL, Barber MD, Walters MD, Falcone T. Anatomy of ilioinguinal and iliohypogastric nerves in relation to trocar placement and low transverse incisions. Am J Obstet Gynecol. 2003;189:1574–8.
31. Bell EA, Jones BP, Olufolabi AJ, Dexter F, Phillips-Bute B, Greengass RA, Penning DH, Reynolds JD. Iliohypogastric-ilioinguinal peripheral nerve block for

post-cesarean delivery analgesia decreases morphine use but not opioid-related side effects. Can J Anaesth. 2002;49(7):694–700.
32. Wehbe SA, Ghulmiyyah LM, Dominique EH, Hosford SL, Ehleben CM, Saltzman SL, Sills ES. Prospective randomized trial of iliohypogastric-ilioinguinal nerve block on post-operative morphine use after inpatient surgery of the female reproductive tract. J Negat Results Biomed. 2008;7:11. doi:10.1186/1477-5751-7-11.

15 Colposcopy

Robert J. Kim

Introduction

Epidemiology

Cervical cancer is the third most common cancer afflicting women worldwide but remains the most common in Eastern Africa, South-Central Asia, and Melanesia. In 2008, there were approximately 530,000 cases worldwide with 85 % occurring within developing countries [1]. In 2010, there were 11,818 cases diagnosed in the USA with 3,939 deaths [2]. While there are multiple factors responsible for reducing the number of cases in the developed world, implementation of screening programs utilizing cervical cytology is most credited. Since the introduction of the Pap smear in the 1940s, cervical cancer deaths have dramatically decreased from 40 per 100,000 women in 1930 to 3 per 100,000 in 1998 [3]. It is estimated that over 80 % of cervical cancers can be prevented with routine screening.

While screening programs have been successful in reducing cervical cancer deaths, we are entering an era of "less is more" in terms of medical costs, resource utilization, and effective triage. There has been renewed focus on the harms of screening and intervention in multiple areas of medicine. With recognition of the role of human papilloma virus (HPV) infection in lower genital tract cancers, there is increased reliance on HPV testing by polymerase chain reaction. The most recent recommendations from the 2012 American Society of Colposcopy and Cervical Pathology (ASCCP) Consensus Guidelines Conference incorporates more HPV testing while decreasing testing intervals in the majority of women. Previous management of many abnormalities included repeat cytology at 6 and 12 months, which have now been replaced with co-testing in 1 year [4].

Prior to the advent of cervical cytology, early medical pioneers developed colposcopy as a screening instrument for cervical cancer. Although screening was eventually replaced by cervical cytology, colposcopy evolved into a diagnostic procedure. Prior to colposcopy, patients with abnormal cytology were subjected to cervical conization for both diagnosis and treatment. Besides being a more invasive and costly tool for diagnosis, conization has been curtailed after the recognition of its negative impact on fertility outcomes including preterm labor and delivery and cervical stenosis [5]. Today, providers perform over two million colposcopies for low grade cytologic abnormalities (e.g., atypical squamous cells of uncertain significance (ASC-US), low grade squamous intraepithelial lesion (LSIL)) in the USA. In 2000, there was an estimated $900 million spent on colposcopy in the USA [6].

R.J. Kim, M.D. (✉)
Department of Obstetrics and Gynecology, John A. Burns School of Medicine, University of Hawaii, 1319 Punahou Street, 8th floor, Honolulu, HI 96826, USA
e-mail: robertjk@hawaii.edu

J.D. Emery and M.F.R. Paraiso (eds.), *Office-Based Gynecologic Surgical Procedures*,
DOI 10.1007/978-1-4939-1414-2_15, © Springer Science+Business Media New York 2015

In an effort to standardize terminology across all lower genital tract disorders affected by HPV, the College of American Pathologists and ASCCP convened to form the Lower Anogenital Squamous Terminology Standardization Project ("LAST"). In 2012, the panel recommended a two-tier grading system so that low grade lesions (e.g., CIN-1, VAIN-1, VIN-1) would be termed LSIL. High grade lesions (e.g., CIN-2-3, VAIN-2-3, VIN-2-3) would be termed HSIL [7]. For the purposes of this chapter, we will continue to use the common conventions of CIN, VAIN, and VIN.

Anatomy

Colposcopy is a technique of visual pattern recognition, which requires practice and exposure to myriad variations in appearance. The enlarged nuclei and cell crowding of dysplastic cells often produce visible changes in epithelial opacity and vascular patterns.

During fetal development, paired Mullerian (paramesonephric) ducts fuse to form the fallopian tubes, uterus, cervix, and upper two-thirds of the vagina. Simple columnar-type cells line the upper tract. This epithelium is one cell layer thick and envelops the stromal core of a single capillary loop. The layer is villous and folded. Non-glycogenated, stratified squamous epithelium lines the lower tract fused to the urogenital sinus. The epithelium is 20–30 cells thick, opaque, and appears flat and smooth. A small rim of columnar epithelium surrounds the external cervical os. As females mature, the vaginal pH decreases from a neutral/basic state to an acidic environment approximating pH 3.0. Consequently, the tips of the columnar epithelial villae undergo rapid cell turnover and "transform" by squamous metaplasia. The valleys between the fronds fill in, and central capillary cores are buried into the subepithelium. In the adult woman, this area termed the transformation zone (TZ) surrounds the external os and extends outward by 2–6 mm or greater [8]. In areas where metaplasia occurs quickly, surface villae coalesce, entrapping mucus-producing columnar cells within crypts creating the classic Nabothian cyst.

Screening

Approximately 10 % of Pap smears will exhibit some degree of abnormality. The Bethesda System for reporting the degree of cervical and vaginal severity was established in 1988, revised in 1991 and 2001 [9]. The link between HPV and cervical cancer was established as early as 1976 [10], and this has led to recent adoption of HPV testing (reflex and co-testing) and vaccine immunization. Since 2001, the ASCCP has convened experts within the field representing the major medical organizations to form guidelines for the standardized management of women with cervical cytologic abnormalities and cervical cancer precursors [11]. The most recent update to the guidelines published in 2012 incorporates increased knowledge of HPV infection and genotyping and clinical experience involving over 1.4 million women [4].

Within these new guidelines are multiple algorithms illustrating recommended triage and management of abnormal cytology. For the same abnormal cytology, management may differ based on patient age, HPV status and type, pregnancy, and previous cytologic history. A smartphone and computer tablet application ("app") is available to aid clinicians navigate these complex algorithms (Fig. 15.1). Colposcopy remains integral to many of these algorithms as hysterectomy is not indicated for cervical dysplasia except in special cases.

Screening Program Success

The health profession's success on limiting cervical cancer deaths is based on a confluence of favorable factors. For one, HPV infection causes the vast majority of cervical cancer cases. This has singled out a clear target for prevention and treatment efforts (i.e., HPV testing, immunization) that is lacking in other gynecologic cancers such as ovarian cancer. Secondly, cervical cancer tends to develop gradually through a series of precursor lesions that are identifiable visually and histologically. Lastly, cervical cancer usually invades adjacent structures with

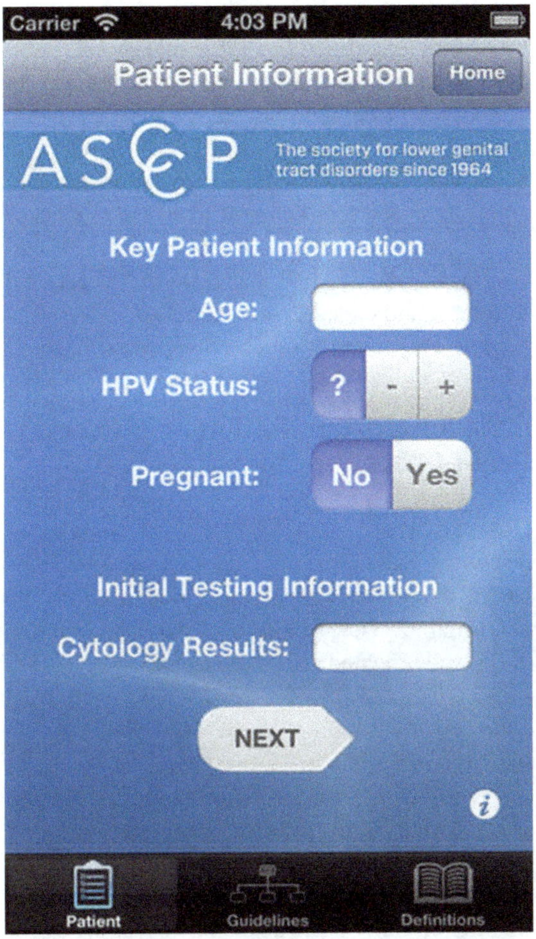

Fig. 15.1 ASCCP application for smartphone and tablets

loco-regional metastases (i.e., pelvic lymph nodes) before metastasizing to distant organs.

Since the link between HPV infection and cervical cancer was made, much of the focus towards preventing cervical cancer is predicated upon the natural history of HPV. Latency, which refers to the onset of HPV infection to the appearance of cervical cancer, often spans 5–10 years. This provides time for providers to detect HPV infection and HPV-related changes. HPV is not a complete carcinogen as very few of the millions of women infected with HPV every year will develop cervical dysplasia. For women who develop low grade dysplasia or cervical intraepithelial neoplasia 1 (CIN-1), approximately 60 % will spontaneously regress, 10–15 % will progress to a higher grade (CIN-2-3), and only 0.3 % will develop cancer if untreated [12]. Even for women with CIN-3, approximately 30 % will spontaneously regress [13].

Prior to the appearance of cancer, there is a natural progression of precursor lesions CIN-1-3 that are detectable in cervical cytology and visually recognizable by colposcopy. This has enabled colposcopy to evolve from a screening tool into a diagnostic one for the entire lower genital tract including the cervix, vagina, vulva, and anus. Pap smears are not intended to diagnose cervical cancer. In fact, the sensitivity of Pap smears for CIN-2-3 may be as low as 55 % and may miss CIN-3 or cancer up to one-third of the time [14]. Likewise, the main benefit of colposcopy is to identify dysplastic cells amenable to treatment before they progress to cancer.

Colposcopy uses illumination and magnification to direct biopsies and treatment through identification of the TZ and abnormal-appearing lesions. Perhaps its greatest contribution is the ability to identify cells responsible for abnormal cytology without resorting to cervical conization. Unfortunately, colposcopy requires access to expensive equipment, trained practitioners, and access to pathology not available in many underdeveloped countries. In these regions, providers have investigated alternative methods using broad-band light sources (e.g., visual inspection with acetic acid) or see-and-treat algorithms.

Brief History of Procedure

Modern comprehensive cervical cancer screening stems from three separate but intertwined paths—the discovery of cervical cytology, colposcopy, and HPV. In 1927, Aurel Babes, a Romanian physician, presented his findings of cervical cancer smears to the Romanian Society of Gynecology. Concurrently Georgios Papanicolaou, a Greek pathologist working at Cornell Medical College, presented his observations using vaginal pool cytology to detect cervical cancer precursors at the Third Race Betterment Conference in Battle Creek, MI in 1928 [15]. Both presentations were met with harsh criticism, but Papanicolaou persevered and teamed up with a gynecologist Herbert Traut to present his findings in 1941 [16]. In 1949, a visiting Canadian scholar, James Ernst Ayre, worked with Papanicolaou and developed the wooden spatula now used today in various forms to directly sample the cervix.

In 1925, Hans Peter Hinselmann, a German gynecologist, worked in the women's ward of a hospital in Altona, a district in the northern city Hamburg. He mounted a fixed binocular instrument on a tripod and created an intense light source reflected by a mirror to study the cervix. He used a variety of solutions including cedar wood oil and 5 % silver nitrate. When he applied 3 % acetic acid, he noted tiny, dot-like tumors and leukoplakia [17]. He expanded his findings to include punctation, ground leukoplakia, and mosaic patterns in 1936. He was imprisoned infamously for war crimes related to the forced sterilization of Gypsy women [15]. Walter Schiller, an Austrian pathologist, introduced the use of iodine to aid visualization of abnormal squamous cells that had lost their glycogen content in 1928.

Many US physicians did not accept colposcopy with its cumbersome equipment and variable impressions. In the USA during the early 1960s, enthusiasm gained momentum among gynecologists and pathologists including Walter Lang and Ralph Richart. The ASCCP was formed in 1964. Adolf Stafl, an early pioneer who fled to the USA from Czechoslovakia, joined Johns Hopkins University. He teamed up with a private practitioner, Joseph Scott, and began importing colposcopes and offering instructional courses [18]. By the 1980s, colposcopy became firmly planted as the gold standard to exclude cervical dysplasia and cancer in women with abnormal cytology. It is now an integral part in the management algorithms for the 2012 Updated Consensus Guidelines.

As early as 1842, epidemiological studies revealed that virginal women did not develop cervical cancer [19]. In the 1960s to early 1970s, much interest focused on the viral theory of cancer with host DNA integration and oncogene expression. Herpes simplex virus 2 (HSV-2) was implicated as the sexually transmitted cause but later concluded to be a confounder of increased sexual activity [20]. In 1976, Meisels and Fortin described the appearance of koilocytes in cervical smears of mild dysplasia indicating the presence of HPV [10]. German pathologist Harold zur Hausen isolated HPV-16 as the first cervical cancer-linked HPV subtype [21]. Since then, there have been 14–15 "high-risk" subtypes of HPV associated with cervical dysplasia and cancer.

Data-Supporting Rationale/Efficacy for In-Office Procedure

Indications

There are seven indications for colposcopy by abnormal cervical cytology established in the 2006 and updated 2012 Consensus Guidelines [4, 22]. Colposcopy is not restricted to abnormal cytology alone and may be used for common indications (Table 15.1).

Diethylstilbestrol (DES) was used from about 1940 to 1970 to prevent adverse pregnancy outcomes in women with previous history of miscarriage. In 1971, Herbst published a report linking in utero DES exposure to vaginal clear cell adenocarcinoma, which prompted the FDA to place a black box warning label later that year

Table 15.1 Indications for colposcopy

Cytology/HPV	Normal (persistent HPV+)
	ASC-US (persistent OR HPV+)
	ASC-H
	LSIL
	HSIL
	AGC
	Cancer
Visible lesions	Genital warts/condyloma
	Abnormal visual/palpable lesions of cervix, vagina, vulva
	Ulcers
	Lichen sclerosus, extra-mammary Paget's disease
Other	In utero DES exposure
	Posttreatment surveillance for CIN-2-3

Source: Adapted from Wright TC et al. [22]

[23]. Today, women with in utero DES exposure are approximately 40+ years or older.

While there are no absolute contraindications to performing colposcopy, it may be limited in the setting of active pelvic infections (i.e., cervico-vaginitis) such as the classic strawberry spots representing dilated capillary loops in Trichomoniasis or thick vaginal discharge of Candidiasis. Late term pregnancy may yield little treatment information in the absence of gross cervical cancer. Severe vulvo-vaginal atrophy may also yield poor diagnostic information.

Training

The main objective of colposcopy is to prevent cervical cancer by finding cancer precursors using directed biopsies. To accomplish this task, colposcopy requires several essential steps that include applying appropriate indications, maximizing visualization, forming an accurate impression, performing directed biopsies, and establishing appropriate follow-up.

While there is some question to its overall effectiveness and accuracy (see section "Effectiveness"), colposcopy performance is dependent upon provider experience. The continued decline in smoking rates in the USA and introduction of the HPV vaccine is anticipated to erode cervical cancer incidence. Most recently, screening intervals have been extended from traditional annual Pap smears to once every 3–5 years in most women. While this is sure to dwindle the number of colposcopies performed today, it places greater emphasis on establishing the correct diagnosis by colposcopy.

Colposcopy is an office-based procedure, so there are no credentialing requirements by hospitals, insurance companies, or malpractice carriers. The American College of Obstetrics and Gynecology (ACOG) suggests performing 30–50 colposcopies under supervision with an additional 80–100 exams to achieve proficiency [24]. The ASCCP estimates that a provider performs 25–100 colposcopies with a minimum of 10 high grade lesions to become competent. In a 30-question survey sent to 485 Ob/Gyn and Family Practice residency program directors, most programs did not meet the minimum number of procedures for its residents [25]. In a study at a university-based Ob/Gyn residency program, increasing level of training correlated with improvement in accurate impression. Overall accuracy was only 32 %, however, and nurse practitioners outperformed resident physicians [26].

As the number of colposcopy procedures diminishes, it is uncertain whether colposcopy will be practiced widely or become concentrated among providers with keen interest and expertise. For those motivated to perform colposcopy, one might consider obtaining additional teaching at postgraduate curricula offered through various organizations of the ASCCP, ACOG, and American Academy of Family Physicians.

Effectiveness

Colposcopy is considered the reference standard for which cervical cytology is measured. Likewise, histology measures the performance of colposcopy as a diagnostic tool. In 1988, a meta-analysis by Mitchell estimated colposcopy performance at a mean-weighted sensitivity of 96 % and specificity of 48 % comparing all abnormal findings to normal tissue. When comparing only high grade results to low grade abnormalities, sensitivity remained high at 85 % with specificity of 69 % [27].

More recently, it has become recognized that studies often overestimate colposcopy performance due to inherent biases of study design. The methods used to obtain tissue histology are variable (e.g., conization versus colposcopic-directed biopsies) and influence the rate of CIN diagnoses. In many studies, verification bias is introduced when only a select group of women at risk for high grade dysplasia undergo biopsy or treatment. Therefore, calculating the true values for sensitivity and specificity is difficult.

Among experienced colposcopists, there seems to be good interobserver agreement for normal epithelium, high grade dysplasia, and cancer. There is more variability for lesser grade lesions of CIN-1-2 [28]. This was confirmed during the ASC-US and LSIL Triage Study (ALTS) trial, when three experienced reviewers examined digitized images with poor-to-fair agreement on impression [29]. Even for high grade lesions, colposcopy may miss over half of CIN-3 initially [30].

A meta-analysis of 32 studies including 7,873 biopsies examined the diagnostic performance of colposcopic-directed biopsies to that of excisional cervical conization or hysterectomy. Limiting the analysis to four pooled studies with lower rates of positive biopsies provided a more accurate reflection of colposcopic performance to a sensitivity of 81.4 % and specificity of 63.3 % [31]. However, Stoler reviewed the findings of the FUTURE I, II, and III trials in 2011 revealing that LEEP conization diagnosed twice as many CIN-2-3 disease versus same day colposcopic-directed biopsies [32].

It is estimated that over half of missed high grade lesions are due to sampling error [33]. Intuitively, performing more biopsies as opposed to a single biopsy decreases the likelihood of missing a high grade lesion. In the ALTS trial, where only women with ASC-US or LSIL cytologic abnormalities were enrolled, there were 408 women with CIN-3 or cancer of which 69.9 % had a colposcopic-directed biopsy of CIN-2 or greater. Sensitivity increased for procedures with two or greater biopsies [34].

Whether it is better to take multiple biopsies from the most abnormal area, biopsy every abnormal finding, or consider "random" biopsies is uncertain [13]. Belinson and colleagues reported the results of their cross-sectional study Shanxi Province Cervical Cancer Screening Study (SPOCCS I) in 2001 (Table 15.2). Among 1,997 women enrolled, the cervix was divided into four quadrants. "Random" biopsies were performed at the squamo-columnar junction (SCJ) if there was no identifiable lesion, and ECC was performed. Among 86 women with CIN-2 or greater, 16 had normal findings in all four quadrants (12 CIN-2, 4 CIN-3) [35]. In their follow-up study SPOCCS II, they analyzed 364 patients with CIN-2 or greater and a satisfactory colposcopy. The diagnosis of CIN-2 or greater was made by colposcopic-directed biopsy in only 208 (57.1 %). The remaining cases were diagnosed by random biopsy in 136 (37.4 %) and ECC in 20 (5.5 %). The yield for random biopsy was greater at 17.6 % when cytology was high grade versus only 2.8 % when cytology was low grade [36].

The utility of ECC has been debated especially in women with low grade abnormalities. In the ALTS trial, the ECC was positive in only 1 % (10/1,119) of women with a negative colposcopy and biopsy. High grade abnormalities of CIN-2 or greater were found by ECC in 3.7 % of 1,119 exams versus 21.7 % by biopsy. Omitting ECC would risk missing 1.1 % (7/653) of women with CIN-2 or greater. In women <40 years old, only 2 % (7/312) were diagnosed with CIN-2 or greater with low grade biopsy versus 13 % (3/23) women >40 years old [37].

The disparity between colposcopic impression and histology may be attributed to the provider's experience in forming an accurate impression and/or performing an adequate biopsy. This does not fully explain the poor performance among experienced colposcopists. It is likely that there are some high grade lesions that do not present with classic findings. Jeronimo and colleagues proposed that different subtypes of HPV may present with different aceto-white

Table 15.2 Shanxi province cervical cancer screening study findings

		Diagnosis	Diagnosis by biopsy method		
Study	*N* (#women)	CIN-2 or worse	Colpo-directed	Random	ECC only
SPOCCS I	1,997	86	60 (69.8 %)	14 (16.3 %)	2 (2.3 %)
SPOCCS II	8,497	364	208 (57.1 %)	136 (37.4 %)	20 (5.5 %)
SPOCCS I&II	10,425[a]	222[b]	141 (63.5 %)	57 (25.7 %)	24 (10.8 %)

Note
[a]Additional 69 women excluded during SPOCCS I follow-up analysis
[b]Only CIN-3 or worse
Source: Adapted from Belinson JL et al. [35] and Pretorius RG et al. [36, 40]

epithelium (AWE). In the ALTS trial, HPV-16 was associated with AWE regardless of whether the lesion was low or high grade. AWE did not seem to be associated with more HPV types or increased number of lesions, suggesting that other subtypes of HPV were less likely to appear [38].

Among 144 cases of CIN-2-3 in the SPOCCS I study, 111 were diagnosed by colposcopic-directed biopsy with impression of CIN-1 or greater. The average epithelial thickness was 321 μm. Among the remaining 33 cases diagnosed by random biopsy due to normal appearance, the average epithelial thickness was a mere 184 μm [39]. Given that some high grade lesions may not demonstrate typical characteristics, it may be reasonable to perform random biopsies and ECC especially in nonpregnant women with high grade cervical cytology [40].

Diagnostic Effectiveness In-Office and Patient Satisfaction

Colposcopy is considered an office-based procedure. The most common reasons for performing colposcopy in a hospital setting is usually related to poor visualization due to patient anxiety, lack of appropriate equipment, or congenital or acquired anatomic distortion. From both a patient and provider's perspective, patient comfort is paramount to performing an adequate colposcopy, obtaining biopsies, and ensuring patient follow-up. Many patients express anxiety over the procedure itself, the diagnosis, and potential findings. Strategies to reduce anxiety may include playing music during the procedure, providing pre-procedural videos, and allowing the patient to watch the procedure via video colposcopy [41]. In a survey conducted from 2007 to 2009 of 245 women undergoing colposcopy, patient satisfaction improved if procedural information was provided during a separate pre-procedural visit with a gynecologist or NP as opposed to during the day of the procedure [42].

The cervix has more stretch than pain receptors. There does not appear to be a significant benefit to the use of oral or topical pain relievers. Younger women and women who experience pain with speculum insertion seem to have increased pain perception during ECC [43]. Distraction techniques (e.g., coughing on cue) has been shown to be equivalent to local anesthesia in a small randomized trial [44].

Necessary Equipment

There are multiple types of colposcopes that employ the same basic principles of illumination and magnification (Fig. 15.2). Most colposcopes have adjustments for gross (often movement of

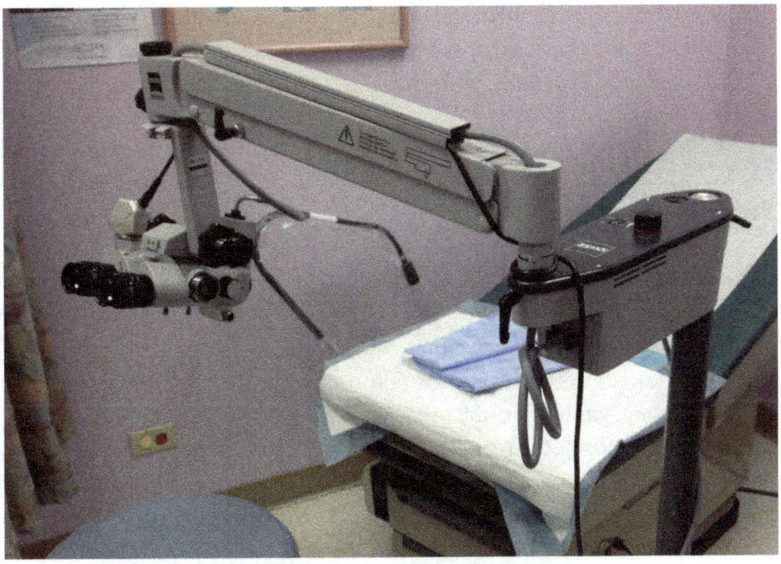

Fig. 15.2 Swing-arm colposcope. Other forms for colposcopes include tilt and roller bases or videoscopes. Note motorized height adjustable exam table

entire colposcope) and fine focusing, magnification, intraocular distance, and green/blue light filter. The most common focal length (distance from lens to cervix) is 300 mm (250-mm near, 400-mm far) to enable vision throughout the entire vaginal length. The provider not only needs to sit close to manipulate the speculum and swabs, but also be far enough away to insert biopsy instruments.

The coaxial light source (usually halogen or xenon) is focused at the same distance as the focal length. Magnification ranges from ×2 to ×40 with the most useful range at ×4 to ×15. Many colposcopes will use a numeric value of ×0.4 for scanning and ×2.5 for detail. Note that as magnification increases, brightness diminishes.

Some colposcopes have beam splitters to divert light to either a video camera, still camera, and/or teaching tube. Many patients find it both informative and anxiety-reducing to watch the procedure on a monitor. Patients watching videos during their procedure may be more likely to comply with recommendations [45]. In addition, the ability to take photographs enables more accurate documentation and comparison for patient records.

Positioning is critical for both patient and provider. A height-adjustable stool and motorized exam table are ideal especially for bulkier or less mobile colposcopes. Cervical punch biopsies may be performed with dual cutting jaws (e.g., Tischler, Burke) or anvil-type (Eppendorfer) instruments. One size does not fit all, so having a variety of instruments including straight and angled, long and short is helpful (Table 15.3) (Fig. 15.3).

Table 15.3 Colposcopic instruments and supplies

Instruments	Vaginal speculum (Graves, Pedersen)
	Endocervical speculum
	Vaginal wall retractor
	Allis clamp or single-tooth tenaculum
	Forceps
	Biopsy (Tischler, baby-Tischler, Kervorkian, Burke, Eppendorfer, Jackson)
	Endocervical curette
Disposables	Cotton-tipped applicator (Fox swabs, Q-tips)
	Gauze
	Cytobrush
	Alcohol wipes
	Sanitary napkin (post-procedure)
Solutions	3–5 % Acetic acid
	Lugol's solution
	Fixative
	Monsel's solution
	Silver nitrate
Other	Ring forceps
	Needle driver
	Absorbable suture (e.g., 2-0 Vicryl)
	Scissors
	Skin hook
	Cervical dilators

Step-By-Step Procedure

Pre-procedure

Prior to the colposcopy procedure, the provider should review the indications for colposcopy to ensure proper guidelines are met. If the Pap smear was performed at another facility, then it is beneficial to request the cytology slides for the pathologist reading the biopsies. Most pathologists will want to corroborate the biopsy results with the cytology. If the patient has any signs or symptoms of cervico-vaginitis, it is beneficial to postpone the visit until this has resolved. Any vaginal creams or douching should be stopped at least 1 day in advance. Relative contraindications to colposcopy include bleeding disorders and anticoagulation therapy so strategies to control bleeding (e.g., discontinuation of anticoagulation) should be implemented prior to the procedure. Colposcopy may be performed in menses if there is light flow.

It is helpful to obtain pertinent patient medical information including last menstrual period, pregnancy and delivery history, and any difficulties with pelvic exams. Prior Pap smear or colposcopy results, previous ablation or conization procedures, and HPV immunization status are important. Modifiable risk factors including previous sexually transmitted diseases, number of sexual partners and practices, and smoking provide opportunity for positive messaging. HIV

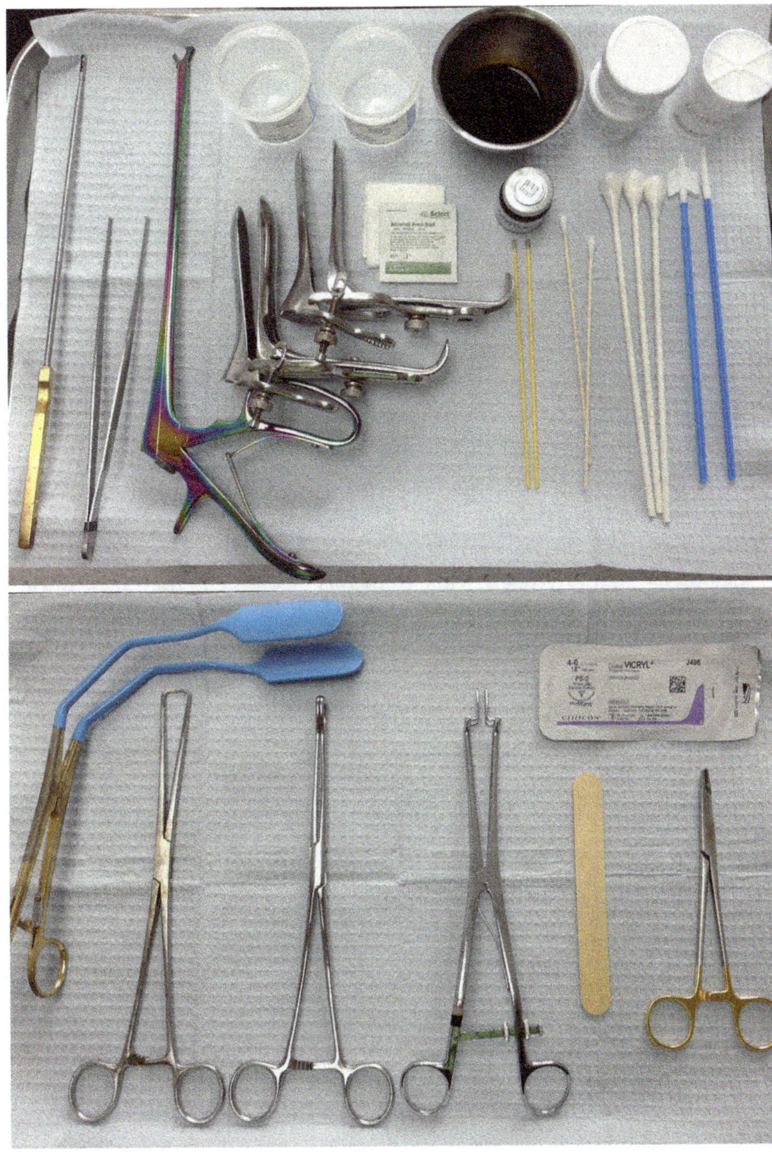

Fig. 15.3 Instrument trays. Main tray is sufficient for most procedures. Accessory tray provides instruments for difficult visualization

status, steroid use, uncontrolled diabetes, and organ transplant history provide additional risk factor information. Most importantly, compliance and social situation should be taken into account especially when establishing a follow-up plan.

Check a spot urine pregnancy test in all premenopausal women unless pregnancy status can be confidently assured. The provider should obtain informed consent. The colposcope and any video equipment and monitors should be turned on to avoid fumbling with plugs and cables during the procedure. Clean all eyepieces, handles, and dials between exams.

Procedure

1. *Position the patient and you so both of you are comfortable*. This may require the lowest setting on a height-adjustable stool with the motorized bed elevated to avoid slouching. The patient should be low enough on the table in dorsal lithotomy position to ensure visualization of an anterior cervix.
2. *Examine the pelvis in the usual fashion* with inspection of vulva, perineum, and anus. You should establish a routine to avoid omitting key parts of the exam. Determine

speculum size. The speculum does not need to be excessively large as an uncomfortable patient will limit your exam. A thorough exam can be performed with a smaller speculum but may require more adjustments to visualize the entire area (see below section "Tips and Tricks Section for Trouble-Shooting").

3. *Obtain a Pap smear (with HPV test if indicated)* if the prior cytology was not performed within the past 2–3 months or is unavailable for review. Cervico-vaginal epithelium may take 6 weeks or longer to regenerate after prior smear or biopsy.
4. *Remove mucus, blood, and discharge using a saline swab.* Examine for leukoplakia, erosions, ulcers, friable or pigmented lesions, or exophytic growths. Some atypical vessels may appear more prominent before they are obscured by dense AWE. At this point, change gloves to avoid gross contamination of the colposcope or place gloves on handles and dials.
5. *Align the colposcope parallel to the shaft of the vagina.* This is where a motorized bed assists in maintaining adequate posture. Start on low magnification ×2 to ×10 to form an overall impression. Avoid focusing on obvious lesions until you have performed a complete survey of the vagina, fornices, and cervix. Increase magnification ×15 to ×20 to inspect vascular patterns. Practice working through the colposcope by passing swabs and instruments without turning away from the colposcopic field.
6. *Apply "vinegar"-soaked swabs to the cervix and vagina.* Patients may describe a cold or burning sensation. Anything greater than 5 % acetic acid may burn the mucosa and cause significant discomfort. Allow at least 30–60 s for the solution to absorb. It is postulated that acetic acid causes swelling in both columnar and abnormal cells. Other theories include reversible coagulation or precipitation of nuclear proteins and cytokeratins. The "light reflex" refers to the white appearance when light is reflected by large, dense nuclei of dysplastic cells rather than transmitted through the 20–30 cell epithelial layer (see section "Findings").
Reapply acetic acid every 3–5 min as lesions will fade over time. This reversal tends to occur slower in high grade dysplasia and cancer. As low grade lesions are confined to the basement membrane, the acetic acid penetration is lower and leads to a less intense white.

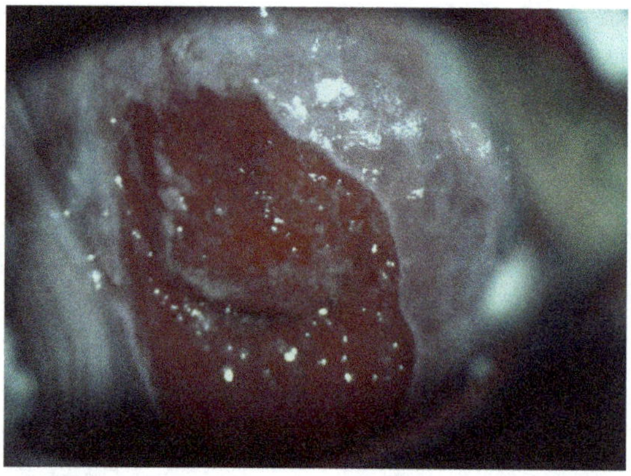

Fig. 15.4 Squamo-columnar junction (SCJ). Clear distinct margin between immature squamous epithelium and glandular ectropion

7. *Identify the SCJ* (Fig. 15.4). If the SCJ is retracted into the canal, insert an endocervical speculum, clear any obstructing mucus, and/or use a moistened Q-tip. If poor visualization is due to cervical stenosis, dilate the cervical os. The endocervical glandular tissue appears grape-like with small fronds and pink-red cobble-stoning. The ectocervical squamous lining appears smooth and gray-pink. The TZ usually extends 2–6 mm from the SCJ but may spread over 1 cm. Many factors impact location including age (e.g., prominent ectropion seen in pre-puberty recedes with age), parity, pregnancy (e.g., ectropion becomes more pronounced with increasing gestational age), previous cervical procedures, menopause, hormonal contraceptives, and vaginal pH. Gland openings and Nabothian cysts are hallmarks of the TZ.

8. *Utilize the green or blue ("red-free") light filter* to enhance border contrast and identify punctations and abnormal vessels as blood will appear black (see section "Findings").
9. *Apply Schiller's test using Lugol's solution* (5 g iodine + 10 g potassium iodide + 100 mL distilled water) to aid or confirm your impression. Glycogen-rich cells absorb iodine and appear mahogany brown or black. Columnar glandular and dysplastic cells often lack glycogen and appear mustard-yellow or saffron colored. Many providers do not perform Schiller's test, but routine practice will enable meaningful use during difficult cases or in vaginal colposcopy. Although it is uncertain whether it is better than acetic acid, Lugol's solution may improve sensitivity and specificity in diagnosing CIN-2-3 from 81.3 % to 91.5 % and 87.3 % to 89 %, respectively [46].
10. *Form your impression.* To make colposcopy less subjective and reproducible between different providers, various physicians have proposed multiple grading systems including Coppleson in the 1960s, Stafl in the 1970s, and more recently by Strander and Shafi and Nazeer in the 2000s. The most familiar grading system was developed by Richard Reid in 1984 using a cumulative total between five signs (thickness, contour, color, vessels, and iodine staining) (Table 15.4) [47]. Unfortunately, most grading systems are inconsistently reproducible or reliable. In the ALTS trial, a modified Reid Colposcopic Index (RCI), which omitted the use of Lugol's solution to account for its diminished use, showed poor agreement (weighted Kappa 0.17) and low sensitivity 37.3 % and specificity of 89.7 % [48]. Of the 3,549 samples, impressions correlated poorly with final pathology independent of provider experience [49]. The RCI, as the other grading systems, are not highly predictive of CIN-3 or greater [50].
11. *Perform endocervical curettage.* ECC is always indicated for high grade abnormalities (Table 15.5). New guidelines do not recommend specific intervention for CIN-1 found on ECC [4]. The benefit of ECC is likely minimal in women <25 years old (see above section "Effectiveness") [51]. Customarily, ECC is performed first but often elicits the most discomfort during the procedure. It should extend approximately 1–2 cm into the canal and curette the endocervix in a circular fashion similar to D&C or endometrial biopsy. Use an endocervical brush to capture any remaining tissue, blood, or mucus as it is less likely to miss disease within the canal. ECC is omitted in pregnant women for concerns of bleeding, infection, and theoretical injury to the gestational sac.
12. *Perform biopsies.* There are no colposcopic findings that are pathognomonic for high grade dysplasia or cancer. All suspicious lesions should be diagnosed by histology (the "gold standard"). If you are uncertain, then perform multiple biopsies. The detection of CIN-3 is improved with two or

Table 15.4 Reid colposcopic index

		Points		
		0	1	2
Criterion	Thickness[a]	Borderline	Definite	–
	Contour[a]	Condyloma micropapillary	Flat	–
	Color	Shiny (white)	Shiny (gray)	Dull
	Vessels	Warty	None	Punctation Mosaicism
	Iodine	Positive	Partial uptake	Negative

Note: Cumulative score of 0–2 = subclinical HPV or CIN-1; 3–5 = CIN-1-2; 6–8 = CIN-2-3
[a]Less predictive and omitted in subsequent criteria
Source: Adapted from Reid R et al. [47]

Table 15.5 Indications for endocervical curettage

Squamous abnormalities	ASC-H
	HSIL
	ASC-US or LSIL without visible lesions
Glandular abnormalities	AGC
	AIS
Other	Unsatisfactory colpo

Source: Adapted from Wright TC et al. [22]

Table 15.6 2011 Colposcopic terminology

Is colposcopy adequate?	Yes or no
	If no, reason:
Is TZ fully visualized?	Yes or no
	If no, reason:
TZ type?	I: All ectocervical
	II: Partial endocervical with some ectocervix seen
	III: All endocervical

Source: Adapted from Bornstein J et al. [55]

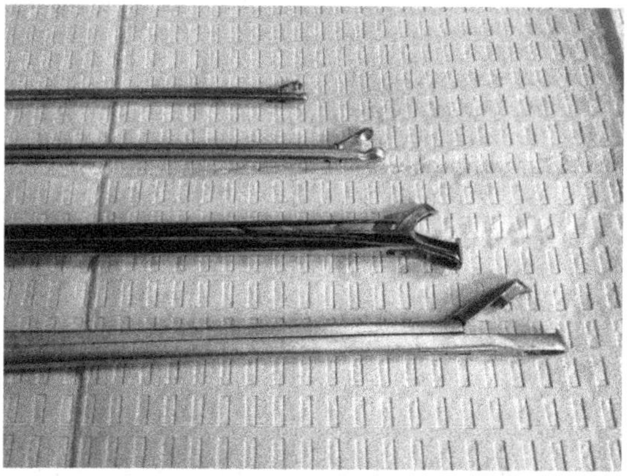

Fig. 15.5 Biopsy instruments. From *top* to *bottom*: Jackson bronchoscopy 2-mm and 4-mm, mini-Tischler, and Tischler biopsy instruments

greater biopsies [52]. Multiple biopsies are not associated with an increased risk of acquiring new HPV infection [53].

Recognize that the epithelium is approximately 1 mm in thickness except in areas of leukoplakia or erosion. This would suggest that use of a smaller biopsy instrument or smaller biopsy with a large instrument should be sufficient for diagnosis while minimizing cervical trauma and bleeding. We favor 2- and 4-mm Jackson biopsy instruments (Fig. 15.5). As a general rule, consider proceeding from posterior to anterior to avoid obscuring your next biopsy site from blood.

While some patients do not experience any pain with biopsy, distraction techniques (e.g., coughing on cue) limit discomfort in most women obviating the need for anesthesia. By convention, the biopsies are labeled by clock face corresponding to the position on the cervix (i.e., anterior is 12 o'clock, right 9 o'clock) and submitted in permanent fixative. Bleeding is achieved with pressure, Monsel's solution, silver nitrate sticks, or suture in extreme cases [54]. Once hemostasis is achieved, remove any excess Monsel's solution, blood, and discharge. The speculum is removed, and pictures are printed if available.

13. *Provide post-procedural instructions*. Most cramping resolves same day but may respond to mild pain relievers (e.g., ibuprofen) as needed. Recommend pelvic rest (i.e., refrain from intercourse, use of tampons, or douching) for 1–3 days minimum. If Monsel's solution was applied, inform her to anticipate a "coffee ground" discharge for a few days. Provide instructions and contact information if she develops excessive bleeding or pain, malodorous discharge, or fever.
14. *Document the findings*. This usually includes the original indication for colposcopy including abnormal cytology and HPV status. According to the updated 2011 International Federation for Cervical Pathology and Colposcopy (IFCPC) group, there are three components to the record (Table 15.6) [55]. This includes whether the colposcopic exam was adequate, the TZ was fully visualized, and TZ type.

The purpose of documentation is for medical, legal, and financial reasons. The record should be clear and consistent using common conventions. Traditionally accepted abbreviations include: transformation zone (TZ), AWE, leukoplakia (L), squamous metaplasia (SM), ectopy (E), punctation

Table 15.7 2011 Colposcopic impression

Impression		Findings: Epithelium	Punctation/ mosaicism	Other
Normal		Squamous original (mature, atrophy)		Deciduosis in pregnancy
		Squamous metaplasia (crypt opening, Nabothian cyst)		
		Columnar (ectopy)		
Abnormal	Grade 1 minor	AWE: thin, geographic border	Fine	Borders: sharp, inner, ridge
	Grade 2 major	AWE: dense, cuffed crypt opening	Coarse	
Suspicion for cancer		Irregular surface		Vessels: atypical, fragile
		Ulceration		Lesion: exophytic, gross
				Necrosis
Non-specific		Leukoplakia		Lugol's staining
		Erosion		

Source: Adapted from Bornstein J et al. [55]

(P), mosaicism (M), atypical vessels (AV), and Nabothian cyst (NC). Paper charting is ideal for drawing your findings. Although some electronic medical record systems have the ability to graphically illustrate your findings, many are cumbersome. This requires the provider to articulate findings in more detail such as coarseness, clock face position, and size dimensions. Use a standard form to ensure no details are missed. Record your impression (e.g., CIN-1), proposed management, and follow-up plan.

15. *Establish a follow-up plan.* For every patient who undergoes biopsy or ECC, schedule an in-person visit within 1–2 weeks to review their recovery, results, questions, and establish a management plan. This patient population tends to be at higher risk of noncompliance, so a follow-up plan is as critical as the performance of colposcopy. This follow-up visit is an opportune time to counsel on smoking cessation and other high-risk behaviors (e.g., contraception).

Findings

Accommodating for interobserver variability, the IFCPC has correlated certain features compatible with a given histologic diagnosis (Table 15.7). The provider must recognize that no visual finding is pathognomic for disease and caution must be exercised in acting upon a colposcopic impression without waiting for histologic confirmation except in certain applications (e.g., "see-and-treat" methods used in underdeveloped countries).

Aceto-white epithelium: This is the most common finding after application of 3–5 % acetic acid and pertains to the "light reflex" (see above **Procedure 6**). Besides location and size, notations include the intensity, contour, and borders of AWE lesions. Aceto-white epithelium is more commonly encountered along the anterior and posterior cervix, but dysplasia is radially distributed [38]. Endocervical glandular cells often appear a faint white after acetic acid application and should not be mistaken for dysplasia.

Low grade disease appears translucent and shiny white, whereas high grade disease is often a dense, dull white. Low grade disease often has diffuse or feathered borders, whereas high grade disease often has sharp, distinct borders, or a well-demarcated area within an area of diffuse AWE (Fig. 15.6). A white patch seen before the application of acetic acid represents leukoplakia, which pertains to hyperkeratosis associated with HPV. Biopsies are recommended to ascertain the degree of abnormality within the underlying epithelium.

Punctation and Mosaicism: These represent changes to the vascular patterns and are the most common vascular findings in cervical dysplasia. It is uncertain whether dysplastic cells stimulate angiogenesis and neovascularization, or whether dysplasia merely influences the existing capillary vessels within columnar epithelium. In normal tissue, the vessels are confined to the stroma underlying the translucent epithelium. In dysplastic tissue, the vessels are within the epithelium. Punctation represents the tips of vascular loops protruding 1–2 mm above the surface, whereas mosaicism represents a haphazard pattern of communicating vessels. Fine punctation and mosaicism usually pertain to low grade disease (Fig. 15.7). Vessels that are >200 μm (0.2 mm) apart create a coarser appearance and are suggestive of more high grade lesions. When mosaic tiles push up between vascular margins, an irregular contour forms usually indicating high grade disease (Fig. 15.8).

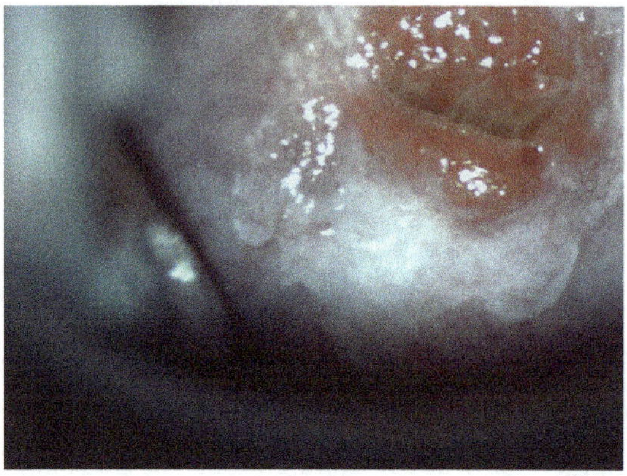

Fig. 15.6 Aceto-white epithelium (AWE). Low grade lesion with flat, thin-white, glass-like appearance and diffuse, feathered borders. Note fine mosaicism forming along posterior left cervical quadrant

Abnormal vessels: Normal vessel patterns appear tree-like, with larger branches giving way to smaller ones. "Atypical" vessels appear irregular with different diameter vessels, abrupt changes in direction, and haphazard arrangements. Often the vessels are widely spaced and may have abbreviated shapes similar to corkscrews, commas, and hairpins. Atypical vessels refer to invasive cancer and are not used to describe punctation or mosaicism. The use of a green or blue filter sharpens the contrast of the vessels to the surrounding epithelium (see above **Procedure 8**) (Fig. 15.9).

Other findings: Ulcerations and erosions may occur from high grade disease and cancer but may represent trauma or infection. Exophytic cauliflower-like growths often pertain to invasive cancer.

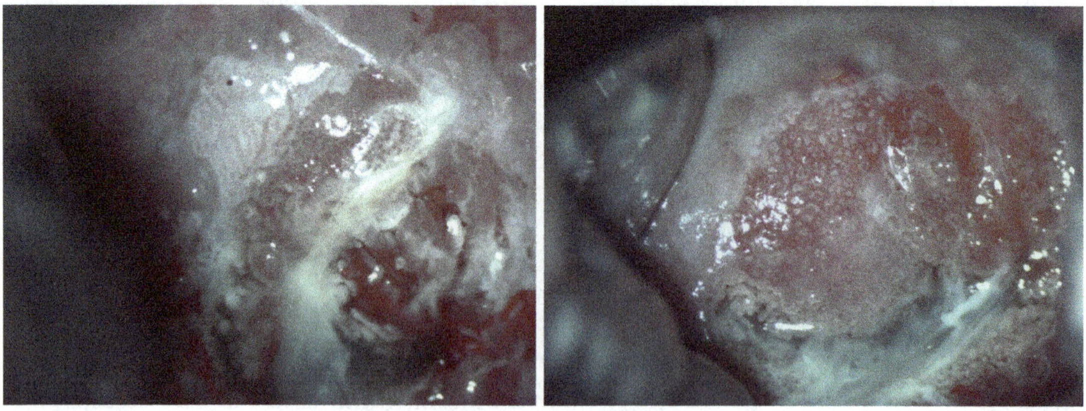

Fig. 15.7 Fine punctation with small, evenly spaced, dot-like vessels. Coarser punctation with larger, irregularly sized and -spaced capillary loop vessels

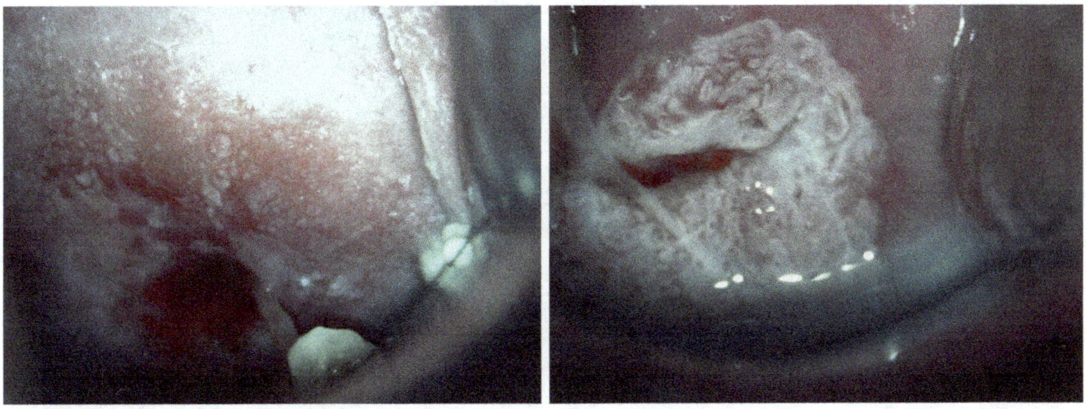

Fig. 15.8 Fine mosaicism with smaller, flatter, more uniform tiling. Coarse mosaicism demonstrates larger, irregular, and raised tiling

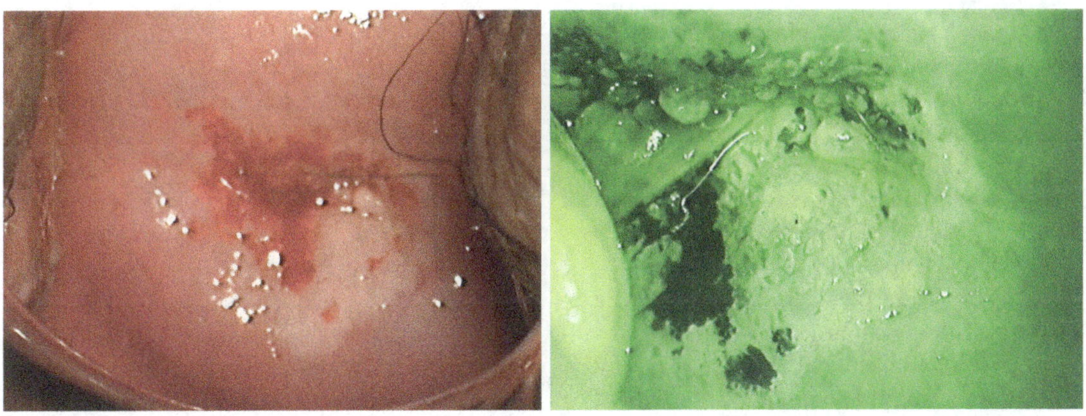

Fig. 15.9 Green-blue filter light. Red blood appears black. Note fine punctations are better appreciated with green filter

Vaginal Colposcopy

Vaginal colposcopy is similar to the cervical procedure with a few exceptions. Dysplastic areas often appear with aceto-white changes and punctation, but rarely does mosaicism appear. Obtaining visualization of the epithelial surface is challenging due to the multiple rugae, folds, and in post-hysterectomy women, the hidden vaginal angles termed "dog ears." Visualization is often achieved by flattening the tissue to make it smooth. This may involve using a larger speculum and/or rotating the speculum to visualize the anterior and posterior surfaces. Ring forceps provide stretch, and hooks may evert tissue. In addition, removal of the speculum allows for good visualization of the vaginal walls as they collapse around the speculum tip.

Lugol's solution may be beneficial to highlight dysplastic changes. Specimens should be labeled by anatomic landmarks (i.e., cuff, fornices, urethra, posterior fourchette). Biopsy all suspicious-appearing polyps or mucosal tags.

Vulvar Colposcopy

Unlike cervical and vaginal colposcopy, this is merely a bright light examination on hair-bearing skin. Low-cost options include handheld

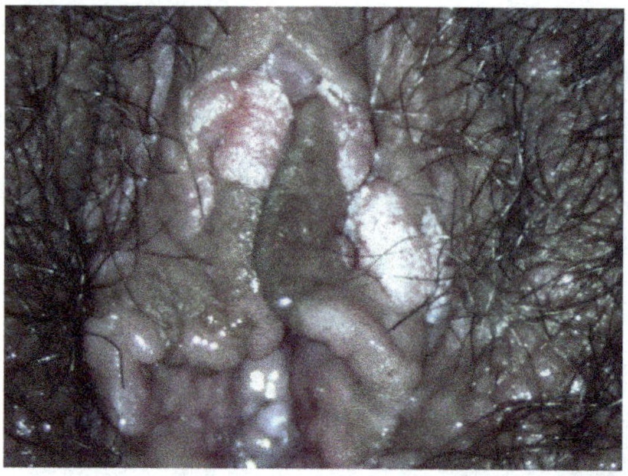

Fig. 15.10 Vulvar changes. Raised white epithelium in HPV-related condyloma

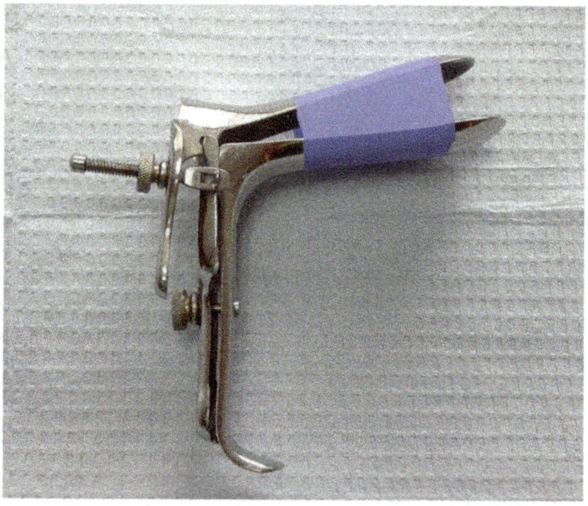

Fig. 15.11 Glove-wrapped speculum. May use ultrasound probe condoms or tongue depressors

lights and magnifying glasses, although the degree of magnification is incomparable. Vulvar colposcopy is usually performed for a grossly visible lesion or persistent vulvar symptoms (e. g., itching, pain) non-responsive to medical treatment. Vulvar colposcopy is rarely performed for abnormal cytologic findings except when cervical or vaginal colposcopy is normal.

Apply 5 % acetic acid in 4″ × 4″ gauze-soaked pads and wait at least 3–5 min. The vulvar skin is keratinized and absorption is slower. The entire vulva, perineum, and anus should be inspected as the entire lower anogenital tract is susceptible to HPV-associated disorders. Acetowhite epithelium is often associated with usual-type VIN (warty-basaloid, undifferentiated), HPV, and hyperkeratosis (e.g., scratching, trauma) (Fig. 15.10). Punctation and mosaicism is not seen on skin. Areas with abnormal vessels and pigmented lesions should be biopsied.

Biopsies may be performed with a 2–4 mm Keyes punch biopsy or scalpel. Unlike the cervix and vagina, biopsy sites must be anesthetized using local injection (e.g., 1 % lidocaine with or without epinephrine) or topical anesthetic (e.g., EMLA cream). Hemostasis is achieved with pressure, silver nitrate, and/or suture. All specimens should be labeled according to anatomic landmarks (i.e., posterior fourchette, labia majora, clitoral hood).

Tips and Tricks Section for Trouble-Shooting

The provider's primary assessment is to determine whether the colposcopic procedure is adequate or inadequate. This depends upon the provider's ability to obtain visualization of the cervix and vagina, and the entirety of the TZ and any lesions. Take care in opening and positioning the speculum to avoid cervical trauma causing pain and/or bleeding especially in a pregnant patient. Sidewall retractors may be used, but if unavailable, a simple glove- or condom-wrapped speculum often works well (Fig. 15.11). Tongue depressors or large cotton swabs rolled into the vaginal fornices provide site-specific visualization. Place a single tooth tenaculum or Allis clamp on the cervix if needed. In difficult cases, the entire cervix may not be seen so consider working in quadrants to ensure a thorough exam.

In the case of a stenotic cervix, perform cervical dilation. Use of misoprostol (e.g., 100 mg oral night prior) [56] may aid visualization, but its utility is debated [57]. Insert an appropriately sized endocervical speculum to see within the canal to visualize a retracted SCJ or proximal lesions. A moistened Q-tip placed into the canal may help prop the endocervical canal open.

Pregnancy often presents a challenging problem due to engorgement of the cervix, expansion of the vagina, and increased mucous discharge. Ideally, pregnant women should undergo colposcopy in the first or early second trimester before the cervix undergoes significant change. There are more management options available earlier in gestation when there is ample time for decision-making before fetal viability. Use a larger speculum and minimize cervical contact to avoid bleeding. If the TZ is not entirely visualized, reexamine the patient in at 14–18 weeks gestation as the SCJ and ectropion often emerges into view. Although ECC is contraindicated in pregnancy, biopsy is not. Biopsy is recommended for areas suspicious for CIN-2 or greater. Adequate hemostasis is often achieved with immediate application of pressure and Monsel's solution into the biopsy crater. We hold a Q-tip impregnated with Monsel's solution adjacent to our biopsy instrument so pressure is applied near simultaneously to our biopsy.

For the postmenopausal woman, the atrophic epithelium is often thin and friable. The subepithelial capillary network appears prominent. Minimal trauma including insertion of a speculum may cause hemorrhage that can obscure findings or be confused for lesions. There are often areas of injury and repair that may appear as AWE. In cases of low grade cytologic abnormalities, consider having the patient apply intravaginal estrogen cream nightly for 2–3 weeks followed by repeat cytology and colposcopy.

The provider should be familiar with different biopsy instruments as one tool does not work for all patients. For a mobile cervix, it may be helpful to stabilize the cervix using a single tooth tenaculum or Allis clamp. The base of the instrument or tooth is usually placed behind the lesion, and the biopsy is performed in a forward motion (i.e., pushing into cervix). If the epithelium is taut, "pinch" the tissue to create a knuckle of tissue to biopsy. For vaginal biopsies, relax the speculum to enable to vaginal tissue to fold. Again, an Allis clamp or forceps may aid creating a knuckle of epithelium to biopsy.

Immediate Procedural and Short-Term Complications

Common risks to all procedures include infection, bleeding, and injury to adjacent structures. Colposcopy is not considered a sterile procedure, and we do not recommend use of prep solutions (e.g., Betadine). The cervix is well-vascularized and infection is extremely unlikely. Delay colposcopy in the setting of acute cervico-vaginitis until the patient has been treated.

The provider should be prepared to handle bleeding during biopsies especially in pregnant women. If available, thickened Monsel's paste (partially dehydrated ferric subsulfate) provides better hemostasis than the more aqueous form found in most prepackaged solutions. While pressure, silver nitrate, and/or Monsel's solution is sufficient for the majority of biopsies, the provider may encounter brisker bleeding requiring more maneuvers. Use gauze to absorb more blood and obtain better visualization. A smaller Q-tip often provides more direct pressure on a bleeding site than a larger cotton swab. A common mistake is continual removal of Q-tips to examine the site of bleeding when sustained pressure will often control hemorrhage and enable clot to form. A ring forceps or Allis clamp may provide compression and aid hemostasis. As a last resort, placing suture (e.g., figure-of-eight) should stop hemorrhage.

While there is concern that cervical conization procedures may affect pregnancy outcomes (see Chap. 16), it is unlikely that colposcopy with biopsies increases adverse risks of preterm labor or delivery [58].

The diagnosis of cervical cytologic abnormality and need for colposcopy may be associated with sexual dysfunction, poor body image, relationships, and depression [59]. Although there does not seem to be any long-lasting effects of colposcopy, up to one-third of women may continue to have a fear of cancer [60].

Summary and Recommendations

Colposcopy is a well-established procedure to evaluate the cervix and vagina for cytologic abnormalities based on visual changes associated with low and high grade dysplasia and cancer. Indications for colposcopy were established in the ASCCP 2006 and recently updated 2012 Consensus Guidelines.

The colposcope consists of high-powered magnification paired with bright illumination and light filters to visualize macroscopic changes after the application of 3–5 % acetic acid and/or Lugol's solution. The provider should note the adequacy of the exam, whether the TZ is entirely visualized, and TZ type. Common nomenclature is used to communicate and compare colposcopic impressions among providers.

The provider should follow an established protocol during the procedure in surveying the lower anogenital tract including the vulva, vagina, and cervix. Avoid fixating on a gross lesion until the entire survey is completed. If visualization is suboptimal, consider working in quadrants. Biopsy abnormal or uncertain lesions. Consider random biopsies and ECC especially in the setting of an older woman with high grade cytologic abnormality. During review of the histology, there should be concordance between the cytology, colposcopic impression, histology, and overall clinical picture. Review your findings with the pathologist if there is discordance. Do not hesitate to refer the patient to a more experienced colposcopist in difficult cases.

References

1. World Health Organization. International agency for research on cancer. Globocan. 2008. http://globocan.iarc.fr/factsheets/cancers/cervix.asp
2. U.S. Cancer Statistics Working Group. United States Cancer Statistics: 1999–2010 incidence and mortality Web-based report. Atlanta, GA: Department of Health and Human Services, Centers for Disease Control and Prevention, and National Cancer Institute; 2013.
3. U.S. Department of Health and Human Services. Healthy people 2010: understanding and improving health. 2nd ed. Washington, DC: U.S. Government Printing Office; 2000.
4. Massad LS, Einstein MH, Huh WK, Katki HA, Kinney WK, Schiffman M, Solomon D, Wentzensen N, Lawson HW. 2012 updated consensus guidelines for the management of abnormal cervical cancer screening tests and cancer precursors. J Low Genit Tract Dis. 2013;17(5 Suppl 1):S1–27.
5. Arbyn M, Kyrgiou M, Simoens C, Raifu AO, Koliopoulos G, Martin-Hirsch P, Prendiville W, Paraskevaidis E. Perinatal mortality and other severe adverse pregnancy outcomes associated with treatment of cervical intraepithelial neoplasia: a meta-analysis. BMJ. 2008;337:a1284.
6. Kim JJ, Wright TC, Goldie SJ. Cost-effectiveness of alternative triage strategies for atypical squamous cells of undetermined significance. JAMA. 2002;287:2382–90.
7. Darragh TM, Colgan TJ, Thomas Cox J, Heller DS, Henry MR, Luff RD, McCalmont T, Nayar R, Palefsky JM, Stoler MH, Wilkinson EJ, Zaino RJ, Wilbur DC. The Lower Anogenital Squamous Terminology Standardization project for HPV-associated lesions: background and consensus recommendations from the College of American Pathologists and the American Society for Colposcopy and Cervical Pathology. Int J Gynecol Pathol. 2013;32(1):76–115.
8. Noller K, Wagner A. Gynecology and obstetrics, Chapter 30, Colposcopy. Baltimore, MD: Lippincott Williams and Wilkins; 2004.
9. Solomon D, Davey D, Kurman R, Moriarty A, O'Connor D, Prey M, Raab S, Sherman M, Wilbur D, Wright Jr T, Young N. The 2001 Bethesda System: terminology for reporting results of cervical cytology. JAMA. 2002;287(16):2114–9.
10. Meisels A, Fortin R. Condylomatous lesions of the cervix and vagina. I. Cytologic patterns. Acta Cytol. 1976;20:505–9.
11. Wright Jr TC, Cox JT, Massad LS, Twiggs LB, Wilkinson EJ. 2001 Consensus guidelines for the management of women with cervical cytological abnormalities. JAMA. 2002;287(16):2120–9.
12. Alonso I, Torné A, Puig-Tintoré LM, Esteve R, Quinto L, Garcia S, Campo E, Pahisa J, Ordi J. High-risk cervical epithelial neoplasia grade 1 treated by loop electrosurgical excision: follow-up and value of HPV testing. Am J Obstet Gynecol. 2007;197(4):359.e1–6.
13. Jeronimo J, Schiffman M. Colposcopy at a crossroads. Am J Obstet Gynecol. 2006;195(2):349–53.
14. Maynard MH, Duarte-Franco E, Rodrigues I, Walter SD, Hanley J, Ferenczy A, Ratnam S, Coutlée F, Franco EL. Canadian Cervical Cancer Screening Trial Study Group. Human papillomavirus DNA versus Papanicolaou screening tests for cervical cancer. N Engl J Med. 2007;357(16):1579–88.
15. O'Connor D. A brief history of lower genital tract screening. J Low Genit Tract Dis. 2007;11(3):182–8.

16. Papanicolaou GN, Traut HF. The diagnostic value of vaginal smears in carcinoma of the uterus. Am J Obstet Gynecol. 1941;42:193.
17. Hinselmann H. Verbesserung der Inspektionsmoglchkeiten von vulva, vagina, and portio. Munchen Med Wchuschr. 1925;72:1733.
18. Baggish MS. Colposcopy of the cervix, vagina, and vulva, Chap 1A: Historical. St. Louis, MO: Mosby, Elsevier Science; 2003. p. 3.
19. Rotkin JD. A comparison review of key epidemiological studies in cervical cancer related to current searches for transmissible agents. Cancer Res. 1973;33:1353.
20. Melnick JL, Adam E, Rawls WE. The causative role of herpes virus type 2 in cervical cancer. Cancer. 1974;34(4 Suppl):1375–85.
21. Dürst M, Gissmann L, Ikenberg H, zur Hausen H. A papillomavirus DNA from a cervical carcinoma and its prevalence in cancer biopsy samples from different geographic regions. Proc Natl Acad Sci U S A. 1983;80:3812–5.
22. Wright Jr TC, Massad LS, Dunton CJ, Spitzer M, Wilkinson EJ, Solomon D. 2006 consensus guidelines for the management of women with abnormal cervical cancer screening tests. J Obstet Gynecol. 2007;197 (4):346.
23. Herbst AL, Ulfelder H, Poskanzer DC. Adenocarcinoma of the vagina: association of maternal stilbestrol therapy with tumor appearance in young women. N Engl J Med. 1971;284(15):878–81.
24. Jordan J. International standards for training in colposcopy. Clin Obstet Gynecol. 1995;38(3):662–5.
25. Spitzer M, Apgar BS, Brotzman GL, Krumholz BA. Residency training in colposcopy: a survey of program directors in obstetrics and gynecology and family practice. Am J Obstet Gynecol. 2001;185(2):507.
26. Baum ME, Rader JS, Gibb RK, McAlister RP, Powell MA, Mutch DG, Gao F, Wright JD. Colposcopic accuracy of obstetrics and gynecology residents. Gynecol Oncol. 2006;103:966–70.
27. Mitchell MF, Schottenfeld D, Tortolero-Luna G, Cantor SB, Richards-Kortum R. Colposcopy for the diagnosis of squamous intraepithelial lesions: a meta-analysis. Obstet Gynecol. 1998;91:626–31.
28. Hopman EH, Voorhorst FJ, Kenemans P, Meyer CJ, Helmerhorst TJ. Observer agreement on interpreting colposcopic images of CIN. Gynecol Oncol. 1995;58 (2):206.
29. Ferris DG, Litaker M. ALTS Group. Interobserver agreement for colposcopy quality control using digitized colposcopic images during the ALTS trial. J Low Genit Tract Dis. 2005;9(1):29.
30. ASCUS-LSIL Triage Study (ALTS) Group. Results of a randomized trial on the management of cytology interpretations of atypical squamous cells of undetermined significance. Am J Obstet Gynecol. 2003;188:1383–92.
31. Underwood M, Arbyn M, Parry-Smith W, De Bellis-Ayres S, Todd R, Redman CW, Moss EL. Accuracy of colposcopy-directed punch biopsies: a systematic review and meta-analysis. BJOG. 2012;119 (11):1293–301.
32. Stoler MH, Vichnin MD, Ferenczy A, Ferris DG, Perez G, Paavonen J, Joura EA, Djursing H, Sigurdsson K, Jefferson L, Alvarez F, Sings HL, Lu S, James MK, Saah A, Haupt RM. FUTURE I, II and III Investigators. The accuracy of colposcopic biopsy: analysis from the placebo arm of the Gardasil clinical trials. Int J Cancer. 2011;128(6):1354–62.
33. Hearp ML, Locante AM, Ben-Rubin M, Dietrich R, David O. Validity of sampling error as a cause of noncorrelation. Cancer. 2007;111(5):275–9.
34. Gage JC, Hanson VW, Abbey K, Dippery S, Gardner S, Kubota J, Schiffman M, Solomon D, Jeronimo J. ALTS Group. Number of cervical biopsies and sensitivity of colposcopy. Obstet Gynecol. 2006;108 (2):264.
35. Belinson J, Qiao YL, Pretorius R, Zhang WH, Elson P, Li L, Pan QJ, Fischer C, Lorincz A, Zahniser D. Shanxi Province Cervical Cancer Screening Study: a cross-sectional comparative trial of multiple techniques to detect cervical neoplasia. Gynecol Oncol. 2001;83(2):439–44. Erratum in: Gynecol Oncol. 2002;Feb;84(2):355.
36. Pretorius RG, Zhang WH, Belinson JL, Huang MN, Wu LY, Zhang X, Qiao YL. Colposcopically directed biopsy, random cervical biopsy, and endocervical curettage in the diagnosis of cervical intraepithelial neoplasia II or worse. Am J Obstet Gynecol. 2004;191 (2):430.
37. Solomon D, Stoler M, Jeronimo J, Khan M, Castle P, Schiffman M. Diagnostic utility of endocervical curettage in women undergoing colposcopy for equivocal or low-grade cytologic abnormalities. Obstet Gynecol. 2007;110(2 Pt 1):288.
38. Guido RS, Jeronimo J, Schiffman M, Solomon D. ALTS Group. The distribution of neoplasia arising on the cervix: results from the ALTS trial. Am J Obstet Gynecol. 2005;193(4):1331.
39. Yang B, Pretorius RG, Belinson JL, Zhang X, Burchette R, Qiao YL. False negative colposcopy is associated with thinner cervical intraepithelial neoplasia 2 and 3. Gynecol Oncol. 2008;110:32–6.
40. Pretorius RG, Belinson JL, Burchette R, Hu S, Zhang X, Qiao YL. Regardless of skill, performing more biopsies increases the sensitivity of colposcopy. J Low Genital Tract Dis. 2011;15(3):180–8.
41. Galaal KA, Deane K, Sangal S, Lopes AD. Interventions for reducing anxiety in women undergoing colposcopy. Cochrane Database Syst Rev. 2011;(12).
42. Hendriksen MT, van Delft KW, Bremer GL, Mertens HJ. Patient satisfaction in treatment for cervical pathology. Oncol Lett. 2011;2(3):439–43.
43. Church L, Oliver L, Dobie S, Madigan D. Ellsworth A Analgesia for colposcopy: double-masked, randomized comparison of ibuprofen and benzocaine gel. Obstet Gynecol. 2001;97(1):5.

44. Schmid BC, Pils S, Heinze G, Hefler L, Reinthaller A, Speiser P. Forced coughing versus local anesthesia and pain associated with cervical biopsy: a randomized trial. Am J Obstet Gynecol. 2008;199(6):641.e1.
45. Takacs P, Chakhtoura N, De Santis T. Video colposcopy improves adherence to follow-up compared to regular colposcopy: a randomized trial. Arch Gynecol Obstet. 2004;270(3):182.
46. Muwonge R, Walter SD, Wesley RS, Basu P, Shastri SS, Thara S, Mbalawa CG, Sankaranarayanan R. IARC Multicentre Study Group on Cervical Cancer Early Detection. Assessing the gain in diagnostic performance when two visual inspection methods are combined for cervical cancer prevention. J Med Screen. 2007;14:144–50.
47. Reid R. Genital warts and cervical cancer: a colposcopic index for differentiating subclinical papillomaviral infection from cervical intraepithelial neoplasia. Am J Obstet Gynecol. 1984;149:815–23.
48. Ferris DG, Litaker MS for the ALTS Group. Prediction of cervical histologic results using an abbreviated Reid Colposcopic Index during ALTS. Am J Obstet Gynecol. 2006;194:704–10.
49. Mousavi AS, Fakour R, Gilani MM, Behtash N, Ghaemmaghami F, Karimi ZM. A prospective study to evaluate the correlation between Reid colposcopic index impression and biopsy histology. J Low Genit Tract Dis. 2007;11:147–50.
50. Massad LS, Jeronimo J, Katki HP, Schiffman M, NIH/ASCCP Research Group. The accuracy of colposcopic grading for detection of high-grade intraepithelial neoplasia. J Low Genital Tract Dis. 2009;13:137–44.
51. Pretorius RG, Belinson JL, Azizi F, Peterson PC, Belinson S. Utility of random cervical biopsy and endocervical curettage in a low-risk population. J Low Genit Tract Dis. 2012;16(4):333–8.
52. Cox JT. More questions about the accuracy of colposcopy: what does this mean for cervical cancer prevention? Obstet Gynecol. 2008;111:1266–7.
53. Castle PE, Wentzensen N, Wheeler CM, Rydzak G, Schiffman M. Effect of the number of biopsies on the subsequent acquisition of new human papillomavirus infections. Obstet Gynecol. 2009;114(5):1057.
54. Martin-Hirsch PL, Kitchener H. Interventions for preventing blood loss during the treatment of cervical intraepithelial neoplasia. Cochrane Database Syst Rev. 1999;1.
55. Bornstein J, Sideri M, Tatti S, Walker P, Prendiville W, Haefner HK. Nomenclature Committee of International Federation for Cervical Pathology and Colposcopy. 2011 terminology of the vulva of the International Federation for Cervical Pathology and Colposcopy. J Low Genit Tract Dis. 2012;16(3):290.
56. Ayensu-Coker L, Sanchez J, Zurawin R, Dietrich JE. Use of misoprostol for management of unsatisfactory colposcopy in the adolescent: a case report and review of the literature. J Pediatr Adolesc Gynecol. 2009;22(5):e139–41.
57. Thanapprapasr D, Wilailak S, Ayudhya NI, Lertkhachonsuk AA, Likittanasombut P, Chittithaworn S, Charakorn C, Weerakiet S. Can vaginal misoprostol effectively increase rate of a satisfactory colposcopy? A randomized double-blind placebo-controlled trial. Jpn J Clin Oncol. 2010;40(3):203–7.
58. Castanon A, Brocklehurst P, Evans H, Peebles D, Singh N, Walker P, Patnick J, Sasieni P, PaCT Study Group. Risk of preterm birth after treatment for cervical intraepithelial neoplasia among women attending colposcopy in England: retrospective-prospective cohort study. BMJ. 2012;345:e5174.
59. Flanagan SM, Wilson S, Luesley D, Damery SL, Greenfield SM. Adverse outcomes after colposcopy. BMC Womens Health. 2011;11:2.
60. Hellsten C, Sjöström K, Lindqvist PG. A 2-year follow-up study of anxiety and depression in women referred for colposcopy after an abnormal cervical smear. BJOG. 2008;115:212–8.

Loop Electro-Excision Procedure (LEEP) 16

Kimberly L. Levinson and Chad M. Michener

Introduction

There are several different procedures, ranging from conservative to aggressive which can be utilized for the treatment of cervical intraepithelial neoplasia. Several outpatient ablative procedures have been well-accepted, easily available, and efficacious. These procedures historically have included electrocoagulation, electrodiathermy, cryosurgery, and laser surgery. The loop electrosurgical excision procedure (LEEP) is an alternative to cryotherapy and laser ablation of the cervix, and may be favored as an excisional procedure that also provides a sample for further pathologic analysis of the cervical tissue. Therefore, as opposed to ablative procedures, the likelihood of missing an invasive cancer is significantly reduced. A cold knife cone biopsy also allows for pathologic diagnosis, however, has significant complications including bleeding (~13 %) as well as cervical stenosis (~17 %). While a cold knife cone may be necessary for certain indications including patients with microinvasive disease or disease within the endocervical canal, a LEEP is a procedure with minimal complications that can performed in a short period of time and still provides a sample for tissue diagnosis [1].

K.L. Levinson, M.D., M.P.H. (✉) • C.M. Michener, M.D.
Department of Obstetrics and Gynecology & Women's Health Institute, The Cleveland Clinic, 9500 Euclid Avenue, Desk A81, Cleveland, OH 44195, USA
e-mail: KLEVINS1@JHMI.EDU; michenc@ccf.org

The combination of an office-based procedure providing additional tissue for pathologic review makes LEEP highly attractive compared with most other modalities for management of cervical dysplasia. Other advantages to LEEP include, but are not limited to, patient comfort, cost, and conservation of medical resources. Additionally, this procedure allows for both diagnosis and treatment to be performed in a single outpatient visit or in a step-by-step approach with colposcopic evaluation prior to performing the LEEP excision [2]. Therefore, depending upon the concern and judgment of the practitioner, risks and benefits of each approach can be weighed, and loss to follow-up does not need to be a limiting factor for the treatment of cervical dysplasia.

Brief History of the Procedure

When the idea of a "pre-cancerous" lesion for cervical cancer first became accepted, many leaders in the field believed that aggressive treatment, including complete removal of the uterus was needed to eradicate the disease. However, over time, less invasive excisional procedures, such as a cold knife cone, became increasingly accepted [3].

The trend continued to shift towards a more conservative approach over time, and after the introduction of colposcopy in the 1970s, several outpatient ablative procedures became increasingly popular as the means to destroy cervical intraepithelial neoplasia. As ablative procedures

J.D. Emery and M.F.R. Paraiso (eds.), *Office-Based Gynecologic Surgical Procedures*,
DOI 10.1007/978-1-4939-1414-2_16,

increased, however, there were an increasing number of invasive cervical cancers that were unrecognized, ultimately leading to delayed treatment. With this outcome, the trend in therapy began to return to excisional procedures requiring anesthesia in an operating room setting [4].

Cartier was one of the first authors to describe the procedure that we now call a LEEP in 1984. At this time, he named the procedure "diathermy loop excision" [5]. This procedure was attractive as it does not require significant technical skill, allows histologic diagnosis, and can be performed in the office setting on an outpatient basis with few complications. Therefore, this technique quickly gained popularity [2]. In 1989, Prendiville and Cullimore described a modified procedure using larger loops. With this modification, the procedure was called a large loop excision of the transformation zone or "LLETZ" [6]. Since that time, the procedure has changed minimally, but has continued to gain popularity both in the United States and Europe. Importantly, this procedure began to be utilized in an office-based setting with minimal complications and comparable results.

Data Supporting Rationale and/or Efficacy of the Procedure In-office (Versus in OR)

We have already highlighted the potential benefits of an office-based excisional procedure over ablative procedures and procedures that require an operating room. LEEP is also beneficial in that it requires minimal equipment, does not cause significant discomfort, takes only a short time to perform, and rarely has significant procedural complications that must be handled in an operating room. For these reasons, a LEEP is an excellent in-office procedure that is not only appealing for patients and physicians, but also has tremendous economic advantages [2].

Several large studies have pointed to the low accuracy of colposcopic biopsies and the possibility of missing an invasive lesion if proceeding directly to ablative procedures. Moreover, studies utilizing a minimum of four ectocervical biopsies by quadrant along with endocervical curettage often show additional lesions in a quadrant with no colposcopic abnormality [7]. This has underscored the importance of providing a pathologic specimen in addition to treating the previously diagnosed dysplastic lesion. In a study by Buxton et al., 47 % of women were found to have a more severe lesion on LEEP than had been identified by colposcopy [8]. Similarly, Chappatte et al. showed only 43 % agreement between biopsy and LEEP specimens in their series and furthermore found that microinvasive carcinoma was missed in approximately 3 % of patients [9]. These findings suggest that it is important to provide further pathologic specimens as part of the treatment of dysplastic lesion, particularly for high-grade lesions. A LEEP is currently the only plausible outpatient procedure that provides a pathologic specimen.

The ability to perform a procedure without general anesthesia is critical for an outpatient, office-based procedure. Several different studies have shown that patients report only minimal discomfort with this procedure when local anesthetic is administered. A study by Wright et al. treated 432 patients as outpatients, using both small and large loop electrodes under local anesthesia. A paracervical block was performed prior to the procedure in this study, and few patients reported any sensation or discomfort. The procedure did not need to be stopped for any patient due to pain [1].

Diagnostic/Therapeutic Effectiveness of In-Office Including Patient Satisfaction

The effectiveness of this procedure has been measured by the absence of any cytologic, histologic, or colposcopic change following treatment via LEEP. Using this definition, early literature described only an 80 % success rate using a small loop 4–48 months following this procedure and 90 % with a large loop after 6–12 months follow-up with a large electrode. Sub-analyses suggested that high-grade disease was as likely to be cured with a LEEP as low-grade disease.

Table 16.1 LEEP outcomes of randomized controlled trials

Author	N	Comparators	Recurrence rate (%)
Mathevet et al. [10]	86	Cold knife cone	3.6
		LEEP	6.9
		Laser	6.9
Mitchell et al. [11]	390	LEEP	13
		Cryotherapy	19
		Laser	13
Alvarez et al. [12]	375	LEEP	7
		Laser	4
Singh et al. [13]	200	LEEP	6
		Cryotherapy	12
Chirenje et al. [14]	400	LEEP	3.6
		Cryotherapy	11.7

Importantly, success rates for patients receiving primary treatment were significantly higher than for those women who had previously failed prior therapy with laser or cryotherapy (94 % vs. 62 %). Furthermore, all of the LEEP failures for women with persistent disease were for grade III lesions whereas persistent grade I and grade II lesions could be cured with LEEP [1].

In subsequent larger series of over 800 patients, 92 % of patients were disease free at ≥6 months after initial treatment, and this increased to 95 % after repeat LEEP. This study also did not show any significant difference in the cure of low- and high-grade lesions [2].

When compared to other procedures, the success rate of LEEP is at least as good as other treatments for cervical dysplasia (Table 16.1) [1, 15]. Even when patients are reported to have positive margins on LEEP specimen or on endocervical curettage (ECC), most women are found to have no residual disease on follow-up evaluation. This may be due to additional tissue destruction via fulguration with electrocautery [3]. Importantly, for those women that do recur, literature suggests that a positive early HPV test (approximately 3 months after LEEP) is strongly predictive of residual or recurrent disease. This may be useful in the follow-up management of patients, particularly those with high-risk disease [16].

In a study by Saidi et al., operative variables of office-based LEEP procedures were compared with those for cold knife cones performed in the operating room. This study showed that LEEPs had significantly less blood loss (mean of 40 cm^3 vs. 195 cm^3), shorter operative time (mean of 5 min with a maximum of 8 min vs. a mean of 22 min), and less postoperative pain (all women undergoing cold knife cone required narcotic medications while women who underwent a LEEP required only naproxen). Furthermore, no patient undergoing a LEEP was hospitalized postoperatively, postoperative bleeding was significantly reduced, and the cost of the procedure was significantly less (mean $550 vs. $2520). These significant differences from the cold knife cone procedure make this a reasonable option for an office-based procedure, and in fact, during this study, the LEEP procedure was successfully moved from a hospital-based procedure to an office-based procedure [17].

Necessary Equipment (Table 16.2)

- Coated speculum
- Smoke evacuation system
- Large cotton swabs
- 3–5 % acetic acid solution and/or Lugol's solution
- Colposcope
- Lidocaine injection (see Table 16.3 for warnings) or spray
- LEEP machine with grounding pad and electrode
- Multi-sized loop electrodes and ball electrode
- Endocervical curettes
- Smooth forceps
- Monsel's solution
- Suture material
- Vaginal packing (such as Kerlex)

Table 16.2 LEEP equipment and procedure steps

Equipment	Steps of procedure
Coated speculum	Obtain patient consent
Smoke evacuation system	Position patient in dorsal lithotomy position and place return electrode
Large cotton swabs	Place speculum and maximize separation of vaginal walls
3–5 % acetic acid solution and/or Lugol's solution	Anesthetize cervix
Colposcope	Choose loop size and select power settings
Lidocaine injection or spray	Activate smoke evacuation system
LEEP machine with grounding pad and electrode	Perform ectocervical excision and orient specimen for pathology
Multi-sized loop electrodes and ball electrode	Change to smaller loop and perform endocervical excision (if indicated)
Endocervical curettes	Change to ball electrode and change settings on machine
Smooth forceps	Cauterize LEEP bed and edges of ectocervix
Monsel's solution	Apply Monsel's (as needed)
Suture material	Give discharge instructions
Vaginal packing (curlex)	

Table 16.3 Lidocaine injection warnings

Pain at injection site
Ringing in ears
Tingling at the tip of the tongue or funny taste in the mouth
Transient heart "racing"

Step by Step of the Procedure (Table 16.2)

Prior to the LEEP, the procedure must be explained including all risks and benefits, and consent should be signed. Additionally, a pregnancy test should be performed and confirmed to be negative, and the physician should ensure that the patient does not have any overt symptoms of vaginitis. If a pregnancy test returns positive, then the physician will need to reevaluate if the procedure is still indicated; if so, additional risks must be discussed with the patient. If the patient does have overt signs of vaginitis, she can be tested and treated, and LEEP can be rescheduled following treatment.

Once consent is signed and pregnancy test is confirmed negative, the procedure can be started. No prophylactic antibiotics are indicated for this procedure, regardless of valvular conditions or prosthetics. The patient is asked to move into the appropriate position, placing her feet into stirrups and lying back into the dorsal lithotomy position. Once positioned appropriately, with her buttocks hanging over the edge of the exam table, the coated speculum is inserted into the patient's vagina.

Next, the cervix is evaluated by colposcopy. Large cotton swabs are used to apply 3–5 % acetic acid solution and/or Lugol's solution to the cervix, and a colposcope is then used to visualize the cervix and identify any acetowhite changes or areas of nonstaining in patients evaluated with Lugol's. The squamocolumnar junction is also identified.

A local anesthetic may then be applied to the cervix. Lidocaine with epinephrine may be used to administer a paracervical block or lidocaine spray may be utilized. This can be performed either by injecting in 2 or 4 places on the cervix. We typically utilize a total of 3–5 mL of 2 % lidocaine with 1:100,000 epinephrine injected at 2, 4, 8, and 10 o'clock.

In order to perform the electro-excision procedure, a grounding pad must be placed on the patient's thigh and the appropriate loop electrode must be selected. The electrosurgical generator should be used in a blend mode (often 80 % cutting 20 % coagulation).

The loop is then carefully positioned close to the cervix. The LEEP may be performed in either a vertical or horizontal fashion. If, for example, the lesion is wide and narrow, it may be best to proceed from right to left (or left to right if the practitioner is left handed). If the lesion is more vertically aligned, then the practitioner can begin the LEEP at the 12 o'clock position on the cervix (at the uppermost part of the lesion) and carry the electrode down to the 6 o'clock position on the cervix.

Prior to touching the cervix, the loop electrode should be activated, and once activated, the energy should not be stopped until the loop electrode has exited the cervical tissue. A LEEP should therefore be performed in one continuous motion. Once activated, the loop should be moved directly into the cervix to the desired depth (Fig. 16.1). Once at the desired depth, the loop should be carried down or across the cervix (at the same depth) until the most distant desired area has been reached. Then the loop should be pulled directly out of the cervical tissue. The LEEP is then complete, and the specimen can be removed with a smooth forceps. An ECC should be performed after the removal of the specimen to ensure that there is no remaining lesion higher up in the endocervical canal.

The cervical bed should be carefully inspected to ensure that there is no bleeding from the site. A 3 or 5 mm ball attachment can be used to cauterize the crater and the edges of the lesion. Electrosurgical settings should be changed to cautery mode for this part of the procedure, and can be set on a range from 50 to 80 W. Pure coagulation mode should be utilized for hemostasis. Monsel's solution may alternatively be used on the cervix or can be used in addition to ball cautery as needed to achieve hemostasis and prevent posttreatment bleeding.

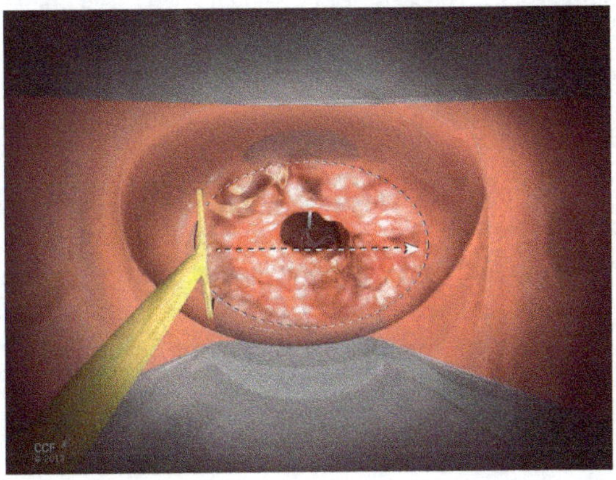

Fig. 16.1 Basic LEEP procedure. The loop electrode is moved steadily across the cervix, here right to left, to excise the abnormal region and transformation zone

Post-treatment Instructions for Patients

Patients are instructed to refrain from strenuous activity for 24–48 h and not to place anything in the vagina for 4 weeks. Tylenol or nonsteroidal anti-inflammatory medications are typically used for discomfort. Patients are instructed to call if heavy vaginal bleeding ensues or if a fever greater than 101.0 °F is noted, especially if related to increasing pelvic pain or vaginal drainage (Table 16.4).

"Tips and Tricks" Section for Troubleshooting

- If a "see and treat" approach is utilized, the limitations, including the possibility of missing a lesion in the canal, should be recognized. This approach is therefore best utilized when a clear lesion is visualized, and the boundaries of the lesion can clearly be identified colposcopically.
- A randomized controlled trial was performed by Paraskevaidis et al. which examined the

Table 16.4 Post-LEEP instructions

Refrain from strenuous activity for 24–48 h
Nothing in the vagina for 4 weeks
Tylenol or nonsteroidal anti-inflammatory medications for discomfort
Call the doctor's office for:
• Heavy vaginal bleeding
• Fever >101.0 °F
• Increasing pelvic pain
• Increasing vaginal discharge

timing of LEEP procedure based on the phase of a woman's menstrual cycle. This study found that women who were in the follicular phase of the cycle experienced significantly less bleeding than those women in the luteal phase of the cycle during the procedure. The mean drop in hematocrit for those women in the follicular phase of the cycle during the procedure was 0.9, whereas the mean drop for those women in the luteal phase was 3. This study therefore suggests that bleeding may be avoided by appropriately timing the procedure with the follicular phase of the women's menstrual cycle [18].

- If a patient is young and desires future fertility, risks specific to future pregnancies must be addressed. Evidence regarding the effect of LEEP on future pregnancy outcome remains controversial. Several large studies suggest that there is an approximately twofold increased risk of preterm delivery following LEEP, as well as an increased incidence of premature rupture of membranes (approximately threefold) [19]. While there are some studies that report no statistical difference in obstetric outcomes, physicians should counsel patients on the possible risks associated given the available data. Additionally, some studies have investigated if there are modifiable aspects of the procedure which may affect obstetric outcomes. In one large retrospective review cone height was found to be a significant predictor of increased risk of premature rupture of membranes. Increasing height of the specimen was associated with greater risk of adverse outcomes [20]. Therefore, if feasible, physicians should attempt to remove a shallow piece of tissue in patients wishing to preserve fertility.
- The size of the loop should be chosen based on the size of the lesion as well as the size of the cervix and the goal of the procedure (Fig. 16.2). Prior to performing a LEEP, the practitioner should have the results of an endocervical curettage (ECC) (performed with the initial colposcopy and biopsies). The pathologic results from this initial evaluation should also play a role in determining which areas on the cervix should be removed. If the patient has a positive ECC, then an additional LEEP specimen (often called a "top hat") can be performed after the initial LEEP to obtain tissue from deeper in the cervical canal (Fig. 16.3). A smaller, often rectangular loop is often selected to excise the endocervical specimen after the initial ectocervical LEEP has been performed.

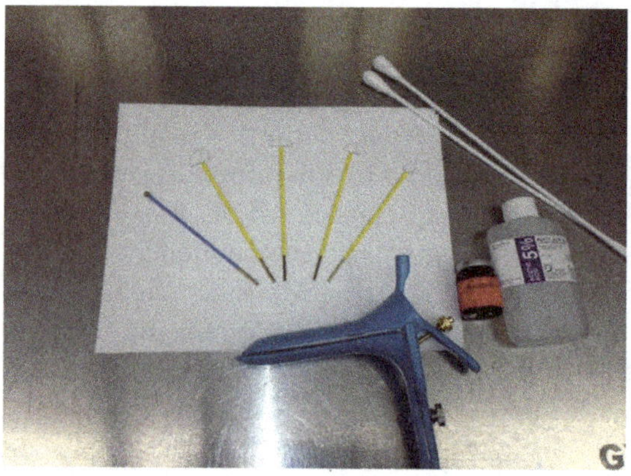

Fig. 16.2 Basic LEEP equipment. Various size loop electrodes, ball electrode, monsel's solution, 5 % acetic acid, large cotton swabs, coated speculum

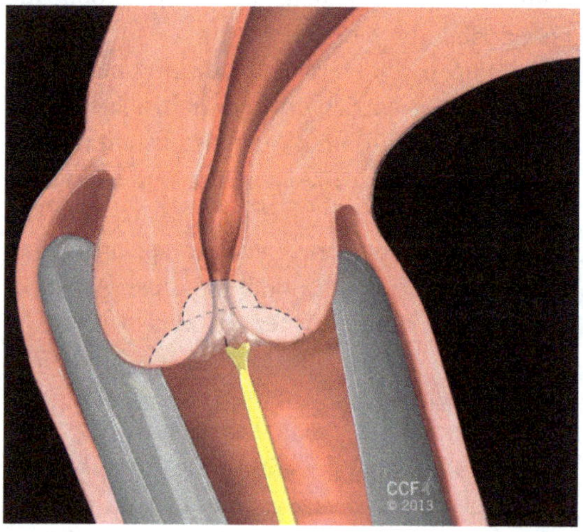

Fig. 16.3 "Tophat" LEEP, sagittal view. The initial ectocervical specimen is obtained with a larger loop followed by removal of an endocervical LEEP with a narrow (usually 1 cm × 1 cm) loop higher up the endocervical canal

- If a paracervical block is being administered, 1 % or 2 % lidocaine with 1:100,000 epinephrine can be utilized. The block is often performed in four quadrants of the cervix (the 2, 4, 8, and 10 o'clock positions) and is injected submucosally. A lidocaine spray can also be utilized as anesthetic and is administered by applying four puffs of 10 % lidocaine to the cervix prior to the procedure. One study that randomized 100 patients compared this spray to paracervical block found that patients who had a spray anesthetic reported significantly less pain than those who received an injection. This therefore may be a beneficial alternative for patients [21].
- The LEEP should ideally be performed in one smooth motion, as described above. This will allow for an optimal size specimen for histologic diagnosis, and will also allow maximum comfort for the patient. If a lesion is in two distinct locations or is too big to be excised as a single specimen, the practitioner should plan the best way to remove the desired tissue in two slightly overlapping segments.
- There are three options for performing a LEEP in women with an IUD. The first option is that the IUD can be removed if it is due to be changed or the patient no longer wants the IUD. Alternatively, the strings of the IUD can be tucked up into the endocervical canal for the procedure, and then be retrieved following the completion of the LEEP. Finally, a hollow plastic tube can be used to cover the strings during the procedure. Although this can at times be difficult to place appropriately, once the tube is protecting the strings, the LEEP can be easily performed around the tubing [22] (Fig. 16.4).
- Performing a LEEP on women with redundant vaginal tissue can be difficult, as the vaginal sidewalls need to remain away from the area of the cautery. Commercially available sidewall retractors, as well as large cotton swabs in the vaginal fornices may be helpful. Although condoms have been used to cover the speculum for colposcopy, caution should be taken to avoid fragmenting the condom with cautery if this technique is utilized.

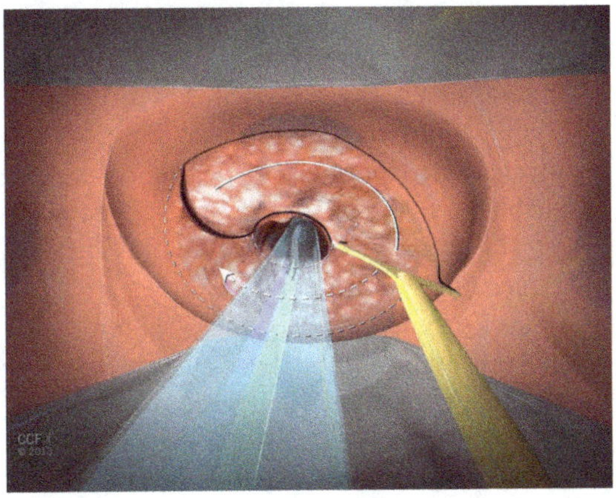

Fig. 16.4 Leep with IUD in place. IUD strings can be placed inside of a hollow plastic tube and LEEP is performed circumferentially around the tube

- All specimens should be oriented for pathologic evaluation. This can be done with either a suture, marking a specific position or with fixation to a solid media, such as paraffin, via colored needles.
- A bridge that sits across the loop electrode can be utilized to minimize the depth of the LEEP specimen excised. This is especially helpful for practitioners who are new to the procedure or for teaching facilities where a practitioner is not accustomed to recognizing the depth of the loop. This bridge prevents the practitioner from exceeding an absolute maximal depth when the loop is buried in the cervical tissue.
- In a randomized trial that compared ball electrocautery to Monsel's solution for hemostasis, the time to hemostasis was statistically significantly shorter for the group of women who received Monsel's solution (90 s vs. 131 s), women reported less pain, and half as many women required alternate means of hemostasis. While these values were all statistically significant, the distinction in the values may not have clinical significance as time to hemostasis was less than 3 min and there was not significant pain with either method [23]. A different randomized trial examined the

benefit of Monsel's solution in addition to electrocautery for hemostasis. This study found that the incidence of severe complications were similar for those women who had electrocautery alone and those who had both electrocautery and Monsel's solution applied to the cervix. However, the duration of bleeding was shorter for women who had Monsel's solution applied [24]. Therefore, the information from these two randomized trials suggests that either ball electrocautery or Monsel's solution can be used to achieve hemostasis, and both may be utilized if bleeding continues after one or the other.

- Suture and packing material should always be available in the office setting in the event of arterial or uncontrolled bleeding. Although hemorrhage is a rare event following a LEEP procedure, having suture available can at times allow for cessation of bleeding; if this does not control the bleeding, then hemostatic agents such as surgical sealant or other local acting hemostasis agents can be considered in addition to packing material. This can be used either to allow pressure over time or to transfer to an operating room for further surgical intervention. If packing is required, a foley catheter should be placed prior to performing packing; Kerlex should then be packed firmly into the vagina with the end of the packing visible at the introitus. If more than one Kerlex is required, the two Kerlex should be tied in a knot so that when removed, all packing material comes out together.

Immediate (Procedural) and Short-term Complications

The most frequent immediate or short-term complication of a LEEP is bleeding, which may occur at the time of the procedure or up to 2 weeks postoperatively [2]. In a large retrospective review of 857 women undergoing a LEEP, 3.4 % of women were found to have bleeding at the time of the procedure, 0.6 % of women experienced bleeding within the first 24 h, and 4.9 % of women experienced bleeding after 24 h but less than 2 weeks following the procedure. The size of the LEEP specimen was predictive of perioperative complications [25].

In the study by Wright et al., bleeding occurred in less than 2 % of patients, on average approximately 4–5 days following the procedure [1]. Similarly, in a larger study by Ferenczy et al., bleeding occurred in approximately 3.5 % of patients with most (2.5 %) occurring at the time of the procedure and was able to be controlled with electrocautery and Monsel's solution with the exception of a single patient who required further intervention [2]. In a study by Lipscomb et al., even in patients with invasive cervical carcinoma diagnosed in the LEEP specimen, studies suggest that rates of both intraoperative and postoperative bleeding were comparable to those women without invasive disease [24].

Post-procedural infection is also a rare but important complication. Studies suggest that this occurs in less than 1 % of patients and can be effectively treated with postoperative antibiotics once diagnosed. Similarly, cervical stenosis is a rare complication that also occurs in approximately 1 % of patients and rarely causes symptoms [2].

Post-treatment Recommendations

Following a LEEP procedure, patients should receive instruction to call their physician for bleeding, fever, or purulent discharge. Patients should then be instructed to return to their physician approximately 2–4 weeks later for an examination of the cervix. At that time, the physician should gently perform a speculum examination to ensure that the cervix is healing well.

In order to monitor patients for persistent or recurrent disease, patients should return for screening 6 months following their procedure. Both cytology and HR-HPV testing should be performed at this time. Studies suggest that HR-HPV testing at 6 months is highly predictive of persistent or recurrent disease with a sensitivity of approximately 90 %, whereas cytology has a sensitivity of only 70 %. However, when cytology and HPV are both performed, studies suggest that there is only a 4.6 % risk of recurrence if both are negative at 6 months, and if both tests continue to be negative 24 months after LEEP, the risk of recurrence is as low as 1.8 %. If either cytology or HPV is positive 6 months after a LEEP procedure, there is a 45–60 % risk of recurrence for cervical dysplasia [26].

Conclusion

Use of LEEP in the office is simple to perform and has clear advantages when performed as an office-based procedure rather than performed in the operating theater. Evaluation of cervix tissue to allow for pathologic evaluation and subsequent treatment is a mainstay of the procedure and it is straightforward with few complications.

References

1. Wright TC, Gagnon S, Richart R, Ferenczy A. Treatment of cervical intraepithelial neoplasia using the loop electrosurgical excision procedure. Obstet Gynecol. 1992;79(2):173–7.
2. Ferenczy A, Choukroun D, Arseneau J. Loop electrosurgical excision procedure for squamous intraepithelial lesions of the cervix: advantages and potential pitfalls. Obstet Gynecol. 1996;87(3):332–7.
3. Richart RM, Wright TC. Outpatient surgery in gynecologic oncology. Curr Opin Obstet Gynecol. 1993;5:318–21.
4. Ferenczy A. Management of the patient with an abnormal Pap smear. In: Balloon SC, editor. Gynecologic oncology. Controversies in cancer treatment. Boston: GK Hall Medical Publishers; 1981. p. 137–47.
5. Cartier R. Practical colposcopy. 2nd ed. Paris: Laboratorie Cartier; 1984. p. 139–56.
6. Prendiville W, Cullimoore NS. Large loop excision of the transformation zone (LLETZ): a new method of management for women with cervical intraepithelial neoplasia. Br J Obstet Gynaecol. 1989;96:1054–60.
7. Pretorius RG, Belinson JL, Burchette RJ, Hu S, Zhang X, Qiao YL. Regardless of skill, performing more biopsies increases the sensitivity of colposcopy. J Low Genit Tract Dis. 2011;15(3):180–8.
8. Buxton EJ, Luesley DM, Shafi JI, Rollason M. Colposcopically directed punch biopsy: a potentially misleading investigation. Br J Obstet Gynaecol. 1991;98:1273–6.
9. Chappatte OA, Byrne DL, Raju KS, Nayagam M, Kenney A. Histological differences between colposcopic-directed biopsy and loop excision of the transformation zone (LLETZ): a cause for concern. Gynecol Oncol. 1991;43:46–50.
10. Mathevet P, Chemali E, Roy M, Dargent D. Long-term outcome of a randomized study comparing three techniques of conization: cold knife, laser, and LEEP. Eur J Obstet Gynecol Reprod Biol. 2003;106 (2):214–8.
11. Mitchell MF, Tortolero-Luna G, Cook E, Whittaker L, Rhodes-Morris H, Silva E. A randomized clinical trial of cryotherapy, laser vaporization, and loop electrosurgical excision for treatment of squamous intraepithelial lesions of the cervix. Obstet Gynecol. 1998;92(5):737–44.
12. Alvarez RD, Helm CW, Edwards RP, Naumann RW, Partridge EE, Shingleton HM, et al. Prospective randomized trial of LLETZ versus laser ablation in patients with cervical intraepithelial neoplasia. Gynecol Oncol. 1994;52:175–9.
13. Singh A, Arthur B, Agarwal V. LEEP versus cryotherapy in CIN. J Obstet Gynaecol India. 2011;61 (4):431–5.
14. Chirenje ZM, Ruskaniko S, Akino V, Mlingo M. A randomized clinical trial of loop electrosurgical excision procedure (LEEP) versus cryotherapy in the treatment of cervical intraepithelial neoplasia. J Obstet Gynaecol. 2001;21(6):617–21.
15. Mathevet P, Chemali E, Roy M, Dargent D. Long-term outcome of a randomized study comparing three techniques of conization: cold knife, laser, and LEEP. Eur J Obstet Gynecol Reprod Biol. 2003;106(2):214–8.
16. Ryu A, Nam K, Kwak J, Kim J, Jeon S. Early human papillomavirus testing predicts residual/recurrent disease after LEEP. J Gynecol Oncol. 2012;23 (4):217–25.
17. Saidi MH, Setzer FD, Sadler K, Farhart S, Akright BD. Comparison of office loop electrosurgical conization and cold knife conization. J Am Assoc Gynecol Laparosc. 1994;1(2):135–9.
18. Paraskevaidis E, Davidson EJ, Koliopoulos G, Alamanos Y, Lolis E, Martin-Hirsch P. Bleeding after loop electrosurgical excision procedure performed in either the follicular or luteal phase of the menstrual cycle: a randomized trial. Obstet Gynecol. 2002;99 (6):997–1000.
19. Bevis KS, Biggio JR. Cervical conization and the risk of preterm delivery. Am J Obstet Gynecol. 2011;205 (1):19–27.
20. Sadler L, Saftlas A, Wang W, Exeter M, Whittaker J, McCowan L. Treatment for cervical intraepithelial neoplasia and risk of preterm delivery. JAMA. 2004;291(17):2100–6.
21. Vanichtantikul A, Charoenkwan K. Lidocaine spray compared with submucosal injection for reducing pain during electrosurgical excision procedure: a randomized controlled trial. Obstet Gynecol. 2013;122(3):553–7.

22. Bailey AP, Darracott MM. Loop electrosurgical excision procedure with an intrauterine device in place. Am J Obstet Gynecol. 2010;203(3):291.e1–3.
23. Lipscomb GH, Roberts KA, Givens VM, Robbins D. A trial that compares Monsel's paste with ball electrode for hemostasis after loop electrosurgical excision procedure. Am J Obstet Gynecol. 2006;194:1591–5.
24. Kietpeerakool C, Srisomboon J, Suprasert P, Cheewakriangkrai C, Charoenkwan K, Siriaree S. Routine prophylactic application of Monsel's solution after loop electrosurgical excision procedure of the cervix: is it necessary? J Obstet Gynaecol. 2007;33(3):299–304.
25. Sutthichon P, Kietpeerakool C. Perioperative complications of an outpatient loop electrosurgical excision procedure: a review of 857 consecutive cases. Asian Pac J Cancer Prev. 2009;10(3):351–4.
26. Kocken M, Helmerhorst TJ, Berkhof J, Louwers JA, Nobbenhuis MA, Bais AG, Hogewoning CJ, Zaal A, Verheijen RH, Snijders PJ, Meijer CJ. Risk of recurrent high-grade cervical intraepithelial neoplasia after successful treatment: a long-term multi-cohort study. Lancet Oncol. 2011;12(5):441–50.

Vulvar Biopsy and Excision/Ablation 17

Sarah Goodrich and Mehdi Kebria

Vulvar Colposcopy and Toluidine Blue Examination

Introduction

Vulvar colposcopy is indicated in several situations. These include to further evaluate visible lesions, or to look for abnormalities when symptoms or testing suggest possible vulvar pathology in the absence of a visible vulvar lesion. For example, colposcopy is warranted in the cases of abnormal cervical cytology with no visible cervical or vaginal findings and in cases of subjective vulvar irritation without gross lesions.

Necessary Equipment

Equipment and materials needed for vulvar colposcopy include:
- 3–5 % Acetic acid
- Gauze pads
- Colposcope

S. Goodrich, M.D. (✉)
Department of Gynecologic Oncology, Cleveland Clinic, 9500 Euclid Avenue, Desk A-81, Cleveland, OH 44195, USA
e-mail: goodris@ccf.org

M. Kebria, M.D.
Department of Obstetrics and Gynecology, Cleveland Clinic, 9500 Euclid Avenue, Desk A-81, Cleveland, OH 44195, USA
e-mail: kebriam@ccf.org

Equipment needed for blue examination includes:
- 1 % Toluidine Blue
- 1 % Acetic acid
- Gauze pads

Procedure

The patient is placed on the examination table in stirrups. Gauze pads are then soaked in acetic acid and placed over the vulva, being certain to adequately cover the interlabial folds and periurethral and perianal areas. The saturated gauze pads should be held to the vulva for a period of 3–5 min to allow the acetic acid to take effect. First, an unaided visual inspection can be carried out and any acetowhite areas noted. Next, the colposcope is used to perform a magnified examination of the vulvar epithelium. Inspection should be performed in an ordered, systematic fashion so as to examine all areas of the vulva. Examination should begin on low magnification, and then higher magnification can be used to look for abnormal vascular patterns. Using the green filter can further help identify abnormal vascular patterns in lesions. Any suspicious areas should be noted and plans made for biopsy.

Additionally, the vulva can be painted with toluidine blue (1 %) and then washed off with acetic acid (1 %) after 2 min. In general, abnormal areas will remain dyed blue and should then be biopsied. In one study, the toluidine blue test

J.D. Emery and M.F.R. Paraiso (eds.), *Office-Based Gynecologic Surgical Procedures*,
DOI 10.1007/978-1-4939-1414-2_17, © Springer Science+Business Media New York 2015

had 92 % sensitivity, 88 % specificity, and 96 % negative predictive value for differentiating Vulvar Intraepithelial Neoplasia (VIN) from nonneoplastic vulvar lesions [1].

Tips and Tricks

- If a colposcope is not available, a magnifying glass can be used.
- Lesions of VIN are typically found in non-hair baring areas of the vulva (87.6 %), and tend to be multifocal (56.6 % of patients) [2].
- The toluidine blue test can be falsely negative in conditions that make the epithelium less able to take up dye—such as severely thickened or ulcerated epithelium. Thus, a negative test in an area with a visible lesion does not rule out the need for biopsy.

Complications

Colposcopy and toluidine blue test of the vulva are well tolerated and are without any significant complications. Patient discomfort is related mostly to positioning and psychological distress.

Vulvar Biopsy and Excision

Introduction

Vulvar biopsy is warranted if an abnormality is noted on examination of the vulva, either unaided visualization or on colposcopic or toluidine blue aided exam. Some characteristics that increase the suspicion of a lesion for malignancy include: asymmetry, irregular borders or color, bleeding, non-healing, changes in the lesion over time, or non-response to treatment (Table 17.1).

Biopsy may be performed via punch or excision. If the lesion is <4 mm in size or if ulcerated, it should be completely excised. If the lesion is larger, the biopsy should be taken from the area that has the most abnormal features. If there are multiple abnormal lesions noted on the vulva, then multiple biopsies should be taken.

Table 17.1 Indications for vulvar biopsy

Subjective persistent irritation or other local symptoms with no gross lesions
Persistent lesion despite standard therapy (i.e., unresolved candidiasis)
Lesions with any of the following features: asymmetrical, irregular border, color variation, rapidly changing lesion, bleeding or non-healing lesion
Vulvar ulceration (non-herpetic)
Pigmented vulvar lesions (i.e., melanoma)
Exophytic growths (i.e., condyloma, acrochordon)
Vulvar dysplasia/VIN

Necessary Equipment

- Sterile gloves
- Skin antiseptic
- Skin marker
- Local anesthetic (1 or 2 % lidocaine with or without epinephrine)
- 30-gauge needle
- Syringe
- Keyes punch (2–5 mm) or scalpel (15-blade)
- Forceps
- Iris scissors
- Gauze pads
- Needle holder
- Small diameter absorbable suture, preferably monofilament
- Silver nitrate
- Items needed for pathology (specimen cup, requisition)

Step by Step of the Procedure

As with any procedure, the first step should involve discussing the steps and rationale for the procedure with the patient and obtaining informed consent. The patient should then be placed in a comfortable position that allows exposure of the area in question, typically in stirrups on the examination table.

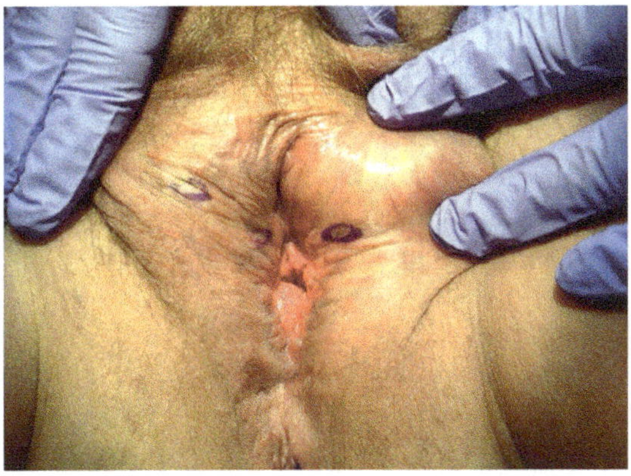

Fig. 17.1 Example of antiseptic cleansing and marking identifiable vulvar lesions to be biopsied

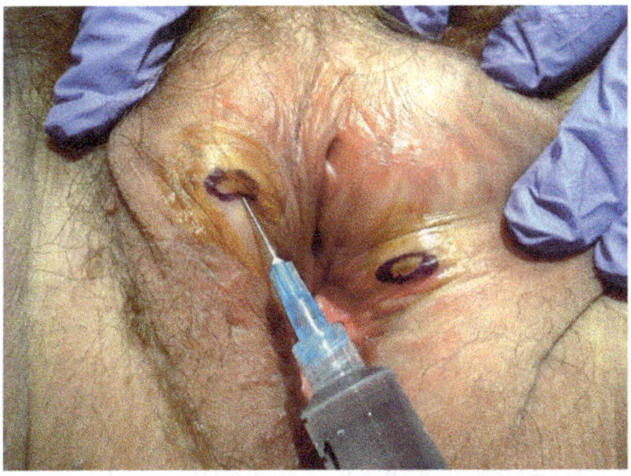

Fig. 17.2 Infiltrating local anesthesia into the dermis below the vulvar lesion for local anesthetic

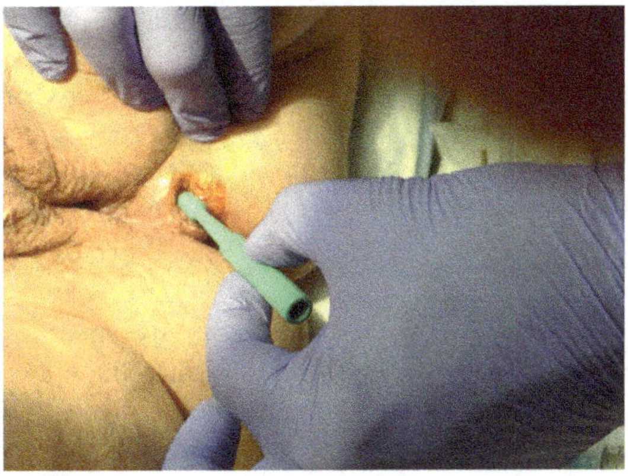

Fig. 17.3 Use of a Keyes punch biopsy to remove a vulvar lesion

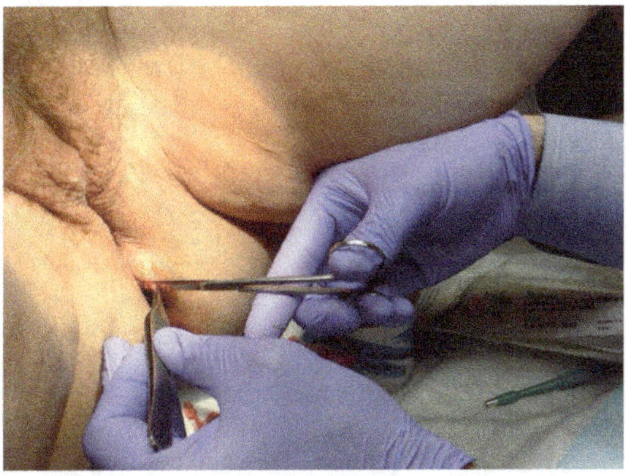

Fig. 17.4 Complete excision of tissue from subdermal layer after use of Keyes punch biopsy

The lesion should be examined and the type of biopsy (punch or excisional) planned. The vulvar skin should be cleansed with antiseptic solution and the site of biopsy marked with a marking pen (Fig. 17.1). Local anesthetic should then be infiltrated into the dermis underlying the lesion, being certain to infiltrate the subcutaneous tissues surrounding the entire area to be excised (Fig. 17.2) Next the biopsy will be performed—either punch or excisional.

If performing a punch biopsy, the most abnormal appearing area should be biopsied. The 2 mm punch biopsy is usually of sufficient size to produce an accurate histologic diagnosis [3]. The skin surrounding the lesion should be placed on stretch and the punch placed perpendicular to the skin over the area to be biopsied (Fig. 17.3) Pressure is applied and the device is twisted until the subcutaneous tissues have been entered. Forceps are then used to elevate the core of tissue and iris scissors are used to transect the base of the specimen (Fig. 17.4) The specimen is then placed in the container to be sent to pathology. Pressure is applied to the wound with gauze pads. Hemostasis can be obtained with pressure or with the use of silver nitrate sticks. If a 3 mm or smaller punch was used, then skin closure is typically not required. If a larger biopsy punch was used, then simple sutures should be placed to reapproximate the skin edges to result in improved patient satisfaction of cosmesis [4].

Excisions are performed if the entire lesion needs to be removed. Langer's lines of skin tension should be identified and the long axis of excision should parallel these lines. Using a 15-blade, an elliptical excision is made around the lesion to be removed. The elliptical excision allows for easier and more cosmetic skin closure. Next, the superior edge of the specimen is grasped with forceps and the specimen is removed from the subcutaneous fat using either the blade or iris scissors. Hold pressure to the skin with gauze pads and place the specimen in the specimen cup. Prior to placing the specimen in the cup, while the specimen is still in anatomic orientation, the superior edge of the specimen can be tagged with a suture to aid the pathologist in reporting margin status. Simple interrupted sutures of a small suture diameter are then used to reapproximate the skin edges.

"Tips and Tricks" Section for Troubleshooting

- Marking the lesion prior to infiltration of anesthetic can help with identification, as injection can change skin contours and make it difficult to identify the area to be excised/biopsied if the lesion is nonpigmented.
- Langer's lines can be identified by gently pinching the skin between the thumb and index finger. Incisions should be placed parallel to these lines for improved cosmesis.
- Using a smaller gauge needle will cause less discomfort to the patient.
- Smaller syringes allow for easier infiltration of local anesthetic.
- After infiltrating the skin with local anesthetic but before proceeding with biopsy, use the needle or forceps to test the adequacy of the patient's anesthesia.
- Punch biopsy instruments are available in sizes from 2 to 10 mm, but typically if using a punch greater than 3 mm a suture will be required to close the excisional site.
- Starting suturing in the middle of the wound and working in either direction can avoid the production of "dog ears" of the wound.

Post-procedure Care

The surgical wound should be kept moist and covered to aid in healing [5]. Applying an ointment to the wound can serve this role, and either petrolatum ointment or an antibiotic ointment, such as bacitracin, may be used for this purpose. One study showed that these two agents had similar results in terms of infection rates, but there was less contact dermatitis with the petrolatum ointment [6]. Sutures can then be removed in 7–10 days, which also gives the physician the opportunity to follow the patient's progress and review pathology reports.

Immediate (Procedural) and Short-Term Complications

As with most surgical procedures, the major complications of vulvar biopsy or excision include pain, bleeding, and infection.

Bleeding during or immediately following the procedure can be controlled with pressure, suture, or with hemostatic agents such as silver nitrate. The risk of hematoma formation can be reduced by the use of pressure dressing and with the application of ice, which also decreases pain [7].

Patients should be instructed to notify the physician's office if the wound becomes erythematous or has purulent discharge. If a cellulitis is noted, oral antibiotics should be initiated and the wound followed. Empiric coverage for streptococcus and staphylococcus should be chosen. If there is concern for methicillin-resistant Staphylococcus aureus (MRSA), cultures should be taken and antibiotic therapy tailored accordingly.

Treatment of Genital Condylomata

Introduction

Vulvar warts are a cutaneous manifestation of infection with the human papillomavirus (HPV). Patients will often seek treatment for removal of these warts due to cosmetic concerns or symptoms (bleeding, pain, or itching). Left untreated, genital warts may regress, increase in size or number, or remain unchanged. It is important that the patient understands that even if visible warts are removed, recurrence is common and thus treatment may be needed again in the future. While there are topical treatments that patients may utilize in their own homes, this section will focus on physician-delivered treatments. Office-based treatments, as opposed to more extensive procedures in the operating room, are typically appropriate for patients with a limited number of warts (≤ 5) of small size [8]. In-office excisional therapy for genital warts follows the same principles as noted above for excising other vulvar lesions. Options for in-office destructive therapy are discussed in the sections below.

Trichloroacetic Acid 80–90 %

Mechanism of action is chemical coagulation of the tissue. This should not be used for lesions that are excessively thick, as the acid may not be able to fully penetrate the lesion. A study comparing trichloroacetic acid (TCA) to cryotherapy noted a 70 % complete clearance rate for cryotherapy, but a 30 % rate of tissue ulceration [9].

Necessary Equipment

- Petroleum jelly or other barrier ointment (optional)
- Small cotton swabs
- TCA (80–90 %)
- Sodium bicarbonate

Step by Step of Procedure

The patient is positioned and the area to be treated is identified. Optionally, the normal skin surrounding the lesion can be coated with a layer of petroleum jelly or another barrier cream. A cotton swab is dipped into the container of TCA and a small amount of TCA then painted onto the lesion. This is repeated until the entire lesion turns white, indicating the solution has dried. This is repeated for all lesions. The patient should not change position or dress until all treatment areas have dried, to avoid contact of normal skin with the acid. The patient will have to return weekly for 6 weeks or until all lesions have resolved.

"Tips and Tricks" Section for Troubleshooting

- Applying a barrier ointment to normal tissues around the warts can prevent unintentional damage to surrounding normal skin
- Excess TCA can be neutralized by washing the area with sodium bicarbonate

Post-procedure Care

- Over the counter pain medication is sufficient
- Loose clothing should be worn
- Keeping the area clean and dry can promote wound healing and prevent infection

Immediate (Procedural) and Short-Term Complications

Pain during and following treatment is a potential complaint. TCA, which is a caustic agent, may result in skin ulceration and chemical burns to healthy tissue near the treatment site. This can result in scarring of the tissues.

Cryotherapy

Cryotherapy is an office procedure that can be used for patients with several lesions. It works by causing lysis of cells. There is discomfort associated with this procedure, and so use of local anesthetic may enhance patient comfort. The study noted above comparing cryotherapy to TCA found that cryotherapy was more successful, with an 86 % complete clearance rate [9].

Necessary Equipment

- 1 % lidocaine (with or without epinephrine; syringe, small gauge needle) (Optional)
- Small cotton swabs
- Liquid nitrogen
- Container for liquid nitrogen

Step by Step of Procedure

The patient is positioned and the area to be treated is identified. A cotton swab is dipped into the container of liquid nitrogen and the swab then placed in contact with the lesion. The swab should remain in contact with the lesion until the entire wart and a 1–2 mm rim of surrounding tissue is enveloped by an ice ball. This is repeated for all lesions. The patient will have to return weekly until all lesions have resolved.

"Tips and Tricks" Section for Troubleshooting

- Avoid over or undertreating with cryotherapy
- Have local anesthetic ready in case the patient is unable to tolerate treatment

Post-procedure Care

- Over the counter pain medication is sufficient
- Loose clothing should be worn
- Keeping the area clean and dry can promote wound healing and prevent infection

Immediate (Procedural) and Short-Term Complications

Each of these modalities is associated with pain or discomfort during or following the treatment. Additionally, excisional procedures carry the risks of bleeding and infection, and long-term complications such as scarring. Further, ablative therapies (such as cryotherapy) may result in permanent changes in skin pigmentation. TCA, which is a caustic agent, may result in skin ulceration and chemical burns to healthy tissue near the treatment site.

Podophyllum Resin 10 or 25 % Solution

Podophyllum resin is a plant base compound and contains antimitotic and mutagenic agents, it is not safe for use during pregnancy [8]. It is available as a 10 % or 25 % solution in a tincture of benzoin.

Necessary Equipment

- Podophyllum Resin 10 or 25 % solution (no more than 0.5 mL total)
- Container
- Small cotton swabs

Step by Step of Procedure

The patient is positioned and the area to be treated is identified. A cotton swab is dipped into the container of podophyllum resin and the solution applied to the lesion. This is repeated for all lesions. Because there is the potential for systemic absorption, and the compound is mutagenic, this treatment is only appropriate for small warts. The patient will have to return weekly until all lesions have resolved.

"Tips and Tricks" Section for Troubleshooting

- Do not treat large areas due to potential for systemic absorption
- If large areas must be treated, use a weaker (10 %) solution
- Do not apply to open wounds

Post-procedure Care

- The patient should wash the vulva 1–4 h after application to help avoid absorption and excessive irritation

– Over the counter pain medication is sufficient
– Loose clothing should be worn
– Keeping the area clean and dry can promote wound healing and prevent infection

Immediate (Procedural) and Short-Term Complications

Complications may include mild skin irritation. However, if large amounts of podophyllum are used or if prolonged skin contact occurs, severe pain and ulceration may result.

Excision

Excision of vulvar warts follows the same principles as excision of other lesions, as noted in an earlier section of the chapter. Excision may be considered if a patient has failed medical therapy. Alternatively, if a patient has numerable or large lesions, excision may be considered as the first-line treatment. However, in this case, lesions are typically so extensive as to necessitate treatment in the operating room for patient comfort.

Conclusion

Many dermatoses can affect the vulva. Thankfully, there are a number of diagnostic and treatment methods that can be employed in the office to aid the practitioner in managing these conditions. Regarding the treatment of vulvar warts, the treatment method selected should be based on the number and size of warts and a discussion with the patient of the risks and benefits of each treatment.

References

1. Joura EA, Zeisler H, Losch A, Sator MO, Mullauer-Ertl S. Differentiating vulvar intraepithelial neoplasia from nonneoplastic epithelial disorders. The toluidine blue test. J Reprod Med. 1998;43(8):671–4.
2. Rodolakis A, Diakomanolis E, Vlachos G, Iconomou T, Protopappas A, Stefanidis C, et al. Vulvar intraepithelial neoplasia (VIN)–diagnostic and therapeutic challenges. Eur J Gynaecol Oncol. 2003;24 (3–4):317–22.
3. Todd P, Garioch JJ, Humphreys S, Seywright M, Thomson J, du Vivier AW. Evaluation of the 2-mm punch biopsy in dermatological diagnosis. Clin Exp Dermatol. 1996;21(1):11–3.
4. Christenson LJ, Phillips PK, Weaver AL, Otley CC. Primary closure vs second-intention treatment of skin punch biopsy sites: a randomized trial. Arch Dermatol. 2005;141(9):1093–9.
5. Hinman CD, Maibach H. Effect of air exposure and occlusion on experimental human skin wounds. Nature. 1963;26(200):377–8.
6. Smack DP, Harrington AC, Dunn C, Howard RS, Szkutnik AJ, Krivda SJ, et al. Infection and allergy incidence in ambulatory surgery patients using white petrolatum vs bacitracin ointment. A randomized controlled trial. JAMA. 1996;276(12):972–7.
7. Telfer NR, Moy RL. Wound care after office procedures. J Dermatol Surg Oncol. 1993;19 (8):722–31.
8. Beutner KR, Reitano MV, Richwald GA, Wiley DJ. External genital warts: report of the American Medical Association Consensus Conference. AMA Expert Panel on External Genital Warts. Clin Infect Dis. 1998;27(4):796–806.
9. Abdullah AN, Walzman M, Wade A. Treatment of external genital warts comparing cryotherapy (liquid nitrogen) and trichloroacetic acid. Sex Transm Dis. 1993;20(6):344–5.

Index

A
Abdominal leak point pressure (ALPP)
  description, 155
  multichannel cystometry, 156
  patient evaluation, 157
  SUI and urethral hypermobility, 155
Abnormal transvaginal ultrasound, 89–90
Abnormal uterine bleeding (AUB)
  definition, 133
  determination, 134
  endometriosis and, 133
  fibroids, 125
  office hysteroscopy, 85–86
  perimenopausal women, 118
  pre and postmenopausal women, 71
  SIS, 75
Aceto-white epithelium (AWE)
  biopsies, 203–204
  description, 203
  low grade lesions, 203, 204
  subtypes, HPV, 196–197
ACLS. *See* Advanced cardiovascular life support (ACLS)
ACOG. *See* The American College of Obstetrics and Gynecology (ACOG)
Advanced cardiovascular life support (ACLS), 15
AIUM. *See* American Institute of Ultrasonography in Medicine (AIUM) guidelines
ALPP. *See* Abdominal leak point pressure (ALPP)
AMA. *See* American Medical Association (AMA)
Ambulatory procedures
  by facility type, 1, 2
  and operating room (OR) setting, 46
  surgery visits and hospital inpatients with procedures, 1, 2
  unrecognized pregnancy, 5
Ambulatory surgery center (ASC)
  anesthesia and analgesia, 13, 46
  diagnostic hysteroscopy, 98
  hysteroscopic procedure, 109
  in-office gynecologic surgical procedures, 102–104, 109
  postmenopausal bleeding, 89
  sterilization, 103
The American College of Obstetrics and Gynecology (ACOG), 16, 21, 104, 109, 195
American Institute of Ultrasonography in Medicine (AIUM) guidelines, 11, 81
American Medical Association (AMA), 16
American Urological Association (AUA) guidelines, 168
Analgesia. *See* Anesthesia
Anesthesia.*See also* Office gynecological proceduresdescription, 13
  guidelines for sedation, 13
  medications, 14–15
  operative hysteroscopy, 121
  procedure, 13
Asherman's syndrome, 72, 77
AUA. *See* American Urological Association (AUA) guidelines
AUB. *See* Abnormal uterine bleeding (AUB)
AWE. *See* Aceto-white epithelium (AWE)

B
Bartholin abscess. *See* Bartholin gland cyst
Bartholin gland cyst
  antibiotic treatment, 60
  differential diagnosis, 60
  and duct, 59
  I&D (*see* Incision and drainage (I&D))
  marsupialization, 65–67
  peri-procedural complications, 67
  procedure checklist, 64, 65
Basic life support (BLS), 15
Botulinum toxin
  anaerobic gram-positive bacterium *Clostridium botulinum*, 180
  trigger point injections (*see* Trigger point injections)

C
Calcium hydroxylapatite. *See* Coaptite
Carbon beads. *See* Durasphere
Cervical cancer
  colposcopy (*see* Colposcopy)
  description, 191
  human papilloma virus (HPV) infection, 191, 192
  late term pregnancy, 195
  malignant cells dissemination, 90
  Shanxi province screening, 196

J.D. Emery and M.F.R. Paraiso (eds.), *Office-Based Gynecologic Surgical Procedures*, DOI 10.1007/978-1-4939-1414-2, © Springer Science+Business Media New York 2015

Cervical cytology
colposcopy, 195
precursor lesions CIN-1-3, 193
screening programs, 191
Cervical intraepithelial neoplasia (CIN), 211
Cervical intraepithelial neoplasia 1 (CIN-1)
colposcopic directed biopsy, 197
endocervical curettage, 201
low grade dysplasia, 193
Cervical intraepithelial neoplasia-2-3 (CIN-2-3), 193, 196, 197
Chronic pelvic pain
in clinical practice, 179
diagnosis and treatment, 179
management, 179
trigger point injections (*see* Trigger point injections)
CIN. *See* Cervical intraepithelial neoplasia (CIN)
CIN-1. *See* Cervical intraepithelial neoplasia 1 (CIN-1)
CIN-2-3. *See* Cervical intraepithelial neoplasia-2-3 (CIN-2-3)
Coaptite
adverse events, 167
calcium hydroxylapatite, 166
description, 166
injections, 167
Coaptite® Injectable Implant Procedure Guide
attached with injection syringe, 172
end injection needle, 171
injection, 172
needle placement, 172
sidekick needle, 171
Colposcopy
anatomy, 192
ASCCP application, smartphone and tablets, 192, 193
beam splitters, 198
The Bethesda system, 192
coaxial light source, 198
findings, 203–205
high and low grade lesions, 192
HPV infection and cervical cancer, 192–193
in-office procedure (*see* In-office procedure)
instruments and supplies, 198
instrument trays, 198, 199
low grade cytologic abnormalities, 191
pap smear, 198
precursor lesions CIN-1-3, 193
procedure, 193–194, 199–203
risk factors, 198
screening instrument, cervical cancer, 191
spot urine pregnancy test, 199
swing-arm, 197
terminology, 202
TZ and abnormal-appearing lesions, 193
vaginal, 205
vulvar, 205–206
Condyloma. *See* Genital condylomata
Cryoablation, 134, 135, 138
Cryotherapy
description, 211, 225
equipment, 226
post-procedure care, 226
procedural and short-term complications, 226
Cystometry
detrusor overactivity, 151, 152
ICI guidelines, 151
procedure, 151
single/multiple catheters, 150–151
variations, 150
volume and pressure, filling, 150
Cystoscopy
air bubble, 146–147
bladder evaluation, 146
blunt obturator, 146
consent, 146
continued device progression, 144
cooling system, 143
distending media, 146
flexible cystoscopes, 144–145
illumination, 145
in-office, 144
left ureteral orifice, 146–147
mignon bulb, 143
post procedural complications, 148
potential device malfunctions, 147–148
right ureteral orifice, 146–147
rigid cystoscope, 144–145
types, 144
urethral dilation, 146–147
variations/developments, 143

D

Detrusor leak point pressure (DLPP), 155
Diagnostic hysteroscopy
abnormal transvaginal ultrasound, 89–90
advantages, 92
bleeding, 98
cervical trauma and false passage creation, 97
contraindications, 90–91
dilatation and curettage (D&C), 87–88
distention media associated, 98
equipment and office setup
diaphragmatic irritation, 94
distention media, management and utilization, 94
initial decision, 93
saline, 93–94
surgeon preference, 93
fiberoptics, 91
FIGO classification system, 85
hysterosalpingography (HSG), 85, 87
hysteroscopically endometrial polyps, 89
hysteroscopic procedure, 94–96
in vitro fertilization (IVF), 87
indications, 85–87
intrauterine device (IUD), 90
Karl Storz rigid hysteroscope, 91–92
levonorgestrel releasing IUD (LNG-IUD), 90
Lippes loop, 90
operative hysteroscopies, 96–97

pain, 97
PALM-COEIN basic classification system, 85, 87, 133
patient preparation, 92–93
pulmonary edema and congestive heart failure, 98
reproduction abnormalities, 85–86
rigid and flexible, 91–92
"space-occupying lesion", 90
submucosal leiomyomata, hysteroscopic resection, 89
tamoxifen, 89
uterine cavity inspection, 87
uterine fibroid embolization (UFE), 88
uterine perforation, 97
vasovagal episode, 97
video monitoring, 91
Dilatation and curettage (D&C), 87–88
DLPP. *See* Detrusor leak point pressure (DLPP)
Durasphere
to bovine collagen, 166
bulking agents, randomized controlled trials (RCT), 165, 166
description, 165
radiologic stability, 166
Durasphere EXP® Office Procedure Guide
peri-urethral injection, 170–171
transurethral injection, 169–170

E
Emergency preparedness, 21
Endocervical curettage (ECC)
description, 201
indications, 201, 202
LEEP, 213, 216
Endometrial biopsy/sampling (EMB/ES)
checklists, 57
curettes and aspirators, 57
endometrial sampling, 57
pelvic infection, 57
peri-procedural complications, 58–59
procedure, 57–58
sufficient vacuum suction, 56–57
Endometrial polyps
abnormal bleeding, 125
benign, 125
cervical polyps, 119
characteristics, 118
diagnostic hysteroscopy, 89
hysteroscopically confirmed, 89
intracavitary masses, 119
office-based hysteroscopic procedures, 126
removal, 129
SIS detection, 72
Essure™ delivery catheter, 102
Ethylene oxide gas sterilization, 13

F
Fentanyl, 48, 121
Fiberoptics, 85, 91
Fibroid resection, 125–126
Flexible cystoscopes, 144–145
Flexible hysteroscope, 93, 95, 122, 128
Foreign bodies, 90, 127

G
GEA. *See* Global endometrial ablation (GEA)
Genital condylomata
cryotherapy, 225–226
equipment, 225
office-based treatments, 225
podophyllum resin, 226–227
post-procedure care, 225
procedural and short-term complications, 225
trichloroacetic acid, 225
vulvar warts, 224
Global endometrial ablation (GEA)
and abnormal uterine bleeding (AUB), 87, 133
complications, 11, 139–141
FDA-approved methods
cervical ripening, 137
endometrial thinning, 135
global endometrial ablation devices, patient selection, 136
gonadotropin-releasing hormone (GnRH) agonist, 135
non-resectoscopic endometrial ablation device comparisons, 137
oral contraceptive pills (OCP), 135
Gynecare ThermaChoice®, 138
and heavy menstrual bleeding (HMB), 133
Her Option® Cryoablation, 138
Hydro ThermAblator®, 138
in-office *vs.* GEA in OR, 134–135
Microwave Endometrial Ablation® system, 139
NovaSure endometrial ablation device, 138
patient selection, 15
pelvic pain, 114
Gynecare ThermaChoice® system, 134, 136–138, 140, 141
Gynecare Versapoint™ resectoscope, 123
Gynecologics
bartholin gland cyst and abscess (*see* Bartholin gland cyst)
ES, 56–59
history, 4
IUDs, 51–56

H
Heavy menstrual bleeding (HMB)
definition, 133
menorrhagia, 133
surgical management, 134, 139
High grade dysplasia
biopsy/treatment, 195
colposcopy, 208
Hydro ThermAblator® (HTA), 134, 136, 141
Hysterosalpingography (HSG)
bilateral tubal occlusion, 105
diagnostic hysteroscopy, 85, 87
hysteroscopic microcoil application, 107

Hysterosalpingography (HSG) (*cont.*)
informed consent, 106
intrauterine device (IUD), 107
pain relief, 106–107
pregnancy and, 105
tubal occlusion rates, 103
Hysteroscopic morcellator, 123–127
Hysteroscopic resectoscope, 123, 125
Hysteroscopic scissors and grasper, 122
Hysteroscopy
distending media, monitoring and management, 108
saline infusion sonogram, 106
sterilization program (*see* Sterilization)
uterine cavity measurement, 109

I
ICS. *See* International Continence Society (ICS)
Ilioinguinal/iliohypogastric nerves
injections, 186–187
local anesthetic agents and steroids, 187
lower abdominal and/or groin pain, 185, 186
pubic symphysis, 186, 187
Incision and drainage (I&D)
excisional biopsy, 63
fistula formation, 60, 63
simple, 60
vestibular glands, 63
vulvar carcinoma, 63
word catheter placement, 64, 66
Informed consent
autonomy, 25, 26
beneficence and non-maleficence, patient care, 25
bioethical framework, 25
core components, 28
definition, 15
disclosure, 27, 29–30
discussion with patients, 16
legal scholars and bioethicists, 27
medical decision-making capacity, 27–29
medical record, 16
modern medical ethics, 26
outpatient gynecologic surgery (*see* Outpatient gynecologic surgery)
outpatient procedures, 26
physicians, 25–27
self-determination, 26–27
understanding, 31
voluntariness, 31
Injections. *See* Peri-urethral bulking agents (PBAs); Trigger point injections
In-office procedure
ASC-US and LSIL Triage Study (ALTS) trial, 196
colposcopy performance, mean-weighted sensitivity, 195
diagnostic effectiveness and patient satisfaction, 197
ECC, 196
indications, 194–195
procedural and short-term complications, 207
SPOCCS I and II, 196, 197
tissue histology, 195
training, 195
International Continence Society (ICS), 149, 152, 154, 156
Intracervical block
anatomy, 40
complications, 42
equipment, 41
procedure, 41
solution, 40
Intrauterine devices (IUDs)
comparison, 61–62
Mirena and Skyla, 52, 53
paracervical block, 53
ParaGard, 52
pelvic infections, 52
peri-procedural complications
expulsion, 55
infection, 54–55
malposition, 55–56
perforation, 55
removal, 56
vasovagal reaction, 54
placement, 53
pregnancy test, 53
procedure checklist, 53
"radio-opaque", 51
"see-and-treat" approach, 90
Intrinsic sphincter deficiency (ISD)
definition, 168
Durasphere, 165
SUI, 166–167
UPP, 154, 155
IUDs. *See* Intrauterine devices (IUDs)

J
Joint Commission on Accreditation of Healthcare Organizations (JCAHO), 12

K
Karl Storz rigid hysteroscope, 91–92
Keyes punch biopsy, 222, 223

L
Leak point pressure
ALPP and DLPP, 155–156
involuntary leakage of urine, 155
ISD, 168
LEEP. *See* Loop elector-excision procedure (LEEP)
Levonorgestrel releasing IUD (LNG-IUD), 90
Lippes loop, 90
Local anesthetics
central nervous and cardiovascular system, 37
chemical structure, 35
clinical properties, 36
complications, 38
dosage, 37
drug allergies and anaphylactic reactions, 37
guidelines, 37
methemoglobinemia, 38

primary properties, 35
receptors, 36
sodium channel blocker, 37
vasoconstrictors, 36
Loop elector-excision procedure (LEEP)
basic LEEP equipment, 216
description, 211
"diathermy loop excision", 212
equipment, 213–214
in-office procedure, 212
with IUD in place, 217
office-based procedure, 211
outpatient ablative procedures, 211–212
patient satisfaction, 212–213
post-treatment, 215, 218–219
"pre-cancerous" lesion, 211
procedure, 214–215
short-term and procedural complications, 218
suture and packing material, 218
"Tophat" LEEP, 216
Lower urinary tract (LUT)
anorectal function, 157
International Consultation on Incontinence (ICI), 150
urodynamic testing, 149
Low grade dysplasia, 193
LUT. *See* Lower urinary tract (LUT)

M

Macroplastique® Procedure Guide
locking adapter onto administration device, 172, 173
needle placement, 172–173
needle priming, squeezing, 172, 174
sliding metal adapter over syringe, 172, 173
winged needle hub and syringe attachment, 172, 174
wings to needle attachment, 172, 174
Marsupialization, bartholin duct
advantages, 66
bartholin cyst, 66–67
word catheter placement, 65
MEA. *See* Microwave Endometrial Ablation (MEA)
Medical director
ACOG and national accrediting institutions, 18
office-based gynecologic surgical practice, 18, 20
office surgical safety checklist, 18–20
Microcoils
Essure™ delivery catheter, 102
hysteroscopic sterilization, 103, 107, 110
placement, 105–107
tubal ostium with "trailing" coils, 112
Microwave Endometrial Ablation (MEA), 134, 136, 139
Midazolam, 47–48
Mignon bulb, 143
Mirena and Skyla IUDs, 52
Morphine, 48
Mosaicism, 204, 205
Multichannel cystometry
ALPP, 156
detrusor overactivity, 152
filling, 150
single-channel, 151
technique, 158
MyoSure® tissue removal system, 124

N

National Patient Safety Foundation, 16, 17
Neuralgia
ilioinguinal/iliohypogastric nerves
(*see* Ilioinguinal/iliohypogastric nerves)
pudendal, 185
Noninvasive uroflowmetry
abnormalities, 153
clinical utility, 152
technique, 157–158
urine flow calculation, 152
uroflow, 152, 153
Nonsteroidal anti-inflammatory drugs (NSAIDs)
preprocedure treatment, 53, 79, 121
surgical intervention, treatment of HMB, 134
Novasure® radiofrequency ablation device, 134, 141

O

OAB. *See* Overactive bladder (OAB)
Occupational Safety and Health Administration
(OSHA), 12
Office-based surgery program
description, 1, 3
laboratory, 5
patient selection, 3–4
physical exam, 4–5
thrombotic risk management, 5–6
Office checklists, 18–20
Office Continuous Flow Operative Hysteroscope, 122
Office gynecological procedures
intracervical block, 40–42
local anesthetics, 35–38
paracervical block, 38–40
pudendal block, 42–44
regional blocks, 45
sedation and analgesia, 45–48
topical anesthetics, 44–45
Office set-up
anesthesia and analgesia (*see* Anesthesia)
documentation, 16–17
equipment, 10–11
informed consent, 15–16
medical assistants (MA) and/or nurses, 10
patient safety (*see* Patient safety)
physician, 10
procedure room set-up, 9, 10
recovery and follow-up, 15
sterilization (*see* Sterilization)
Operative hysteroscopy
abnormal uterine bleeding, 118
anesthesia, 121
bimanual pelvic examination, 119
cervical lacerations, 128
dilutional hyponatremia, 128
endocervical polyps, 118

Operative hysteroscopy (*cont.*)
endometrial cavity and polyps, 118, 119
fibroid resection, 125–126
fluid deficit, 129
hypoosmolality, 128
imaging, 119
infection, 129
infertility complaints, 118
informed consent, 120
instrumentation, 122–125
intrauterine adhesions, 118
introitus and perineal skin, thermal injures, 128
mechanical and traumatic type, 127
office-based, 126–127
patient selection, 120
perforation, 127
polypectomy, uterine septum, 128
polyp resection, 125
preop preparation, 121
submucosal type I leiomyoma, 118
vagina and cervix visualization, 118
OSHA. *See* Occupational Safety and Health Administration (OSHA)
Outpatient gynecologic surgery
experience with new device/procedure, 32
sedation for, 32
Overactive bladder (OAB), 157

P
PALM-COEIN basic classification system, 85, 87, 133
Pap smears
CIN-2-3, 193
colposcopy, 198
culture swab, 5
Paracervical block
anatomy, 38
cervical manipulation, 53
complications, 40
equipment, 38
procedure, 38–39
solution, 38
Patient autonomy
beneficence, non-maleficence and justice, 25
consent process, 26
healthcare, 25
physicians, 25–26
self-determination, 25, 27
Patient education, 16, 21, 93, 168
Patient preparation, sterilization
contraindications, 104–105
counseling, 105
endometrial atrophy, 106
endometrial pathology, 106
high microcoil placement rate, 106
hormonal management, 106
HSG confirmation, 105
informed consent, 105–106
initial screening, 104
intrauterine device (IUD), 107
long-acting reversible contraception (LARC), 104
misoprostol, 106
post-procedural issues, 106–107
pretreatment with medications, 106
Patient safety
checklists, 18, 20, 21
competency and credentialing, 21–22
emergency preparedness, 21
medical director, 18–20
Patient satisfaction, 197
Pelvic floor muscle spasm
Botox and placebo group, 184
botulinum toxin, 182–183
description, 182
in gynecology, 182, 183
symptoms, 183–184
Pelvic inflammatory disease (PID)
bacterial contamination, IUD insertion, 54
description, 4
significant hydrosalpinx, 98
Pelvic pain. *See* Chronic pelvic pain
Peri-urethral bulking agents (PBAs).*See also* Stress urinary incontinence (SUI)antimicrobials, 168
AUA guidelines, 168
carbon beads (Durasphere), 165–166, 169–171
coaptation after urethral bulking, 169
coaptite (calcium hydroxylapatite), 166–167, 171–172
cross-linked bovine collagen, 164
description, 163
equipments, 168
ethylene vinyl alcohol copolymer, 164
FDA-approved agents, 169, 170
injection therapy, 165
local anesthetics, 168
macroplastique, home-based pelvic floor exercises, 165
midurethral and bladder neck placement, 168–169
patient characteristics and indications, 168
pediatric vesicoureteral reflux, 164
prior to urethral bulking, 169
short-and long-term complications, 173
silicone (macroplastique), 167–168, 172–173
treatments, 164
PID. *See* Pelvic inflammatory disease (PID)
Podophyllum resin
description, 226
equipment, 226
post-procedure care, 226–227
procedural and short-term complications, 226, 227
Polyp resection, 125
Post-void residual (PVR)
patient/equipment factors, 151
poor detrusor contractility/outlet obstruction, 151–152
ultrasonic techniques/catheterization, 151
Preoperative evaluation. *See* Pre-procedure patient evaluation
Pre-procedure patient evaluation
advantages, 1
ambulatory surgery visits and hospital inpatients discharges, 1, 2
by facility type, ambulatory surgery visits, 1, 2
office-based surgery (*see* Office-based surgery program)

2014 Physician Fee Schedule Search, National Payment Amount, 1, 2
Pressure-flow study
abdominal and bladder pressure measurements, 153
detrusor muscle ability, 154
indications, 154
measurements, 154
patients evaluation, 158–159
Propofol, 48
Pudendal block
anatomy, 42
complications, 44
equipment
transperineal, 43–44
transvaginal, 43
procedure
transperineal, 43
transvaginal, 42–43
solution, 42
Pudendal neuralgia
chronic pelvic pain, 185
computed tomography/ultrasound guidance, 185
etiologies, 185
posterior approach, 185
traditional vaginal approach, 185
Punctuation and mosaicism, 204
PVR. *See* Post-void residual (PVR)

R
Regional anesthesia, 35, 37, 40, 49
Reid colposcopic index, 201
Repeat botulinum toxin injections, 184–185
Rigid cystoscope, 144–145
Rigid hysteroscope
for office hysteroscopy, 91–93, 95–96, 107, 109, 122
procedure, 95–96
sterilization, 107

S
Saline infusion sonohysterography (SIS)
abnormal/inconclusive transvaginal sonographic results, 74
advantages and complications, 81
Asherman's syndrome, 72, 77
cervical dilators, 79
contraindications, 75
description, 71
diagnostic hysteroscopy with endometrial biopsy, 73–74
distention, uterine cavity, 74
endometrial abnormalities, 71
enlarged uteri/uteri, 80
equipment, 77, 79
fibroid, woman with infertility, 72, 75
HSG, 72
indications, 75
malignant cell dissemination, 76
office hysteroscopy, 74
patient preparation and selection, 79, 80
polyp, perimenopausal woman with menorrhagia, 72–74
sagittal view and 3D rendering, 71, 72
suspected endometrial pathology, 71
thickenend endometrium, patient with postmenopausal bleeding, 77, 78
transcervical catheter placement and optimal acquisition, 79
TVUS, 71
woman with dysmenorrhea and menorrhagia, fibroid, 72, 76
Saline ultrasonography. *See* Saline infusion sonohysterography (SIS)
Sedation and analgesia, gynecologic procedures
"conscious sedation", 45
intra-procedure
emergency equipment, 47
monitoring, 46–47
personnel, 47
pharmacologic agents
fentanyl, 48
Midazolam, 47–48
morphine, 48
propofol, 48
post-procedure, 48
pre-procedure
contraindications, 46
evaluation, 45–46
informed consent, 46
risk factors, 46
"See-and-treat" approach, 90, 215
Sexually transmitted infections (STI), 4, 54, 55
Shanxi Province Cervical Cancer Screening Study (SPOCCS I), 196
Silicone (macroplastique), 167–168
Sonohysterography. *See* Saline infusion sonohysterography (SIS)
SPOCCS I. *See* Shanxi Province Cervical Cancer Screening Study (SPOCCS I)
Steam sterilization, 12
Sterilization
ambulatory surgery center (ASC), 102
black positioning marker, 111
complications, 113–114
cost advantages, 104
data supporting transfer, 103
delivery catheter, 111
description, 11
determination factors, 12
equipment and personnel, 107–109
equipment needed, 109, 110
Essure™, 102, 104, 112
ethylene oxide gas, 13
hospital stay, 104
hysterosalpingography (HSG), 103
hysteroscopic, 101–102
maintenance and equipment, 104
monitored anesthesia care, 109
office hysterocope disassembly, 12
operating room (OR), 102

Sterilization (*cont.*)
- patient preparation (*see* Patient preparation, sterilization)
- physician adoption, 103
- placement failure rate, 103
- polyethylene terephthalate (PET) fibers, 102
- procedure, 103, 109, 110
- proper cleaning, 12
- protocols, 11
- "sounding the uterus", 109
- steam, 12
- steris systems, 13
- trailing coils, 111–112
- tubal occlusion, confirmation, 102, 114
- tubal ostia, 103
- tubal ostium, 111

Steris systems, 13
STI. *See* Sexually transmitted infections (STI)
Stress urinary incontinence (SUI)
- description, 156, 163
- low pressure injection system, 164
- minimal inflammatory and fibrotic response, 163
- treatment, 156
- urodynamic testing, 156–157

Submucosal bulking agents, 163
Submucosal fibroids
- polyps, 120
- preoperative assessment, 119
- submucosal type I leiomyoma, 118
- types, 126
- ultrasound, 119
- uterine leiomyomata, classification, 126
- uterine septum correction, 127

Surgical risks, 1, 101
Swing-arm colposcope, 197

T

TCA. *See* Tricloroacetic acid (TCA)
ThermaChoice® system, 134, 136–138, 140, 141
Thrombotic risk management
- "certified" interpreters, 6
- description, 5
- preparation, 6

Toluidine blue examination. *See* Vulvar colposcopy
"Tophat" LEEP, 216
Transurethral bulking, 170
Transvaginal ultrasonography (TVUS)
- pelvic cavity evaluation, 71
- and SIS, 71–72

Tricloroacetic acid (TCA), 225, 226
Trigger point injections
- botulinum neurotoxin, 181
- botulinum toxin, 180
- comparison of, local anesthetic agents, 180
- complications, 182
- hypersensitive areas in body, 179
- ilioinguinal/iliohypogastric nerves, 185–187
- informed consent, 180
- Iowa trumpet needle, 180, 181
- mechanisms, 180
- myofascial, 179
- pelvic floor muscle spasm (*see* Pelvic floor muscle spasm)
- pudendal neuralgia, 185
- repeat botulinum toxin injections, 184–185
- sterile technique, 180–181
- transvaginal approach, 181
- vaginismus (*see* Vaginismus)
- vulvodynia, 184

Truclear Hysteroscopic Morcellator, 124
Tubal occlusion
- bilateral, 105, 107, 112
- confirmation, 114
- contraception, 3
- contralateral proximal, 105
- hysteroscopic, 87
- incomplete, 102
- rates, 103

Tubal ostia, 103, 106–109, 111
TVUS. *See* Transvaginal ultrasonography (TVUS)

U

UPP. *See* Urethral pressure profile (UPP)
Urethral function testing
- leak point pressure, 155–156
- UPP, 154–155

Urethral pressure profile (UPP), 154–155
Urethral pressure profilometry, 159
Urge urinary incontinence (UUI), 157
Urinary incontinence, 163
Urodynamics. *See* Urodynamic testing
Urodynamic testing
- bladder filling and storage, 150–151
- complications, 159
- components, 150
- emptying/voiding, bladder, 151–154
- equipment and setup, 157, 158
- indications, 149–150
- International Continence Society (ICS), 149
- LUT function, 149
- multichannel cystometry, 158
- noninvasive uroflowmetry, 157–158
- OAB/UUI, 157
- physiology, 149
- pressure-flow study, 158–159
- SUI, 156–157
- urethral function testing (*see* Urethral function testing)
- urethral pressure profilometry, 159
- videourodynamics, 159

Uterine fibroid embolization (UFE), 88
Uterine perforation, 97
UUI. *See* Urge urinary incontinence (UUI)

V

Vaginal colposcopy, 205
Vaginismus
- Botox and placebo group, 184
- botulinum toxin, 182
- definition, 182
- in gynecology, 182, 183
- symptoms, 183–184

Vaginoscopic technique, 85, 96
Valsalva leak point pressure (VLPP), 168
Vasovagal episode, 97
Vasovagal syncope, bradycardia, 4
Versapoint (TM) hysteroscopic system, 123
Videourodynamics, 159
VIN. *See* Vulvar intraepithelial neoplasia (VIN)
VLPP. *See* Valsalva leak point pressure (VLPP)
Voluntariness, informed consent, 31
Vulva
  biopsy and excision (*see* Vulvar biopsy and excision)
  colposcopy (*see* Vulvar colposcopy)
  genital condylomata (*see* Genital condylomata)
Vulvar biopsy and excision
  antiseptic cleansing and marking, vulvar lesion, 223
  description, 222
  equipment and indications, 222
  infiltrating local anesthesia into dermis, 223
  Keyes punch biopsy, vulvar lesion, 223
  Langer's lines, skin tension, 224
  post-procedure care, 224
  procedural and short-term complications, 224
Vulvar colposcopy, 205–206
  complications, 222
  description, 221
  equipment and procedure, 221–222
Vulvar intraepithelial neoplasia (VIN)
  and AWE, 206
  nonneoplastic vulvar lesions, 222
Vulvar warts excision, 227
Vulvodynia, 184

W
Word catheter placement, 64, 66

CPSIA information can be obtained
at www.ICGtesting.com
Printed in the USA
LVHW061615311019
635974LV00003B/27/P

9 781493 914135